Gene Therapy: Biological Aspects and Applications

Gene Therapy: Biological Aspects and Applications

Edited by **Harvey Summers**

New Jersey

Published by Foster Academics,
61 Van Reypen Street,
Jersey City, NJ 07306, USA
www.fosteracademics.com

Gene Therapy: Biological Aspects and Applications
Edited by Harvey Summers

International Standard Book Number: 978-1-63242-196-8 (Hardback)

Printed in the United States of America.

Contents

Preface

Due to new discoveries, gene therapy has gained a lot of popularity in recent years. Issues in the past which were troubling scientists and practitioners are now being easily resolved. The growth of secure and effective gene transfer and development in the field of cell therapy has now brought new ways to deal with varied diseases. The book aims at compiling information from different resources about various biological gene therapy tools, the important subjects covered are cancer gene therapy – biological concepts in the design of multifunctional non-viral delivery systems, gene therapy based on fragment C of tetanus toxin in ALS, lentiviral gene therapy vectors, transposons for non-viral gene transfer and retroviral genotoxicity.

The information contained in this book is the result of intensive hard work done by researchers in this field. All due efforts have been made to make this book serve as a complete guiding source for students and researchers. The topics in this book have been comprehensively explained to help readers understand the growing trends in the field.

I would like to thank the entire group of writers who made sincere efforts in this book and my family who supported me in my efforts of working on this book. I take this opportunity to thank all those who have been a guiding force throughout my life.

Editor

Gene Therapy Tools: Biological

Cancer Gene Therapy – Key Biological Concepts in the Design of Multifunctional Non-Viral Delivery Systems

Cian M. McCrudden and Helen O. McCarthy

Additional information is available at the end of the chapter

1. Introduction

The importance of gene therapy strategies for the treatment of malignancies is highlighted by the fact that there are (at the time of writing) 823 cancer gene therapy clinical trials worldwide that are actively, or have yet to begin recruiting patients (www.clinicaltrials.gov - accessed November 2012). The potential of the delivery of genetic material for therapeutic purposes has long been recognised, but to this point, has yet to be successfully translated. Strategies that have proved promising in the *in vitro* setting have stumbled when exposed to the complexities of the *in vivo* environment. Classically involving the delivery of plasmid DNA (pDNA) that encodes a therapeutic protein product, the field of gene therapy has evolved to encompass not only delivery of therapeutic DNA, but also micro- (miRNA), short hairpin- (shRNA) and small interfering RNAs (siRNA) and oligodeoxynucleotides (ODNs) [1]. Despite the evolution of the technology for altering the genotype of target cells and tissues, the problem of overcoming the biological barriers that limit the efficacies of these technologies remains. These barriers exist at both systemic and local levels. To date, the only approved nucleic acid-based treatments for clinical use are an antisense ODN for the treatment of cytomegalovirus retinitis [2], and pegaptanib sodium (Macugen), an RNA aptamer targeted against VEGF-165 and used to treat age-related macular degeneration [3]. This chapter will focus on the biological barriers faced by non-viral vectors for gene therapy, strategies that have been employed to overcome these barriers, and will conclude by documenting the state of the art technologies being used to propel non-viral gene therapies forward.

1.1. Non-viral gene therapy

Delivery of genetic material for therapeutic use from virus-like particles has received considerable attention, and has generated extensive knowledge. The molecular evolution of viruses over the aeons has produced DNA-delivering organisms of incomparable efficiency. The use of 'gutted' viruses that lack virulence properties and replicative capacity is the most efficient method of genetic material delivery [4], and modified viruses have been used extensively in gene therapy; commonly employed viruses include adenovirus, retrovirus, vaccinia virus and herpes simplex virus [5]. The allure of viral gene therapy was hindered however, when a clinical trial patient died four days after receiving adenoviral therapy for treatment of ornithine transcarbamylase deficiency [6]. The negative press that this generated, along with other disadvantages of viral gene therapy (including generation of immune response, possibility of proto-oncogene activation, production costs, and limitations in deliverable gene size) have necessitated the generation of alternative gene therapy strategies [7].

Despite some success when naked DNA has been delivered *in vivo* (naked pDNA has been effectively delivered to the liver in mice and rats [8] by tail vein injection), pDNA for gene therapy is conventionally delivered complexed with materials with suitable physical characteristics. pDNA's hydrophilicity and anionic nature impair the uncomplexed molecule's passage through the lipophilic plasma membrane [1,9,10]. Non-viral gene therapy strategies usually involve wrapping of the nucleic acid to be delivered in a protective envelope that neutralises the negative charge of the DNA. A range of compounds has been used to envelop pDNA, including cationic lipids, polymers and peptides.

Cationic lipids were among the first compounds complexed with pDNA for non-viral gene delivery. Felgner reported that N-[1-(2,3-dioleyloxy)propyl]-N,N,N-trimethylammonium chloride (DOTMA) formed lipid-DNA complexes based on the interaction between the positively charged lipid and the negatively charged phosphates of the DNA. The lipoplexes so-formed were capable of delivering DNA to cells *in vitro* [11]. Numerous cationic lipids have since been reported to neutralise, condense and encapsulate pDNA, including dioctadecyla-midoglycylspermine (DOGS) [12],[1,2-bis(oleoyloxy)-3-(trimethylammonio)propane] (DO-TAP) [13] and 3β[N-(N', N'-dimethylaminoethane)-carbamoyl] cholesterol (DC-Chol) [14]. Variations on a theme, these lipids behave similarly to innate biological lipids [15]. The addition of co-lipids such as cholesterol and dioleoylphosphatidylethanolamine (DOPE) can improve transfection efficiency [16]. Recent developments in the field have seen a 1-palmito-yl-2-oleoyl-sn-glycero-3-ethylphosphocholine (EPOPC):cholesterol liposome with folate electrostatically-associated used to deliver HSV-tk suicide gene therapy to SCC-VII xenografts, which resulted in considerable tumour growth delay [17]. In a magnetofection method, intravenous delivery of superparamagnetic iron oxide lipid nanoparticles in combination with an Nd-Fe-B magnet placed externally in the tumour locality resulted in improved IGF-1R shRNA delivery to A549 xenografts [18].

Cationic polymers have been used to condense and deliver genetic material, including poly(l-lysine) (PLL), polyethylenimine (PEI), chitosan and polyamidoamine (PAMAM) [7]. PLL incorporated into a spider silk-based nanoparticle with a tumour-homing peptide was recently reported to deliver a luciferase plasmid to MDA-MB-231 xenografts following intravenous administration [19]. A novel triblockpoly(amido amine)-poly(ethylene glycol)-poly-l-lysine (PAMAM-PEG-PLL) nanocarrier successfully delivered Bcl-2 siRNA and elicited knockdown of the same in A2780 ovarian carcinoma cells *in vitro* [20]. Heparin-PEI nanogels were used to reintroduce heparin sulphate 6-O-endosulfatase 1 (HSulf-1) to ovarian SKOV-3 xenografts, which resulted in anti-angiogenesis, induction of apoptosis and suppression of cell proliferation [21], while a PEI-poly(hydroxyethyl glutamine) (PEI-PHEG) copolymer successfully delivered pGL3 pDNA by intratumoural administration to Lewis Lung Carcinoma xenografts in C57BL/6 mice [22].

Cationic peptides that are capable of neutralising, condensing and wrapping pDNA have also been used as non-viral delivery vehicles [23]. These cell-permeating peptides were designed to interact with cell membranes similarly to viral fusion proteins. GALA, a synthetic peptide designed to interact with lipid bilayers at an acidic pH, was observed to aid in the delivery of DNA to cells [23]. A derivative, termed KALA, through presence of positively charged lysine residues, is capable of condensing and delivering DNA unaided [24], and improved gene delivery ten-fold in hepatoma [25] and also in HEK293T and HepG2 cells [26]. The cell-penetrating peptide TAT and fusogenic peptide HA2 were used to improve pDNA delivery by gelatin-silica nanoparticles [27]. Recent developments in the field have seen the development of multi-domain peptidic biomimetic vectors tailored to overcome the various biological barriers that gene delivery vehicles encounter *in vivo*, including degradation by serum nucleases, endosomal entrapment and nuclear localization. One such designer biomimetic vector was used to deliver tumour-related apoptosis inducing ligand (TRAIL) [28] and inducible nitric oxide synthase (iNOS) pDNA to ZR-75-1 breast cancer cells *in vitro* [29].

Non-viral strategies for gene therapy have several advantages over traditional viral approaches, including reduced cost and ease of large-scale production, as well as avoidance of the virulence commonly associated with viral delivery. However, non-viral gene delivery systems suffer from lower potency of transfection ability, resultant of lower ability to traverse the various obstacles faced upon administration [7].

2. Extracellular barriers to gene delivery

2.1. The skin

The most fundamental barrier that the human body possesses is its skin. The stratum corneum is the skin's outermost layer, and provides an imposing barrier to gene delivery [30]; the densely packed cornified cells of this layer protect the body from a range of foreign material. The skin is not a commonly used route for gene therapy approaches, but it is an attractive route for local targeting of dermatological ailments [31]. However, skin nucleases, and in particular DNAse 2, active at the skin and in the stratum corneum, degrade topically-applied nucleic acids [32]. An appropriate and potent delivery mechanism could open the door to gene therapy strategies for the treatment of skin conditions and malignancies, including xeroderma pigmentosum (a cancer-linked disorder that has shown promise in preclinical gene therapy approaches [33]), when replacement of the defective XPC gene is in keratinocytes would be therapeutically beneficial [34].

Introduction of micron-sized pores to the skin using minimally-invasive silicone microneedles allowed for the delivery of a 'non-viral gene vector-mimicking' charged fluores cent nanoparticle [35,36]. A needle-free injection device successfully delivered luciferase pDNA to porcine skin, resulting in higher protein expression than conventional hypodermic needle administration [37], while subcutaneous melanoma xenografts were targeted for gene therapy using a hybrid electro-microneedle; delivery of 20 μg interleukin-12 pDNA to the skin, followed by eight 50 ms pulses delivering 70V/0.5 cm from the electrode to improve transfection resulted in a significant improvement in survival of tumour-bearing mice [38]. Most recently, researchers from Northwestern University reported the generation of siRNA-carrying nanoparticles (spherical nucleic acid nanoparticle conjugates (SNA-NCs)) that are capable of penetrating nude mouse and human skin, whilst maintaining their RNA interference potential [36]. The nanoparticles comprise gold cores surrounded by a dense shell of highly oriented, covalently immobilised siRNA and could be delivered topically, avoiding the need for disruption of the skin. As the skin is unmolested, the authors propose that the miniscule nature of the SNA-NCs permit dermal crossing, a theory that is currently under investigation.

2.2. Barriers to systemic gene therapies

Needle-administered systemic therapeutics bypass the skin, but encounter further extracellular barriers before reaching their site of action. The various administration routes (intravenous, -muscular, -ocular, -nasal) present their own unique impediments to nucleic acid delivery. Intravenously- [39] and intramuscularly-administered [40] therapies are subject to nuclease degradation from the point of entry. Conversely, naked uncomplexed anti-respiratory syncytial virus (RSV) siRNA was almost as effective as that complexed with TransIT-TKO transfection reagent when nasally-administered in mice [41], suggesting that nasally-administered gene therapies may not be as prone to nuclease insult. The compartmental nature of the eye, and ease of access to it simplifies avoidance of similar barriers in ocular gene therapy delivery [42]. pDNA complexed with poly(d,l-lactic-co-glycolic) acid (PLGA) and dimethyldioctadecylammonium bromide (DDAB) produced nanoparticles capable of traversing one of the most inhospitable of barriers, the gastric mucus [43]. For simplicity, this chapter will focus on the barriers faced by intravenously delivered therapies, as this route has the potential to target almost all tissues of the body.

The complexing of DNA into lipo- or polyplex nanoparticles in non-viral delivery can effectively protect the pDNA from nuclease degradation [44] (although, paradoxically, cationic and anionic lipoplexes can hinder pDNA delivery by electroporation [45]). Whilst in the circulation, however, non-viral agents can be subject to non-specific binding by serum proteins, which can result in aggregation or dissociation of nanoparticles, resultant of the generally positive charges of the nanoparticles and the negative charge of circulatory proteins [1]. Positive charge is essential to ensure interaction of the nanoparticle with its target cell, however the mononuclear phagocytic system (MPS) eliminates foreign hydrophobic particles from the circulation [7] by opsonisation. The MPS was neutralised in mice by pretreatment with polyinosinic acid (a synthetic nucleic acid strand) before therapeutic measles virus treatment; this led to competitive inhibition of the scavenging of particles by macrophages, and improved virus delivery to and efficacy at SKOV3 xenografts [46]. Aggregation of nanoparticles can cause embolization of microvessels, and non delivery of the therapeutic to target [1].

The differential in ionicity between gene therapy formulation and the extracellular space poses another obstacle for nanoparticles, which can lead to colloidal instability [44]. The issue of non-specific interaction between nanoparticles and plasma proteins has been addressed by the coupling of hydrophilic molecules to the nanoparticle. The most commonly employed candidate is poly(ethylene glycol) (PEG), whose anionicity has led to reduced aggregation and improved transfection ability [47]. PEG has been incorporated into a myriad of non-viral gene therapy strategies. Recently, polyacridine peptide nanoparticles were PEGylated and found to persist in the mouse circulation for up to nine hours, compared to non-PEGylated nanoparticles, which were inactive within five minutes [48], while biodegradable dextran nanogels were PEGylated and analysed for their siRNA delivering prowess [49]. Particulate gene therapies are also subject to entrapment by the mononuclear phagocyte system (reticuloendothelial system - RES), when they are captured and held in the spleen or liver [50], which was responsible for the inactivation of adenoviral vectors that have been used as viral gene therapeutics [51]. Avoidance of non-specific biomolecular interaction, referred to as 'stealth' [1], is a prerequisite for successful gene delivery. Functionalisation of non-viral gene therapies with agents such as PEG to facilitate RES avoidance will be discussed in subsequent sections.

Assuming a gene therapeutic persists in active form in the circulation and the target tissue is reached, extravasation from the circulation is imperative. The architecture of normal vasculature ensures that transport of macromolecules out of the circulation is difficult. One characteristic of tumour vasculature, however, is its propensity to leakiness, an attribute that can be exploited by gene therapies. It is unsurprising that siRNA lipoplexes that target RAN GTPase were delivered more effectively, and evoked more impressive anti-tumour effects in highly vascularised xenografts than in xenografts with poorer vascularity [52]. The leaky vessel phenomenon, known as the enhanced permeability and retention (EPR) effect, has been utilised to enable the delivery of pDNA-containing particles in various malignancies [53]. The utilization of EPR will be further discussed below. The angiogenic tumour vasculature was itself targeted in a murine dorsal air sac assay; siRNA targeting Ago2 was complexed into cationic liposomes and intravenously administered. The authors successfully delivered the interfering RNA to the angiogenic vessels, and reported tumour regression, presumed to be resultant of anti-angiogenesis in their model [54].

Perhaps the most intimidating vascular obstacle that a gene therapy can face is the blood-brain barrier, where tight junctions between endothelial cells of the capillaries limit the passage of molecules much more than at other capillary sites in the body. One of the most exciting techniques available to the gene therapy researcher is the use of ultrasound-targeted microbubble destruction (UTMD); nucleic acid contained within a gas-filled microbubble is administered, before exposure to ultrasonic waves at a frequency that exceeds the resonance frequency of the microbubbles, causing their destruction and leading to increased capillary and cell membrane permeability [55]. This technology was used to deliver pDNA for the green fluorescent protein (GFP) reporter gene across the mouse blood-brain barrier [56], and presents new possibilities for overcoming this most daunting of circulatory barriers.

2.3. Cellular barriers to gene delivery

2.3.1. The cell membrane and endocytosis

Specific targeting of gene vectors to ensure delivery to the target tissue will be discussed in a subsequent section. The nanoparticle's nucleic acid cargo determines the site to which delivery is required; plasmid DNA must be delivered to the nucleus to affect transcription, while siRNA need only reach the cytoplasm to interfere with translation [57]. The most elemental impediment to entry into the animal cell is the lipid bilayer membrane. The cell membrane can be breached using physical means in certain circumstances to allow delivery of naked pDNA. These methods include electroporation (local destabilization of the cell membrane using an electric pulse), sonoporation (membrane destabilization using ultrasound) or laser irradiation (introduction of transient pores in the membrane using a lens-focussed laser beam). The application of these methods is limited, however, by inaccessibility to most tissues [58].

Condensation and neutralization of nucleic acids into nanoparticles abrogates the two fundamental properties of pDNA that preclude its cellular entry, namely its large size and negative charge [1]. Particles of excessive size can aggregate and cause embolization of narrow capillaries, as mentioned above. Nanoparticles for gene delivery tend to be sub-200 nm for this reason. However, *in vivo* delivery of fluorescently labelled liposomes of up to 400 nm diameter has been reported [59]. Particle size also appears to dictate the pathway that performs internalization of complexes; 200 nm particles have entered cells by clathrin-dependent routes, 300 nm particles by caveolae-mediated pathways [7]. Optimization of the net charge (or zeta/ζ potential) of delivery vehicle/nucleic acid complex of lipid/polymer/peptide and pDNA complexes is achieved by the electrostatic interaction between the negatively charged phosphate residues present in the pDNA and the positively charged nitrogen in the vehicle. The net charge of the resultant particle can be increased by increasing the vehicle (nitrogen) to pDNA (phosphate) ratio (known as N:P ratio) [1]. The negative charge of serum proteins can thwart the therapeutic potential of nanoparticles; this can be overcome by increasing the N:P ratio of complexes above that sufficient to condense the pDNA. Altering the net charge of the nanoparticles can significantly alter the array of plasma proteins that interact with the particles. Similar liposomal particles with charges of -9.0, -11.4 and -27.4 were incubated with human plasma, and the interacting proteins were identified; 117 proteins were found bound to particles of all three charges, while 12, 6 and 15 plasma proteins interacted uniquely with the three particle charge types respectively [60]. Kim and coworkers reported that hyperbranched polysiloxysilane nanoparticles with a moderate positive charge (46 mV) were more efficient gene delivery agents than analogous particles with a high positive charge (64 mV) [61]. Clearly, nanoparticle size and charge are parameters that require optimization for appropriate cell membrane breaching. Phosphonium-based vectors (as opposed to nitrogen-based) are also being explored for their gene delivery potential; preliminary studies have revealed that phosphonium-based vectors condensed DNA at lower charge ratios than corresponding nitrogen-based vectors [62].

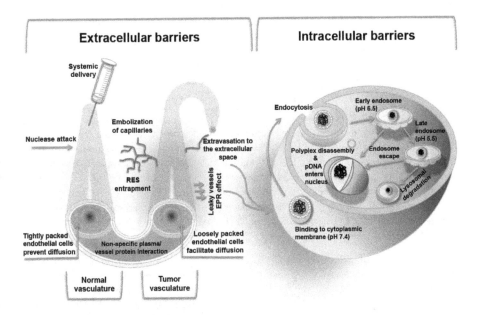

Figure 1. Summary of the extra- and intracellular barriers faced by non-viral gene therapies following systematic delivery. Based on [1].

Electrostatic interaction between the cationic nanoparticle and the anionic cell membrane that facilitate association between the cell and nanoparticle was assumed to result in endocytosis of the nanoparticle, although the machinery of internalization appears to be material- and cell type-dependent. Endocytotic access to cells is by pinocytosis in the majority of cases, rather than by phagocytosis [9]. A mechanism of endocytosis was clarified by Payne and colleagues, who followed the intracellular trafficking of PEI- and Lipofectamine™-complexed nucleic acids in mammalian cells, and reported that endocytosis relied upon cell surface heparin sulphate proteoglycans (HSPG) and was dependent on dynamin- and flotillin, rather than clathrin- and caveolin-dependent mechanisms [63]. On the other hand, nanoparticles formed from pDNA complexed with PEG-CK$_{30}$ were endocytosed after interaction with cell surface nucleolin, a process that was reliant on the activity of lipid rafts [64]. A recent study reported by a team at the University of Groningen very elegantly showed lassoing of PEI- and Lipofectamine™-complexed pDNA by syndecan- and actin-rich filaments of HeLa cells, presumed to be filopodia and retraction fibers; the nanoparticles then 'surf' along the filopodia, or the filopodia are retracted toward the cell body, thereby facilitating HSPG-mediated endocytosis [65].

2.3.2. Endosomal escape

The result of endocytic cellular entry is endosomal entrapment. Endosomes are a range of membrane-bound organelles that include early, late and recycling endosomes that are responsible for the short-term storage and sorting of endocytosed materials, including macromolecules and pathogens (including viruses). Once material is endocytosed, it is either evicted from the cell by the recycling endosome, or the complex process of endosome maturation ensues, late endosomes fuse with lysosomes, and active degradation of endosome cargoes occurs [66]. Macromolecules that are unable to escape the endosome are bound for lysosomal degradation.

The mechanism of endosomal escape by non-viral vectors is dependent on the complexing material used. Cationic lipids appear to interact with the anionic endosomal membrane, resulting in ion pair formation and consequent transformation to inverted hexagonal phase (H_{II}), causing disruption of the endosomal membrane. Alternatively, an inversion of the endosomal membrane as a result of electrostatic interactions has been proposed, which would instigate nucleic acid cargo being deposited in the cytoplasm. When polymeric materials are used to complex pDNA, the polymers themselves absorb protons in the endosome (proton-sponge effect), leading to chloride ion influx, increased osmotic pressure and water flow into the endosome, resulting in endosome rupture [7].

The fusogenic lipid DOPE is frequently used as a co-complexing agent due to its inherent ability to facilitate endosomal escape; conformational change from lipid bilayer to an inverted hexagonal structure is triggered by the sub-physiological pH of the endosome, and causes endosomal membrane disruption and escape of nucleic acid cargo [67]. Viral membrane proteins have provided inspiration for the non-viral gene delivery researcher. Influenza viruses escape the endosome with the help of hemagluttinin A2 (HA2), while the adenoviral protein, penton, assists adenovirus endosome escape. Glycoprotein H from herpes simplex virus induced 30-fold improvement of transfection by lipoplexes in human cell lines [68]. Conformational changes of these proteins consequential of the acidic environment in the endosome facilitate viral particle escape from the endosome; the more hydrophobic conformation that they adopt at low pH permits membrane fusion and disruption [1].

Synthetic fusogenic peptides are increasingly being used to improve transfection in non-viral systems. The conformational status of GALA is responsive to pH, adopting alpha-helical status in acidic environments, and in that sense, mimics the endosomal escape route favoured by viruses [69]. Derivatives of GALA such as GALAdelE3, YALA [70], and KALA [24] have all shown promise as endosome escaping agents. Similarly, two endosomal escape peptides, INF7 and H5WYG, improved endosome escape of PEG-based vectors by up to 100-fold [71].

2.3.3. Nuclear envelope penetration

The final obstacle faced by pDNA gene therapies is the nuclear envelope, a barrier punctuated with nuclear pores impermeable to molecules greater than 70 kDa, or roughly 10 nm in diameter [72]. Liposomal fusion with the nuclear membrane that facilitates direct cargo transfer from vector to nucleus has been reported [73]. Mitotic division temporarily disrupts the nuclear membrane's barrier properties, which can allow pDNA transgene entry [9]. The nuclear pores can be more actively targeted for penetration by the use of nuclear localization signalling (NLS) peptides or DNA targeting sequences (DTS). NLSs are short clusters of basic amino acids (such as lysine) that bind to importins, receptors that facilitate cytoplasm-nuclear transport [74]. Active transport of macromolecules through nuclear pore complexes causes expansion of the pores to approximately 30 nm in diameter [75]. The nuclear localization peptide SV40 from Simian virus 40 was used to improve the delivery of luciferase gene-carrying liposomes to neuroblastoma cells [76], while NLSs from adenovirus E1a, the transcription factor c-myc, mouse FGF3, and the DNA repair protein PARP have all been used to guide transgene delivery to the nucleus [74]. Some of the recently employed nuclear envelope penetration strategies are summarised in Table 1.

3. Evading the immune system

As mentioned previously, although viruses are masters of nucleic acid delivery, alternative delivery mechanisms are being sought to avoid the pitfalls associated with viral systems. Fundamentally, viruses remain foreign pathogens, agents that the human body has evolved to protect itself from. Of the commonly employed viral vectors, adenoviral, adenovirus-associated vectors and lentivirus vectors all produce immune responses in mice and humans, with antibodies often being produced against both the packaging vector as well as the transgene product. Exposure to viral particles triggers the adaptive immune response. Pinocytosis of viral particles by immature dendritic cells elicits maturation of the dendritic cells into mature antigen-presenting cells that present antigens in major histocompatability complexes (MHCs). Activation of T cells by antigen presentation leads to both the destruction of the antigen-presenting cells, and the recruitment and activation of B cells, responsible for antibody production [84].

Attempts to avoid provocation of immunologic responses have been made by the viral gene therapist that include deletion or nullification of viral coding genes and elimination of pathogenic genes, or use of targeting strategies to ensure avoidance of the immune cells. Additionally, pharmacological immunosuppression has been used extensively to avoid the neutralization of various viral gene therapy strategies [85].

3.1. DNA-mediated immune responses

It is generally accepted that non-viral gene therapy strategies elicit fewer immune responses than their viral counterparts, although certain facets of non-viral complexes mark them as targets for immune system intervention [86]. An early report into immune responses induced by non-viral gene therapy revealed cytokine induction (TNFα and IL-1β) by PEI/DNA complexes; the extent of immune induction was determined by the route of delivery, aerosol proving less detrimental than intravenous [87]. In mice, lipoplex administration evoked complement activation and induction of IFN-γ, TNF-α, IL-6, and IL-12. These effects

NLS	Sequence	Summary	Result	Ref
TAT	Ac-GCGYGRKKRRQRRRG-NH$_2$	PEG-based vector with DNA binding peptide	Up to 15-fold increase in CHO cell transfection	[77]
NLS-1 NLS-2 NLS-3	DPKKKRKV DPKKKRKVDPKKKRKV DPKKKRKVDPKKKRKV-DPKKKRKV	Inclusion of NLS peptides in Lipofectamine liposomes for transfection into human and rat mesenchymal stem cells	Roughly two-, four- and six-fold enhancement of luciferase expression respectively	[78]
I-NLS	Iodinated-PKKKRKV	Iodinated NLS was complexed with pDNA and PEI. Luciferase transfection was assessed in MCF-7 breast cancer cells	130-fold improvement in transfection compared to absence of NLS. Iodination improved nuclear localization	[79]
Human surfactant protein C promoter	318 nucleotides PCR amplified from genomic DNA	Sequence cloned into promoterless plasmid and microinjected into cytoplasm of MLE-12 cells.	Fluorescent in situ hybridization revealed nuclear localization in 25-30% of injected cells compared to control (0%). Specific to alveolar type II epithelial cells	[80]
Triamcinolone acetonide (TA)	N/A	TA was conjugated to PEI (various molecular weights) and nuclear localization determined	Low molecular weight PEI/TA efficiently targeted the nucleus	[81]
Dexamethasone	N/A	Polyplexed (PEI) with pLuciferase	10 – 100-fold increase in transfection efficiency	[82]
Trans-cyclohexane-1,2-diol	N/A	Amphipathic alcohol that collapses nuclear pore cores allowing macromolecule uptake	Improved Lipofectamine 2000-mediated gene transfection to 293T cells in vitro, but was not reproducible in vivo	[83]

Table 1. Recent strategies employed to aid the delivery of non-viral gene therapies to the nucleus.

were independent of N:P ratio or the cationic lipid complexed with the pDNA [88]. Although observed immune responses tend to be dose-dependent, dose reduction to avoid immune induction consequently also lessens the transfection ability of the complexes, stressing the narrow therapeutic index of non-viral gene therapies [89].

It is well established that immune responses in non-viral therapies is resultant of the presence of unmethylated CpG motifs in the bacterial backbone of the plasmid. In mammals, roughly 75% of CpG motifs are methylated to 5'-methycytosine, whereas in bacteria they are usually unmethylated [89]. Recognition of unmethylated CpG motifs by Toll-like receptor 9 on immune cells causes activation of mitogen-activated protein kinases and NF-κB [90]. As well as eliminating an immune response, evidence exists to suggest that removal of unmethylated CpG motifs can increase the duration of transgene expression [91,92]. PEI-based delivery of CpG-rich pDNA was associated with a reduction in lung compliance, while delivery of CpG-diminished pDNA was not [93]. Furthermore, methylation of CpG motifs in pDNA largely reversed the immunostimulatory activity of lipoplexes and polyplexes in C57BL/6 mice [94].

Numerous strategies have been investigated to abrogate immune responses upon non-viral gene therapy administration. Liu and colleagues encapsulated various anti-inflammatory agents into DOTAP/pLuciferase liposomes, and termed the resultant complex a 'safeplex'. Safeplexes carrying dexamethasone, prednisone, indomethacin, tetrandrine and gliotoxin inhibited TNFα expression compared to that seen in the absence of anti-inflammatory. Importantly, the complexing of dexamethasone into the safeplex did not affect the complex's ability to deliver its pDNA cargo [89]. Delivery of oligonucleotides to inhibit cytokine (NFκB) translation using non-viral carriers has also been proposed as a mechanism of counteracting the host's immune response to non-viral therapies [95].

Lipid-protamine-DNA complexes (LPDs) were used to deliver a PCR amplicon of the luciferase gene rather than a bacterial plasmid containing the luciferase gene. Luciferase translation was as efficient from the PCR amplicon as from the plasmid when both were complexed with LPD, but the immune response evoked by the PCR fragment complex was three-fold less potent than that evoked by the plasmid complex (determined by TNFα and IL-12 expression) [96].

The immune response can be avoided by the removal of unnecessary bacterial DNA that contains the immunological CpG motifs, bacterial origin of replication, as well as genes for plasmid antibiotic resistance that are not required for transgene expression. First reported in 1997, minicircles are gene delivery vehicles that lack prokaryotic nucleic acid, and were produced by the thermo-responsive activity of λ integrase [97]. Minicircles were more potent reporter gene deliverers than their parental pDNA in melanoma and colon carcinoma cell lines by lipofection and electroporation [98]. Minicircles complexed with PEI also delivered the GFP gene more potently than similarly complexed pDNA [99]. The potency of minicircles has been improved by tethering minicircle liposomes to the TetR nuclear targeting device [100].

A further improvement on the immunologically inert minicircles has recently been mooted. Tightly-wound miniknot vectors are the result of DNA minicircle treatment with DNA topoisomerase II, and are proposed to be more resistant to physical damage (strand breaks) that can linearise (thereby reducing/removing efficacy) pDNA and minicircles. DNA delivery methods such as aerosol inhalation, jet-injection, electroporation, particle bombardment and ultrasound DNA transfer can subject DNA to stresses that might cause damage [101].

3.2. Carrier-mediated immune responses

It is important to note that immune responses to non-viral gene therapy are not solely resultant of bacterial CpG motifs. An impressive study from Kyoto University highlighted the immune responses that can be generated by liposomes. Using CpG-free pDNA in lipoplexes, the authors demonstrated activation of IFNβ, TNFα and IL-6 in macrophages from TLR9 knockout mice. The extent of the immune response (as determined by *in vitro* cytokine induction) was dependent on the cationic lipid content of the complex. The reactions elicited by the cationic lipids can be summarised as Lipofectamine 2000 > Lipofectamine Plus > DOTMA/DOPE > DOTMA/cholesterol [102]. The inertness of DOTMA/cholesterol as delivery vehicle was supported further *in vivo*, when CpG-free pDNA lipoplexes provoked no IL-6 or IFNβ induction after intravenous injection in mice [103]. The targeting of nucleic acid cargoes to specific cells/tissues (to be discussed shortly) could also remedy the immune response by preventing the transfection of non-target cells, and in particular, the antigen-presenting cells [85].

The continuing evolution of the non-viral gene therapy field has led to the development of transposon-based delivery strategies, including Sleeping Beauty, Tol2, and piggyBac. These systems appear to deliver DNA as efficiently as viruses, and provoke extended transgene product expression, whilst maintaining the low immunogenicity and other risk factors associated with viral gene delivery [104]. It is anticipated that the momentum of non-viral gene therapy research will lead to the development of vehicles and cargoes that will rival the viral gene therapy field.

4. Targeting in non-viral systems

The optimal gene delivery vector will protect its payload from degradation in the circulation, enable extravasation from the bloodstream, traverse cellular membranes, facilitate endosomal disruption to deliver the payload to either the cytoplasm, or if necessary, transport to the nucleus. The optimal vector should also be non-immunogenic, as discussed above. Design of such vectors obviously presents a huge challenge. Furthermore, for vectors that accomplish extra- and intracellular barrier and immune system avoidance, there is the added layer of complication that targeting presents. Frequently in cancer studies, the payload to be delivered is a therapeutic designed to over-express a protein or knockdown a gene to manifest an anti-cancer effect. In order to spare normal tissue damage, widespread toxicity, and to achieve a clinically viable therapeutic product, targeting has become an essential in the quest for a perfect vector.

4.1. Enhanced permeation and retention effect

Exploitation of the tumour microenvironment presents an obvious option in the targeting strategies employed by many delivery systems. The enhanced permeation and retention effect (EPR), which was mentioned briefly above, is a phenomenon whereby there is defective architecture in blood vessels, extensive angiogenesis, increased vascular permeability and an impaired function of the mononuclear phagocytic system [105-107]. The consequences of these tumour-specific physiological changes is that macromolecules > 40 kDa selectively 'leak' out of the blood vessels and extravasate into the interstitial tumour tissue [108,109].

Particle size is an important factor for utilizing the EPR effect. Studies have shown that nanoparticles up to 400 nm in diameter can permeate across tumour vessels [59,110]. However, circulation times can also play a key role in successful tumour transduction, with a minimum of 6 h required for the EPR effect to occur [111]. The EPR effect has been exploited not only in chemotherapy drug design but also in gene delivery. In one such example, poly-glycerolaminne (PG-Amine) dendrimers were complexed with siRNA and delivered intravenously to mice bearing luciferase tagged mammary tumours; after 24 h, there was a 69% reduction in luciferase activity [112]. The authors also reported that there was clear evidence of accumulation of the complexes in the tumours but not in any other organs, which can be attributed to the EPR effect. In order for continuous knockdown of luciferase, it was determined that injections would be needed every four days [112].

There are however, a number of problems if the EPR effect is the sole mechanism for targeting in cancer gene therapy. One such problem is tumour size. Tumours that are larger than 1 cm in diameter develop hypoxic regions that are characterised by a lack of blood vessels, therefore the EPR effect becomes redundant in these resistant regions. Evans blue dye and albumin were used to generate a synthetic macromolecule delivery of which showed that although selective, in tumours larger than 3 cm, the dye accumulated solely in the peripheral regions and not in the central core [113]. One method to increase the EPR in solid tumours is through the use of nitric oxide donors in combination with macromolecular delivery. Endogenous nitric oxide (NO) has an effect on blood flow, angiogenesis and metastatic potential [114-116]. From a therapeutic perspective there are conflicting reports as to whether it is better to enhance or inhibit nitric oxide within tumours [117]. From an enhancement perspective, studies within our own group using iNOS (inducible NO synthase) gene therapy have shown the cytotoxic and radio-chemo sensitizing affects through the generation of μM levels of NO [118,119]. The controlled generation of high levels of nitric oxide as the gene therapy has several anti-cancer advantages, including a genotoxic effect through oxidation, deamination and alkylation of DNA, reduction of the efficiency of DNA repair proteins such as Poly ADP Ribose Polymerase, inhibition of the transcription of hypoxia inducible factor and the anti-apoptotic factor NF-kB which reduces many other pro tumourigenic factors such as MMP1, 3, 9, VEGF, survivin and BCL2 [120]. Derivatives of NO such as peroxynitrite (ONOO) have also been shown to potentiate the EPR effect. Wu and colleagues showed that this was also linked to activation of MMPs, which are known to enhance vascular permeability and angiogenesis through the degradation of matrix proteins [121]. One of the main ways of enhancing the EPR effect is through NO donors, which have been utilised in combination with chemotherapy drugs. For example nitroglycerin has been delivered with vinorelbine and cisplatin in patients with non-small cell lung cancer in a randomised phase II trial. Results showed a response rate of 73% in those patients that received the nitroglycerin plus chemotherapy, compared to 42% in the chemotherapy only arm. The improved effects were attributed to the known anti-cancer effects of NO and an improvement in drug delivery to the tumour tissue, i.e. the EPR effect [122]. With respect to gene therapy, the delivery of the iNOS gene would most certainly enhance the EPR effect in solid tumours although consideration must be given to the amount of NO generated. As gene expression is dependent on successful nuclear transport of the plasmid, it would be very difficult to predict and indeed control. With NO gene therapy, it is therefore essential to target the expression of the gene to the target tissue to gain the maximum therapeutic benefit.

Another problem in EPR targeting comes about with what is commonly termed the 'PEG dilemma'. This is essentially a trade-off between circulation time and efficacy of nucleic acid delivery. Many nanoparticles are PEGylated to increase circulation time, avoid clearance by the reticuloendothelial system (RES) and evade an immune response. As previously stated, if the EPR effect is to be exploited in solid tumours, a long circulation time is needed and PEG represents a possible solution. However, the physiochemical properties of many delivery systems are altered when PEG is introduced; this is particularly the case when the cargo is nucleic acids such as siRNA or DNA. In order for nucleic acids to be successful they must be delivered to the correct intracellular destination. PEG not only reduces the overall charge of the nanoparticles, which in turn lowers the cellular uptake, but also impairs disruption of the endosome. Therefore if PEGylation is to be used to enable EPR targeting, novel systems must be developed that can overcome the intracellular barriers to effective nucleic acid delivery.

4.2. Targeting ligands

One method of targeting is via the incorporation of targeting ligands that bind to cell-surface receptors. This approach is dependent upon possession of the knowledge of which receptor or combinations of receptors are hyperactivated on the cancer cell surface. One such example is the asialoglycoprotein receptor (ASGPr) which, although present on the surface of normal hepatocytes, is overexpressed in hepatocarcinoma cells. The ligand asialofetuin has been attached to a novel lipopolymeric nanoparticle to deliver the immunostimulatory IL-12 cytokine in the treatment of hepatocellular carcinoma. Following intratumoural administration of the targeted nanoparticles, the authors showed survival in 75% of mice treated with targeted nanoparticles compared to 38% in the non-targeted nanoparticles. This indicates that the presence of the ASGPr targeting ligand improves intracellular internalization via receptor-mediated endocytosis. Following systemic delivery of either nanoparticle type, luciferase expression in the liver and lungs was assessed. Luciferase expression was 10-fold higher in the livers of those mice that received targeted nanoparticles. However, there was also gene expression in the lung with no significant differences between targeted and non-targeted nanoparticles which indicates that further formulations may be necessary, and that evaluation of gene expression in all the organs is necessary to confirm appropriate targeting [123].

Another useful targeting ligand for cancer gene therapy is transferrin. Transferrin is overexpressed in many malignancies including breast, bladder and lung [124-126]. The differential expression of the transferrin receptor and its extracellular location make it an ideal target for systemic targeting. Systemic delivery of transferrin covalently linked to polyethylenimine has not only shown effective tumour targeting *in vivo*, but it can also shield the positive charge of the nanoparticles [127]. Studies by Kircheis showed that a lower molecular weight of PEI was less toxic and that the incorporation of 25% of the negatively charged lipophilic transferrin ligand gave an almost neutral zeta potential with a significant reduction in aggregation of erythrocytes. *In vivo* this translated into lower toxicity, one log greater gene expression than transferrin-free nanoparticles and a 'shielding' effect to bypass organs such as the lung and target the tumour [127].

Identification of overexpressed receptors can also lead to the development tumour targeting peptides. Using phage display methods, the T7 peptide (HAIYPRH) was identified and shown to specifically bind to the human transferrin receptor, with competitive studies indicating that T7 bound at a different site to transferrin [128]. This T7 peptide has recently been utilised for targeted co-delivery of the chemotherapy drug doxorubicin (DOX) together with the human TRAIL gene (Tumour necrosis factor Related Apoptosis-Inducing Ligand) to target gliomas which are known to overexpress the transferrin receptor [129]. DOX was conjugated with a pH linker (for endosomal release) to T7-modified dendigraft poly-L-Lysine dendrimers which then condensed the pORF-hTRAIL DNA [129]. *In vitro* and *in vivo* evaluations revealed targeting via the transferrin receptor and accumulation of the nanoparticles in gliomas following systemic delivery with a synergistic effect. In addition, the targeted T7 nanoparticles induced much less off site toxicity while inducing a significant anti-tumour effect [129].

Other targeting ligands of note include the epidermal growth factor receptor that is upregulated in a number of solid tumours such as breast, prostate, colorectal, and ovarian [130]. Although some anti-cancer strategies are designed to prevent EGFR activation via small molecule inhibitors such as gefitinib or antibodies such as Cetuximab [131], an alternative is to exploit the differential expression of EGFR. Thiol functionalisation to attach the mouse EGF ligand to PEGylated branched PEI (25 kDa) has shown excellent *in vivo* targeting to hepatocellular carcinoma. Biodistribution studies illustrate quite clearly that there is significantly more expression of the luciferase gene in both Huh-7 and HepG2 HCC tumours compared to other organs following intravenous injection of the complexes [132]. The authors also found that any distribution of the DNA to the liver was exclusively in the Kupffer cells and not the epithelial cells, indicative of degradation.

The EGF-PEG-PEI system has also been used to selectively deliver synthetic double stranded RNA (poly IC) [133]. Typically dsRNA is found in virally infected cells and an associated response involves the induction of apoptosis and recruitment of inflammatory cytokines [134,135]. Delivery of poly IC with PEI_{25}-PEG-EGF killed up to 85% of EGFR-over-expressing glioblastoma multiform cells *in vitro* via apoptosis after 1 hour [133]. This cytotoxic effect was significantly enhanced when the PEI was partially replaced with a PEI-Mellitin conjugate, which improved endosomal disruption, enabling greater delivery of the dsRNA to the cytoplasm. In addition, the intratumoural delivery of (poly IC) PEI-PEG-EGF+PEI-Mel complexes completely eradicated the intracranial tumours for more than 1 year [133]. Further studies have revealed that with further formulation of the delivery vehicle (Linear PEI-PEG 2 kDa-EGF), systemic delivery of poly IC can significantly reduce A431 tumour growth *in vivo* [136]. Similar to transferrin, polypeptides for EGFR have been isolated and used effectively in cancer gene therapy. Phage display revealed an 11 amino acid sequence (YHWYGYTPQNVI) termed GE11 that has shown specificity to the EGFR after both *in vitro* and *in vivo* studies [137]. Furthermore, when the GE11 peptide was conjugated to PEI and compared with EGF-PEI, it was found that the latter enhanced mitogenic activity, which is clearly undesirable in the cancer environment. The authors indicate that due to this lack of mitogenic activity, the GE11 ligand is safer *in vivo*, and delivery of the luciferase gene intra-venously revealed an 18-fold increase in luciferase expression in human hepatoma SMMC-7721 tumours compared to non-targeted PEI [137].

The fibronectin attachment protein of mycobacterium has also been utilised as a targeting ligand to the fibronectin molecule on epithelial cell membranes [138]. The Fab receptor was conjugated to chitosan-DNA nanoparticles and delivered via an air jet nebuliser to enhance gene expression in the lung epithelium. Again using the luciferase reporter gene, studies re-vealed that there was a 16-fold increase in gene expression over the non-targeted chitosan nanoparticles [138]. Another example of exploitation of differential expression is in glioma brain capillary endothelial cells that have an upregulation of the lipoprotein receptor-related protein-1. The angiopep-2 peptide ligand (TFFYGGSRGKRNNFKTEEY) has been success-fully conjugated to a polyamidoaminedendrimer (PAMAM) with a PEG spacer and studies showed that cellular uptake of the nanoparticles was targeting ligand dose-dependent, and that targeting to the brain was achieved following intravenous delivery [139]. The angiopep targeting system has also been utilised to achieve a therapeutic efficacy in the delivery of PAMAM-PEG-Angiopep/pORF-TRAIL to glial tumours [140]. The administration of these modified nanoparticles yielded an average survival time of 69 days compared to 30 days in the parental PAMAM-PEG/pORF-TRAIL nanoparticle-receiving mice [140].

There are of course numerous examples of systemic targeted delivery employing such li-gands. The message that is apparent from all of these studies is that if there is enough infor-mation on the expression of a certain receptor, then the incorporation of its targeting ligand into cationic non-viral systems can significantly enhance tumour-targeted accumulation of the nucleic acid.

4.3. Affibody targeting

Affibodies are small stable alpha helical proteins that lack disulphide bonds, have a low mo-lecular weight and are essentially designed to mimic the action of antibodies. An original affibody protein scaffold is used as a template from which combinatorial phage libraries can be generated and subsequently ligand-specific affibodies can be selected from using phage display technology. Such protein scaffolds have been generated from bacterial surface recep-tors such as the IgG binding domains of staphylococcal protein A (SPA). The 58 amino acid Z domain from staphylococcal protein A (SPA) is one such scaffold that has been used as a template for ligand specific affibodies [141,142].

With respect to cancer targeting, high affinity affibodies have been generated for Human Epi-dermal Growth Factor Receptor 2 [143], Epidermal Growth Factor Receptor [144], Insulin-like Growth Factor-1 Receptor [145] and Platelet Derived Growth Factor Receptor β [146]. Using radio-labelling, all of the affibodies have been shown to accumulate in tumours *in vivo* with an impressive level of specificity following systemic delivery. The affinity of the affibodies is an important factor and ideally should be in the nanomolar range for effective targeting. For ex-ample, the affinity levels of affibody $Z_{HER2:4}$ are 50 nmol/L [147] whereas using a one step affin-ity maturation process, Orlova and colleagues were able to generate the $Z_{HER2:342}$ affibody which has an affinity level of 22 pmol/L [143]. The increased affinity translated into a 4-fold increase in tumour uptake of $Z_{HER2:342}$ four hours post-injection with clear contrast in imaging and stability at least up to 24 h post-injection. With respect to the first generation EGFR affibodies, the affinity was in the 150 nM range [148] which is sub optimal for effective systemic targeting. A similar one step maturation procedure for the EGFR affibody showed that affinity could be significantly improved whereby $Z_{EGFR1907}$ had a K_d of 5.4 nM. Furthermore, there was significant uptake of the indium-111-labeled affibody $Z_{EGFR1907}$ in A431 tumours and EGFR-expressing organs *in vivo* compared to the non-EGFR-affibody Z_{taq} [144].

Translational applications of these 2nd generation affibodies to date include therapeutic tools for diagnostic and imaging purposes to aid in the identification of molecular drug targets and for the stratification of cancer patient populations. However these highly stable, selective proteins are undoubtedly going to have a huge role in the advancement of targeted non-viral systems in cancer gene therapy. Recently a peptide chimera was designed that consisted of the cell penetrating peptide TAT (T), the DNA condensing motif Mu and the HER2 affibody (AF). The position of the AF was critical to ensure targeting functionality given that the affibody must be able to fold properly. Prior to synthesis, ITASSER software was employed to predict functionality based upon peptide design with a linker between TAT-MU and AF that was helical and should therefore ensure stability of the domains [149]. Studies with the purified recombinant TAT-Mu-AF showed that this ternary complex could condense DNA, confer protection from degradation by DNase I and offer stability in serum [150]. Using GFP DNA complexed at a 1:8:2 ratio, there was little uptake of the complexes in the HER2-null MDA-MB-231 cell line and green fluorescence in the HER2-expressing MDA-MB-453, SK-OV-3 and SK-BR-3 cell lines that was proportional to HER2 receptor density. Furthermore, the complexes were non-toxic and functional when injected intra-tumourally into the HER2 positive MDA-MB-453 breast tumours *in vivo* [150]. Unfortunately these ternary complexes as yet have not been administered intravenously, which is the ultimate test of functionality, given the range of extracellular barriers previously discussed. Nevertheless, this ternary peptide system holds a lot of promise in the next generation of targeted peptide/protein delivery systems for non-viral gene therapy.

PEGylated liposomes have also been synthesised conjugated to the $Z_{EGFR:1907}$ affibody with a cysteine residue at the C-terminus to form sterically stabilised affibody liposomes (SAL) [151]. Although the SAL system was loaded with the drug mitoxantrone (MTO), other macromolecules such as nucleic acids could be applied to this system. The MTO-SAL nanoparticles were tested for cytotoxicity on EGFR-expressing A431 and MDA-MB-468 cell lines with MCF-7 as a negative control. Results indicated that the MTO-SAL nanoparticles had no effect on the viability of the EGFR-negative MCF-7 cell line (IC50 value > 100 μM, compared with an IC50 of 18 μm for MTO alone), while the EGFR-expressing A431 (2.8 μM) and MDA-MB-468 (6.8 μM) cell lines were as sensitive to MTO-SAL nanoparticles as they were to MTO only (IC50 1.3 μM and 3 μM respectively) [151]. Taken together, these data suggest that SAL specifically delivered its MTO payload to the EGFR-expressing cells, and that EGFR-null cells were protected from MTO-induced cytotoxicity by the SAL vehicle. These studies illustrate that cysteine-modified affibodies can be targeting ligands on liposomal delivery vehicles. Furthermore, by ensuring that receptor-mediated endocytosis occurs via the affibodies, a protective effect is conferred on non-expressing receptor tissue which is highly attractive for the delivery of cytotoxic nucleic acids.

Another example of the use of the $Z_{HER2:342}$ affibody [143] is in a multifunctional biopolymer system that comprises several discrete functions [152]. This system consists of a fusogenic peptide (FP) sequence H5WYG [153], a DNA-condensing and endosomolytic domain (DCE) with repeating sequences of arginine and histidine, a M9 nuclear localization domain (NLS) [154] and a C-terminal $Z_{HER2:342}$ affibody [143]. What is particularly striking about this delivery system is that the authors have designed it taking into account all of the intracellular barriers, and with the use of discrete motifs, have attempted to overcome each hurdle to successful gene delivery. Engineered within this delivery system is also cathepsin D enzyme substrate (CS) to enable cleavage of the targeting motif from the rest of the vector in late endosomes [152]. The DNA sequence for FP-(DCE)3-NLS-CS-TM was cloned into an inducible expression system and the recombinant biopolymer was expressed and extracted using affinity and size exclusion chromatography [152]. The functionality of each discrete motif was proven and competitive inhibitor binding and transfection studies clearly indicated that the affibody ensured receptor-mediated endocytosis *in vitro* [152]. Transfection efficiency of 21% was achieved in the SKOV-3 HER2-expressing cell line, while efficiencies of only 0.1 and 2% were achieved in the non-expressing PC-3 and MDA-MB-231 prostate and breast cancer cell lines, respectively. *In vivo* delivery and evaluation of the immune response are critical for the future development of such smart biopolymer systems. Nevertheless, this study illustrates that high affinity affibodies can be functional in recombinant delivery vectors, thus enabling receptor targeting to occur.

4.4. Transcriptional targeting

Of course it may not be necessary to have a targeted delivery system to achieve expression of a desired gene in a particular tissue. Many tumours have a differential expression of a particular transcription factor that can be exploited and used to restrict gene expression to a particular site. Several promoters that are either tissue- or tumour-specific have been developed that can circumvent the issues surrounding targeting delivery systems. For example the differential expression in telomerase activity between tumour and normal tissue together with the identification of the minimal components necessary for telomerase activity has enabled the use of the human telomerase reverse transcriptase and the template containing telomerase (hTERT and hTER) promoters to control gene expression. Studies by Dufès et al showed that systemic delivery of polypropylenimedendrimers complexed with a TNFalpha-expressing plasmid under the control of hTER and hTERT gave regression of solid carcinomas in xenografts with 100% survival with no obvious signs of toxicity [155]. The hTERT promoter has also been used in a dual reporter system with the human alpha fetoprotein (hAFP) promoter to drive expression of MicroRNA-26a (MiR-26a), a known tumour suppressor downregulated in hepatocellular carcinoma (HCC) [156]. The dual promoter system significantly increased MiR-26a expression and reduced viability *in vitro* and *in vivo* compared to single promoter or constitutively driven MiR-26a constructs in the HCC cell lines [156].

Insulin-like Growth Factor 2 (IGF2) is involved in cellular proliferation and differentiation, but is also overexpressed in a variety of tumours such as bladder carcinoma [157]. IGF2 has a total of four promoters with P3 and P4 promoters responsible for IGF2 expression during foetal and tumour development [158]. P3 and P4 have been utilized to drive expression of the cytotoxic Diphtheria Toxin A gene both as a single promoter system and a dual promoter construct termed P4-DTA-P3-DTA [159]. Part of the rationale for this was related to the differential activation of both P3 and P4 regulatory sequences in human tumours, so a dual system would ensure induction of DTA in a larger population of tumours. Using PEI as the delivery vehicle, bladder carcinoma studies have revealed that P4-DTA-P3-DTA was superior *in vitro* and *in vivo* in both heterotropic and orthotopic bladder tumour models [159]. Similar studies have also been performed in glioma models utilising the cancer-specific H19 promoter in tandem with the P4-IGF2 promoter to selectively control DTA expression [160]. These dual systems have to-date focused on accessible tumours where intratumoural injection would suffice, but only systemic delivery of such systems will fully validate the transcriptional control afforded by these promoters.

Many cancers have the propensity to metastasize to bone, and such tumours acquire osteomimetic characteristics in order to adapt and thrive in the local bone environment. Disseminated bone deposits are resistant to conventional therapies and are particularly difficult to target. Osteocalcin is the most abundant noncollagenous bone matrix protein and is involved in the regulation of bone formation and resorption [161-163]. Osteocalcin is also overe-xpressed in a range of cancers including ovarian, lung, brain, breast and prostate [164-166]. The transcription factor largely responsible for activating the osteocalcin promoter is the master transcription factor RUNX2. RUNX2 is also highly expressed in tumours that metastasise to bone, and therefore widespread activation of the human osteocalcin (hOC) promoter should be achieved, regardless of the heterogeneous tumour microenvironment. The hOC promoter has been utilized to drive inducible nitric oxide synthase (iNOS) expression [167,168]. Commercially available liposomes were used as a delivery vehicle for the hOC-iNOS construct. This resulted in exquisite specificity for androgen-independent prostate cancer cells *in vitro*, coupled with cytotoxicity comparable to that of constitutively expressed iNOS. *In vivo* data also confirmed the potency of hOC-iNOS gene therapy in a mouse xenograft model of human prostate (PC-3) cancer. Multiple intra-tumoural injections slowed tumour growth dramatically and led to some complete responses. On average, tumour growth was delayed by 59 days compared to vector only controls. This data from these studies supports the premise that tumour-specific promoters can effectively drive iNOS monotherapy giving long term tumour control. Future work within this group is now focused on systemic delivery of hOC-iNOS gene therapy. The hOC promoter has also been delivered systemically to control expression of TK in a replication-defective adenovirus (Ad-hOC-TK) and early viral genes in a replication competent adenovirus (Ad-hOC-E1) [169]. The authors found that vitamins C and D_3 significantly increased the activity of the hOC promoter and that triple therapy with Ad-hOC-E1, vitamin D_3 and vitamin C resulted in complete regression in 38% of renal cell carcinomas *in vivo* following a single intravenous injection [169].

Targeting to a desired tissue is quite often the stumbling block to systemic cancer gene therapy. For the delivery of DNA, targeting can be achieved through the use of promoter sequences. The success of this method of targeting is reliant upon prior knowledge of a difference in transcription factor expression between the target and normal tissue. A delivery system could therefore be designed to condense the DNA, traverse cell membranes, disrupt endosomes and actively transport the payload to the nucleus without the added biophysical complications of having an external targeting motif. Such a delivery system would in theory deliver the DNA to all tissue, but the DNA would only be transcribed and translated where the desired transcription factor is present, namely the target tissue.

5. Multifunctional delivery

An understanding of the key biological barriers is critical to the success of a multifunctional delivery vehicle. Perhaps one of the most multifaceted delivery vehicles is the Multifunctional Envelope-type Nano Device MEND system [170]. The authors describe this as a 'programmed packaging' system whereby each part of the system is designed to carry out a specific function in a time-controlled manner. In this system the nucleic acid is condensed with a cationic polymer, wrapped in a lipid envelope which is then functionalised with PEG or other targeting ligands [170]. It is quite clear that PEGylated MEND did have a longer circulation time and was not rapidly cleared from the liver. These are ideal extracellular delivery characteristics, but unfortunately this translated into a much lower gene expression. Therefore circumvention of the 'PEG dilemma' could be achieved via the attachment of targeting ligands to receptors that are known to be over-expressed on tumour cells coupled with the attachment of a cleavable PEG that exploits either intracellular or tumour-specific characteristics. Figure 2 contains a representation of a MEND that highlights some of the nucleic acids that have been delivered and functionalisation strategies that have been used.

The avoidance of an immune response to non-viral strategies can also be greatly improved by use of MENDs as delivery devices. Delivery of pDNA to mice by a MEND resulted in differential expression of almost 1600 genes; PEGylation of the MEND reversed the altered expression of many of these genes. Gene Ontology analysis revealed that in general, the up-regulated genes were associated with "immune response," "response to biotic stimulus," "defence response," and related processes. The expression of IL-6, but not IFNα (commonly activated cytokines, as discussed above), were lower in the PEGylated MEND group compared with the non-PEGylated [171]. PEGylation has been shown to limit endosomal escape of gene delivery complexes [172]; inclusion of GALA in the MEND facilitated endosomal escape, and diminished the previously elevated IFNα levels [171]. A MEND functionalised with a PEG-peptide-DOPE conjugate (PPD) was stable in the systemic circulation after intravenous delivery (thereby benefiting from PEG's stabilising characteristic), while it also potently delivered its pDNA cargo to HT1080 fibrosarcoma cells (MMP-rich), but not to HEK293 human embryonic kidney cells (MMP-deficient), thereby avoiding PEG's limiting characteristic [173]. Cleavage of PEG by MMPs facilitates the targeting of tumour tissues which are high in MMPs.

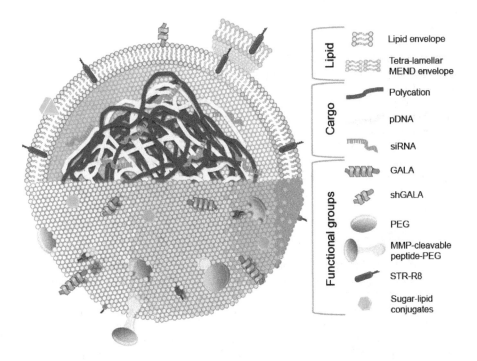

Figure 2. Simplified amalgamation of multifunctional envelope-type nano devices (MENDs) that have been employed for non-viral gene therapy development. pDNA cargoes encoding proteins such as luciferase [173-175] and GFP [176] have been delivered, as well as siRNA targeting luciferase [177,178] and ACTB [179]. MEND polycations are generally PLL [174,178] or protamine [173,175,176]. Lipid envelopes usually comprise DOTAP, DOPE and cholesterol [177,179,180], but can also include CHEMS [174,178]. Tetra-lamellar MEND envelopes comprise DOPE/cholesterol inner and DOPE/phosphatidic acid outer layers [176]. Functionalisation of MENDS with GALA/short GALA [179], STR-R8 [174,176,178], PEG and MMP-cleavable PEG [170,173,177] and sugar-lipid conjugates [175] have all been reported. Based on [181].

The fundamental limitation associated with non-viral gene therapies is their low transfection ability, compared with viral systems [1]. pDNA condensed using poly-L-lysine and incorporated into a MEND that comprised DOPE, cholesterylhemisuccinate and an octa-arginine (R8) peptide (DOPE/CHEMS/STR-R8) transfected HeLa and A549 cells as efficiently as an adenovirus vector. Moreover, the parity of transfection efficiency was achieved without negatively impacting cell viability, as was the case with adenovirus and Lipofectamine™, and evoked its therapeutic benefit following transdermal delivery in mice [181]. The R8 peptide has been used similarly to deliver proteins directly to cells [182].

A tetra-lamellar MEND (T-MEND) was nano-engineered that envelops the cationically-condensed pDNA in distinct functional layers to target the distinct barrier membranes faced by a nanoparticle. The pDNA-containing core was wrapped in a nucleus-fusogenic lipid membrane, which was in turn wrapped in an endosome-fusogenic lipid membrane that was modified with a high density of octa-arginine. Upon endocytosis into the cell, the T-MEND's outermost membrane fuses with the endosomal membrane, releasing the nucleus-fusogenic lipid membrane-bound pDNA core from the endosome into the cytoplasm. The nuclear membrane is then overcome by fusion of the inner nucleus-fusogenic lipid membrane with the nuclear membrane, facilitating transport of the pDNA core into the nucleus. Despite the complexity of the particles, the fully-formed T-MEND produced particles of 163 nm diameter, and zeta potential of 54.5mV. Unsurprisingly, the T-MEND facilitated impressive pLuciferase delivery *in vitro* [176]. This exciting T-MEND was further functionalised by addition of fusogenic KALA to the outer and inner membranes, which improved transfection 20-fold [183]. To the authors' knowledge, systemic delivery of multi-layered MENDs is yet to be reported. Caution must be advised, as promising *in vitro* findings do not always translate into impressive *in vivo* developments.

6. Conclusion

It is apparent that the field of non-viral gene delivery is making significant progress in the quest for the ideal gene delivery vehicle. What is also evident is that the most successful systems are designed to overcome many biological barriers and as a consequence the traditional single function systems are now rendered obsolete. Viruses are nature's perfect delivery vehicle and provide the inspiration to many non-viral gene therapy researchers in the design of state of the art multi-faceted vehicles. Through a greater understanding and appreciation of the biological barriers to systemic gene delivery, non- viral gene therapy researchers are on the cusp of creating a variety of highly efficient vehicles that will revolutionise cancer gene therapy.

Author details

Cian M. McCrudden and Helen O. McCarthy

School of Pharmacy, Queen's University Belfast, Northern Ireland, UK

References

[1] Miyata K, Nishiyama N, Kataoka K. Rational design of smart supramolecular assemblies for gene delivery: chemical challenges in the creation of artificial viruses. Chem Soc Rev 2012 Apr 7;41(7):2562-2574.

[2] Temsamani J, Pari GS, Guinot P. Antisense approach for the treatment of cytomegalovirus infection. Expert Opin Investig Drugs 1997 Sep;6(9):1157-1167.

[3]   Ng EW, Shima DT, Calias P, Cunningham ET,Jr, Guyer DR, Adamis AP. Pegaptanib, a targeted anti-VEGF aptamer for ocular vascular disease. Nat Rev Drug Discov 2006 Feb;5(2):123-132.

[4]   Thomas CE, Ehrhardt A, Kay MA. Progress and problems with the use of viral vectors for gene therapy. Nat Rev Genet 2003 May;4(5):346-358.

[5]   Young LS, Searle PF, Onion D, Mautner V. Viral gene therapy strategies: from basic science to clinical application. J Pathol 2006 Jan;208(2):299-318.

[6]   Marshall E. Gene therapy death prompts review of adenovirus vector. Science 1999 Dec 17;286(5448):2244-2245.

[7]   Wang T, Upponi JR, Torchilin VP. Design of multifunctional non-viral gene vectors to overcome physiological barriers: dilemmas and strategies. Int J Pharm 2012 May 1;427(1):3-20.

[8]   Herweijer H, Wolff JA. Progress and prospects: naked DNA gene transfer and therapy. Gene Ther 2003 Mar;10(6):453-458.

[9]   Khalil IA, Kogure K, Akita H, Harashima H. Uptake pathways and subsequent intracellular trafficking in nonviral gene delivery. Pharmacol Rev 2006 Mar;58(1):32-45.

[10] Lam AP, Dean DA. Progress and prospects: nuclear import of nonviral vectors. Gene Ther 2010 Apr;17(4):439-447.

[11] Felgner PL, Gadek TR, Holm M, Roman R, Chan HW, Wenz M, et al. Lipofection: a highly efficient, lipid-mediated DNA-transfection procedure. Proc Natl Acad Sci U S A 1987 Nov;84(21):7413-7417.

[12] Behr JP, Demeneix B, Loeffler JP, Perez-Mutul J. Efficient gene transfer into mammalian primary endocrine cells with lipopolyamine-coated DNA. Proc Natl Acad Sci U S A 1989 Sep;86(18):6982-6986.

[13] Leventis R, Silvius JR. Interactions of mammalian cells with lipid dispersions containing novel metabolizable cationic amphiphiles. Biochim Biophys Acta 1990 Mar 30;1023(1):124-132.

[14] Gao X, Huang L. A novel cationic liposome reagent for efficient transfection of mammalian cells. Biochem Biophys Res Commun 1991 Aug 30;179(1):280-285.

[15] Balazs DA, Godbey W. Liposomes for use in gene delivery. J Drug Deliv 2011;2011:326497.

[16] Kurosaki T, Kitahara T, Teshima M, Nishida K, Nakamura J, Nakashima M, et al. Exploitation of De Novo helper-lipids for effective gene delivery. J Pharm Pharm Sci 2008;11(4):56-67.

[17] Duarte S, Faneca H, Lima MC. Folate-associated lipoplexes mediate efficient gene delivery and potent antitumoral activity in vitro and in vivo. Int J Pharm 2012 Feb 28;423(2):365-377.

[18] Wang C, Ding C, Kong M, Dong A, Qian J, Jiang D, et al. Tumor-targeting magnetic lipoplex delivery of short hairpin RNA suppresses IGF-1R overexpression of lung adenocarcinoma A549 cells in vitro and in vivo. Biochem Biophys Res Commun 2011 Jul 8;410(3):537-542.

[19] Numata K, Reagan MR, Goldstein RH, Rosenblatt M, Kaplan DL. Spider silk-based gene carriers for tumor cell-specific delivery. Bioconjug Chem 2011 Aug 17;22(8): 1605-1610.

[20] Patil ML, Zhang M, Minko T. Multifunctional triblock Nanocarrier (PAMAM-PEG-PLL) for the efficient intracellular siRNA delivery and gene silencing. ACS Nano 2011 Mar 22;5(3):1877-1887.

[21] Liu P, Gou M, Yi T, Qi X, Xie C, Zhou S, et al. The enhanced antitumor effects of bio-degradable cationic heparin-polyethyleneimine nanogels delivering HSulf-1 gene combined with cisplatin on ovarian cancer. Int J Oncol 2012 Jul 18.

[22] Chen J, Tian H, Kano A, Maruyama A, Chen X, Park TG. In vitro and in vivo gene delivery using polyethylenimine-poly(hydroxyethyl glutamine) as a non-viral carrier. J Control Release 2011 Nov 30;152 Suppl 1:e134-6.

[23] Li W, Nicol F, Szoka FC,Jr. GALA: a designed synthetic pH-responsive amphipathic peptide with applications in drug and gene delivery. Adv Drug Deliv Rev 2004 Apr 23;56(7):967-985.

[24] Wyman TB, Nicol F, Zelphati O, Scaria PV, Plank C, Szoka FC,Jr. Design, synthesis, and characterization of a cationic peptide that binds to nucleic acids and permeabilizes bilayers. Biochemistry 1997 Mar 11;36(10):3008-3017.

[25] Han J, Il Yeom Y. Specific gene transfer mediated by galactosylated poly-L-lysine into hepatoma cells. Int J Pharm 2000 Jul 20;202(1-2):151-160.

[26] Chen S, Zhuo RX, Cheng SX. Enhanced gene transfection with addition of a cell-penetrating peptide in substrate-mediated gene delivery. J Gene Med 2010 Aug;12(8): 705-713.

[27] Ye SF, Tian MM, Wang TX, Ren L, Wang D, Shen LH, et al. Synergistic effects of cell-penetrating peptide Tat and fusogenic peptide HA2-enhanced cellular internalization and gene transduction of organosilica nanoparticles. Nanomedicine 2012 Aug; 8(6):833-841.

[28] Mangipudi SS, Canine BF, Wang Y, Hatefi A. Development of a genetically engineered biomimetic vector for targeted gene transfer to breast cancer cells. Mol Pharm 2009 Jul-Aug;6(4):1100-1109.

[29] McCarthy HO, Zholobenko AV, Wang Y, Canine B, Robson T, Hirst DG, et al. Evaluation of a multi-functional nanocarrier for targeted breast cancer iNOS gene therapy. Int J Pharm 2011 Feb 28;405(1-2):196-202.

[30] Zhang L, Li L, Hoffmann GA, Hoffman RM. Depth-targeted efficient gene delivery and expression in the skin by pulsed electric fields: an approach to gene therapy of

skin aging and other diseases. Biochem Biophys Res Commun 1996 Mar 27;220(3): 633-636.

[31] Foldvari M, Babiuk S, Badea I. DNA delivery for vaccination and therapeutics through the skin. Curr Drug Deliv 2006 Jan;3(1):17-28.

[32] Fischer H, Scherz J, Szabo S, Mildner M, Benarafa C, Torriglia A, et al. DNase 2 is the main DNA-degrading enzyme of the stratum corneum. PLoS One 2011 Mar 1;6(3):e17581.

[33] Menck CF, Armelini MG, Lima-Bessa KM. On the search for skin gene therapy strategies of xeroderma pigmentosum disease. Curr Gene Ther 2007 Jun;7(3):163-174.

[34] Warrick E, Garcia M, Chagnoleau C, Chevallier O, Bergoglio V, Sartori D, et al. Preclinical corrective gene transfer in xeroderma pigmentosum human skin stem cells. Mol Ther 2012 Apr;20(4):798-807.

[35] Coulman SA, Barrow D, Anstey A, Gateley C, Morrissey A, Wilke N, et al. Minimally invasive cutaneous delivery of macromolecules and plasmid DNA via microneedles. Curr Drug Deliv 2006 Jan;3(1):65-75.

[36] Zheng D, Giljohann DA, Chen DL, Massich MD, Wang XQ, Iordanov H, et al. Topical delivery of siRNA-based spherical nucleic acid nanoparticle conjugates for gene regulation. Proc Natl Acad Sci U S A 2012 Jul 24;109(30):11975-11980.

[37] Babiuk S, Baca-Estrada ME, Foldvari M, Baizer L, Stout R, Storms M, et al. Needle-free topical electroporation improves gene expression from plasmids administered in porcine skin. Mol Ther 2003 Dec;8(6):992-998.

[38] Lee K, Kim JD, Lee CY, Her S, Jung H. A high-capacity, hybrid electro-microneedle for in-situ cutaneous gene transfer. Biomaterials 2011 Oct;32(30):7705-7710.

[39] Kawabata K, Takakura Y, Hashida M. The fate of plasmid DNA after intravenous injection in mice: involvement of scavenger receptors in its hepatic uptake. Pharm Res 1995 Jun;12(6):825-830.

[40] Mumper RJ, Duguid JG, Anwer K, Barron MK, Nitta H, Rolland AP. Polyvinyl derivatives as novel interactive polymers for controlled gene delivery to muscle. Pharm Res 1996 May;13(5):701-709.

[41] Bitko V, Musiyenko A, Shulyayeva O, Barik S. Inhibition of respiratory viruses by nasally administered siRNA. Nat Med 2005 Jan;11(1):50-55.

[42] Colella P, Cotugno G, Auricchio A. Ocular gene therapy: current progress and future prospects. Trends Mol Med 2009 Jan;15(1):23-31.

[43] Dawson M, Krauland E, Wirtz D, Hanes J. Transport of polymeric nanoparticle gene carriers in gastric mucus. Biotechnol Prog 2004 May-Jun;20(3):851-857.

[44] Wiethoff CM, Middaugh CR. Barriers to nonviral gene delivery. J Pharm Sci 2003 Feb;92(2):203-217.

[45] Mignet N, Vandermeulen G, Pembouong G, Largeau C, Thompson B, Spanedda MV, et al. Cationic and anionic lipoplexes inhibit gene transfection by electroporation in vivo. J Gene Med 2010 Jun;12(6):491-500.

[46] Liu YP, Tong C, Dispenzieri A, Federspiel MJ, Russell SJ, Peng KW. Polyinosinic acid decreases sequestration and improves systemic therapy of measles virus. Cancer Gene Ther 2012 Mar;19(3):202-211.

[47] Finsinger D, Remy JS, Erbacher P, Koch C, Plank C. Protective copolymers for nonviral gene vectors: synthesis, vector characterization and application in gene delivery. Gene Ther 2000 Jul;7(14):1183-1192.

[48] Kizzire K, Khargharia S, Rice KG. High-affinity PEGylated polyacridine peptide polyplexes mediate potent in vivo gene expression. Gene Ther 2012 Jul 12.

[49] Naeye B, Raemdonck K, Remaut K, Sproat B, Demeester J, De Smedt SC. PEGylation of biodegradable dextran nanogels for siRNA delivery. Eur J Pharm Sci 2010 Jul 11;40(4):342-351.

[50] Xu Z, Smith JS, Tian J, Byrnes AP. Induction of shock after intravenous injection of adenovirus vectors: a critical role for platelet-activating factor. Mol Ther 2010 Mar; 18(3):609-616.

[51] Stone D, Liu Y, Shayakhmetov D, Li ZY, Ni S, Lieber A. Adenovirus-platelet interaction in blood causes virus sequestration to the reticuloendothelial system of the liver. J Virol 2007 May;81(9):4866-4871.

[52] Li L, Wang R, Wilcox D, Zhao X, Song J, Lin X, et al. Tumor vasculature is a key determinant for the efficiency of nanoparticle-mediated siRNA delivery. Gene Ther 2012 Jul;19(7):775-780.

[53] Acharya S, Sahoo SK. PLGA nanoparticles containing various anticancer agents and tumour delivery by EPR effect. Adv Drug Deliv Rev 2011 Mar 18;63(3):170-183.

[54] Tagami T, Suzuki T, Matsunaga M, Nakamura K, Moriyoshi N, Ishida T, et al. Anti-angiogenic therapy via cationic liposome-mediated systemic siRNA delivery. Int J Pharm 2012 Jan 17;422(1-2):280-289.

[55] Geis NA, Katus HA, Bekeredjian R. Microbubbles as a vehicle for gene and drug delivery: current clinical implications and future perspectives. Curr Pharm Des 2012;18(15):2166-2183.

[56] Huang Q, Deng J, Xie Z, Wang F, Chen S, Lei B, et al. Effective gene transfer into central nervous system following ultrasound-microbubbles-induced opening of the blood-brain barrier. Ultrasound Med Biol 2012 Jul;38(7):1234-1243.

[57] Gary DJ, Puri N, Won YY. Polymer-based siRNA delivery: perspectives on the fundamental and phenomenological distinctions from polymer-based DNA delivery. J Control Release 2007 Aug 16;121(1-2):64-73.

[58] Kawakami S, Higuchi Y, Hashida M. Nonviral approaches for targeted delivery of plasmid DNA and oligonucleotide. J Pharm Sci 2008 Feb;97(2):726-745.

[59] Yuan F, Dellian M, Fukumura D, Leunig M, Berk DA, Torchilin VP, et al. Vascular permeability in a human tumor xenograft: molecular size dependence and cutoff size. Cancer Res 1995 Sep 1;55(17):3752-3756.

[60] Capriotti AL, Caracciolo G, Cavaliere C, Foglia P, Pozzi D, Samperi R, et al. Do plasma proteins distinguish between liposomes of varying charge density? J Proteomics 2012 Mar 16;75(6):1924-1932.

[61] Kim WJ, Bonoiu AC, Hayakawa T, Xia C, Kakimoto MA, Pudavar HE, et al. Hyperbranched polysiloxysilane nanoparticles: surface charge control of nonviral gene delivery vectors and nanoprobes. Int J Pharm 2009 Jul 6;376(1-2):141-152.

[62] Hemp ST, Allen MH,Jr, Green MD, Long TE. Phosphonium-containing polyelectrolytes for nonviral gene delivery. Biomacromolecules 2012 Jan 9;13(1):231-238.

[63] Payne CK, Jones SA, Chen C, Zhuang X. Internalization and trafficking of cell surface proteoglycans and proteoglycan-binding ligands. Traffic 2007 Apr;8(4):389-401.

[64] Chen X, Shank S, Davis PB, Ziady AG. Nucleolin-mediated cellular trafficking of DNA nanoparticle is lipid raft and microtubule dependent and can be modulated by glucocorticoid. Mol Ther 2011 Jan;19(1):93-102.

[65] Rehman ZU, Sjollema KA, Kuipers J, Hoekstra D, Zuhorn IS. Nonviral Gene Delivery Vectors Use Syndecan-Dependent Transport Mechanisms in Filopodia To Reach the Cell Surface. ACS Nano 2012 Aug 8.

[66] Mercer J, Schelhaas M, Helenius A. Virus entry by endocytosis. Annu Rev Biochem 2010;79:803-833.

[67] Farhood H, Serbina N, Huang L. The role of dioleoyl phosphatidylethanolamine in cationic liposome mediated gene transfer. Biochim Biophys Acta 1995 May 4;1235(2): 289-295.

[68] Tu Y, Kim JS. A fusogenic segment of glycoprotein H from herpes simplex virus enhances transfection efficiency of cationic liposomes. J Gene Med 2008 Jun;10(6): 646-654.

[69] Subbarao NK, Parente RA, Szoka FC,Jr, Nadasdi L, Pongracz K. pH-dependent bilayer destabilization by an amphipathic peptide. Biochemistry 1987 Jun 2;26(11): 2964-2972.

[70] Haas DH, Murphy RM. Design of a pH-sensitive pore-forming peptide with improved performance. J Pept Res 2004 Jan;63(1):9-16.

[71] Moore NM, Sheppard CL, Barbour TR, Sakiyama-Elbert SE. The effect of endosomal escape peptides on in vitro gene delivery of polyethylene glycol-based vehicles. J Gene Med 2008 Oct;10(10):1134-1149.

[72] Melchior F, Gerace L. Mechanisms of nuclear protein import. Curr Opin Cell Biol 1995 Jun;7(3):310-318.

[73] Kamiya H, Fujimura Y, Matsuoka I, Harashima H. Visualization of intracellular trafficking of exogenous DNA delivered by cationic liposomes. Biochem Biophys Res Commun 2002 Nov 8;298(4):591-597.

[74] Martin ME, Rice KG. Peptide-guided gene delivery. AAPS J 2007 Feb 9;9(1):E18-29.

[75] Dworetzky SI, Lanford RE, Feldherr CM. The effects of variations in the number and sequence of targeting signals on nuclear uptake. J Cell Biol 1988 Oct;107(4):1279-1287.

[76] Aronsohn AI, Hughes JA. Nuclear localization signal peptides enhance cationic liposome-mediated gene therapy. J Drug Target 1998;5(3):163-169.

[77] Moore NM, Sheppard CL, Sakiyama-Elbert SE. Characterization of a multifunctional PEG-based gene delivery system containing nuclear localization signals and endosomal escape peptides. Acta Biomater 2009 Mar;5(3):854-864.

[78] Hoare M, Greiser U, Schu S, Mashayekhi K, Aydogan E, Murphy M, et al. Enhanced lipoplex-mediated gene expression in mesenchymal stem cells using reiterated nuclear localization sequence peptides. J Gene Med 2010 Feb;12(2):207-218.

[79] Wang HY, Li C, Yi WJ, Sun YX, Cheng SX, Zhuo RX, et al. Targeted delivery in breast cancer cells via iodine: nuclear localization sequence conjugate. Bioconjug Chem 2011 Aug 17;22(8):1567-1575.

[80] Degiulio JV, Kaufman CD, Dean DA. The SP-C promoter facilitates alveolar type II epithelial cell-specific plasmid nuclear import and gene expression. Gene Ther 2010 Apr;17(4):541-549.

[81] Ma K, Hu M, Xie M, Shen H, Qiu L, Fan W, et al. Investigation of polyethylenimine-grafted-triamcinolone acetonide as nucleus-targeting gene delivery systems. J Gene Med 2010 Aug;12(8):669-680.

[82] Mi Bae Y, Choi H, Lee S, Ho Kang S, Tae Kim Y, Nam K, et al. Dexamethasone-conjugated low molecular weight polyethylenimine as a nucleus-targeting lipopolymer gene carrier. Bioconjug Chem 2007 Nov-Dec;18(6):2029-2036.

[83] Griesenbach U, Wilson KM, Farley R, Meng C, Munkonge FM, Cheng SH, et al. Assessment of the nuclear pore dilating agent trans-cyclohexane-1,2-diol in differentiated airway epithelium. J Gene Med 2012 Jul;14(7):491-500.

[84] Wu TL, Ertl HC. Immune barriers to successful gene therapy. Trends Mol Med 2009 Jan;15(1):32-39.

[85] Arruda VR, Favaro P, Finn JD. Strategies to modulate immune responses: a new frontier for gene therapy. Mol Ther 2009 Sep;17(9):1492-1503.

[86] Niidome T, Huang L. Gene therapy progress and prospects: nonviral vectors. Gene Ther 2002 Dec;9(24):1647-1652.

[87]   Gautam A, Densmore CL, Waldrep JC. Pulmonary cytokine responses associated with PEI-DNA aerosol gene therapy. Gene Ther 2001 Feb;8(3):254-257.

[88]   Tousignant JD, Gates AL, Ingram LA, Johnson CL, Nietupski JB, Cheng SH, et al. Comprehensive analysis of the acute toxicities induced by systemic administration of cationic lipid:plasmid DNA complexes in mice. Hum Gene Ther 2000 Dec 10;11(18): 2493-2513.

[89]   Liu F, Shollenberger LM, Huang L. Non-immunostimulatory nonviral vectors. FA-SEB J 2004 Nov;18(14):1779-1781.

[90]   Krieg AM. CpG motifs in bacterial DNA and their immune effects. Annu Rev Immunol 2002;20:709-760.

[91]   de Wolf HK, Johansson N, Thong AT, Snel CJ, Mastrobattista E, Hennink WE, et al. Plasmid CpG depletion improves degree and duration of tumor gene expression after intravenous administration of polyplexes. Pharm Res 2008 Jul;25(7):1654-1662.

[92]   Mitsui M, Nishikawa M, Zang L, Ando M, Hattori K, Takahashi Y, et al. Effect of the content of unmethylated CpG dinucleotides in plasmid DNA on the sustainability of transgene expression. J Gene Med 2009 May;11(5):435-443.

[93]   Lesina E, Dames P, Flemmer A, Hajek K, Kirchner T, Bittmann I, et al. CpG-free plasmid DNA prevents deterioration of pulmonary function in mice. Eur J Pharm Biopharm 2010 Mar;74(3):427-434.

[94]   Whitmore M, Li S, Huang L. LPD lipopolyplex initiates a potent cytokine response and inhibits tumor growth. Gene Ther 1999 Nov;6(11):1867-1875.

[95]   Sakurai H, Kawabata K, Sakurai F, Nakagawa S, Mizuguchi H. Innate immune response induced by gene delivery vectors. Int J Pharm 2008 Apr 16;354(1-2):9-15.

[96]   Hofman CR, Dileo JP, Li Z, Li S, Huang L. Efficient in vivo gene transfer by PCR amplified fragment with reduced inflammatory activity. Gene Ther 2001 Jan;8(1):71-74.

[97]   Darquet AM, Cameron B, Wils P, Scherman D, Crouzet J. A new DNA vehicle for nonviral gene delivery: supercoiled minicircle. Gene Ther 1997 Dec;4(12):1341-1349.

[98]   Kobelt D, Schleef M, Schmeer M, Aumann J, Schlag PM, Walther W. Performance of High Quality Minicircle DNA for In Vitro and In Vivo Gene Transfer. Mol Biotechnol 2012 Apr 1.

[99]   Zhang C, Liu H, Gao S, Huang W, Wang Z. Polyethylenimine and minicircle DNA based gene transfer. Sheng Wu Gong Cheng Xue Bao 2010 Jun;26(6):772-779.

[100] Vaysse L, Gregory LG, Harbottle RP, Perouzel E, Tolmachov O, Coutelle C. Nuclear-targeted minicircle to enhance gene transfer with non-viral vectors in vitro and in vivo. J Gene Med 2006 Jun;8(6):754-763.

[101] Tolmachov OE. Tightly-wound miniknot vectors for gene therapy: a potential improvement over supercoiled minicircle DNA. Med Hypotheses 2010 Apr;74(4): 702-704.

[102] Yasuda S, Yoshida H, Nishikawa M, Takakura Y. Comparison of the type of liposome involving cytokine production induced by non-CpG Lipoplex in macrophages. Mol Pharm 2010 Apr 5;7(2):533-542.

[103] Yoshida H, Nishikawa M, Yasuda S, Mizuno Y, Toyota H, Kiyota T, et al. TLR9-dependent systemic interferon-beta production by intravenous injection of plasmid DNA/cationic liposome complex in mice. J Gene Med 2009 Aug;11(8):708-717.

[104] Meir YJ, Wu SC. Transposon-based vector systems for gene therapy clinical trials: challenges and considerations. Chang Gung Med J 2011 Nov-Dec;34(6):565-579.

[105] Matsumura Y, Oda T, Maeda H. General mechanism of intratumor accumulation of macromolecules: advantage of macromolecular therapeutics. Gan To Kagaku Ryoho 1987 Mar;14(3 Pt 2):821-829.

[106] Maeda H, Wu J, Sawa T, Matsumura Y, Hori K. Tumor vascular permeability and the EPR effect in macromolecular therapeutics: a review. J Control Release 2000 Mar 1;65(1-2):271-284.

[107] Maeda H, Matsumura Y. EPR effect based drug design and clinical outlook for enhanced cancer chemotherapy. Adv Drug Deliv Rev 2011 Mar 18;63(3):129-130.

[108] Yuan F. Transvascular drug delivery in solid tumors. Semin Radiat Oncol 1998 Jul; 8(3):164-175.

[109] Dreher MR, Liu W, Michelich CR, Dewhirst MW, Yuan F, Chilkoti A. Tumor vascular permeability, accumulation, and penetration of macromolecular drug carriers. J Natl Cancer Inst 2006 Mar 1;98(5):335-344.

[110] Hobbs SK, Monsky WL, Yuan F, Roberts WG, Griffith L, Torchilin VP, et al. Regulation of transport pathways in tumor vessels: role of tumor type and microenvironment. Proc Natl Acad Sci U S A 1998 Apr 14;95(8):4607-4612.

[111] Matsumura Y, Maeda H. A new concept for macromolecular therapeutics in cancer chemotherapy: mechanism of tumoritropic accumulation of proteins and the antitumor agent smancs. Cancer Res 1986 Dec;46(12 Pt 1):6387-6392.

[112] Ofek P, Fischer W, Calderon M, Haag R, Satchi-Fainaro R. In vivo delivery of small interfering RNA to tumors and their vasculature by novel dendritic nanocarriers. FASEB J 2010 Sep;24(9):3122-3134.

[113] Fang J, Qin H, Nakamura H, Tsukigawa K, Shin T, Maeda H. Carbon monoxide, generated by heme oxygenase-1, mediates the enhanced permeability and retention effect in solid tumors. Cancer Sci 2012 Mar;103(3):535-541.

[114] Tozer GM, Everett SA. Nitric oxide in tumor biology and cancer therapy. Part 2: Therapeutic implications. Clin Oncol (R Coll Radiol) 1997;9(6):357-364.

[115] Tozer GM, Everett SA. Nitric oxide in tumour biology and cancer therapy. Part 1: Physiological aspects. Clin Oncol (R Coll Radiol) 1997;9(5):282-293.

[116] Wink DA, Vodovotz Y, Cook JA, Krishna MC, Kim S, Coffin D, et al. The role of nitric oxide chemistry in cancer treatment. Biochemistry (Mosc) 1998 Jul;63(7):802-809.

[117] Xu W, Liu LZ, Loizidou M, Ahmed M, Charles IG. The role of nitric oxide in cancer. Cell Res 2002 Dec;12(5-6):311-320.

[118] Worthington J, Robson T, O'Keeffe M, Hirst DG. Tumour cell radiosensitization using constitutive (CMV) and radiation inducible (WAF1) promoters to drive the iNOS gene: a novel suicide gene therapy. Gene Ther 2002 Feb;9(4):263-269.

[119] Worthington J, McCarthy HO, Barrett E, Adams C, Robson T, Hirst DG. Use of the radiation-inducible WAF1 promoter to drive iNOS gene therapy as a novel anti-cancer treatment. J Gene Med 2004 Jun;6(6):673-680.

[120] Bonavida B, Khineche S, Huerta-Yepez S, Garban H. Therapeutic potential of nitric oxide in cancer. Drug Resist Updat 2006 Jun;9(3):157-173.

[121] Wu J, Akaike T, Hayashida K, Okamoto T, Okuyama A, Maeda H. Enhanced vascular permeability in solid tumor involving peroxynitrite and matrix metalloproteinases. Jpn J Cancer Res 2001 Apr;92(4):439-451.

[122] Yasuda H, Yamaya M, Nakayama K, Sasaki T, Ebihara S, Kanda A, et al. Randomized phase II trial comparing nitroglycerin plus vinorelbine and cisplatin with vinorelbine and cisplatin alone in previously untreated stage IIIB/IV non-small-cell lung cancer. J Clin Oncol 2006 Feb 1;24(4):688-694.

[123] Diez S, Migueliz I, Tros de Ilarduya C. Targeted cationic poly(D,L-lactic-co-glycolic acid) nanoparticles for gene delivery to cultured cells. Cell Mol Biol Lett 2009;14(2): 347-362.

[124] Yang DC, Wang F, Elliott RL, Head JF. Expression of transferrin receptor and ferritin H-chain mRNA are associated with clinical and histopathological prognostic indicators in breast cancer. Anticancer Res 2001 Jan-Feb;21(1B):541-549.

[125] Seymour GJ, Walsh MD, Lavin MF, Strutton G, Gardiner RA. Transferrin receptor expression by human bladder transitional cell carcinomas. Urol Res 1987;15(6):341-344.

[126] Kondo K, Noguchi M, Mukai K, Matsuno Y, Sato Y, Shimosato Y, et al. Transferrin receptor expression in adenocarcinoma of the lung as a histopathologic indicator of prognosis. Chest 1990 Jun;97(6):1367-1371.

[127] Kircheis R, Wightman L, Schreiber A, Robitza B, Rossler V, Kursa M, et al. Polyethylenimine/DNA complexes shielded by transferrin target gene expression to tumors after systemic application. Gene Ther 2001 Jan;8(1):28-40.

[128] Lee JH, Engler JA, Collawn JF, Moore BA. Receptor mediated uptake of peptides that bind the human transferrin receptor. Eur J Biochem 2001 Apr;268(7):2004-2012.

[129] Liu S, Guo Y, Huang R, Li J, Huang S, Kuang Y, et al. Gene and doxorubicin co-delivery system for targeting therapy of glioma. Biomaterials 2012 Jun;33(19):4907-4916.

[130] Hynes NE, MacDonald G. ErbB receptors and signaling pathways in cancer. Curr Opin Cell Biol 2009 Apr;21(2):177-184.

[131] Brand TM, Iida M, Li C, Wheeler DL. The nuclear epidermal growth factor receptor signaling network and its role in cancer. Discov Med 2011 Nov;12(66):419-432.

[132] Wolschek MF, Thallinger C, Kursa M, Rossler V, Allen M, Lichtenberger C, et al. Specific systemic nonviral gene delivery to human hepatocellular carcinoma xenografts in SCID mice. Hepatology 2002 Nov;36(5):1106-1114.

[133] Shir A, Ogris M, Wagner E, Levitzki A. EGF receptor-targeted synthetic double-stranded RNA eliminates glioblastoma, breast cancer, and adenocarcinoma tumors in mice. PLoS Med 2006 Jan;3(1):e6.

[134] Saunders LR, Barber GN. The dsRNA binding protein family: critical roles, diverse cellular functions. FASEB J 2003 Jun;17(9):961-983.

[135] Parker LM, Fierro-Monti I, Reichman TW, Gunnery S, Mathews MB. Double-stranded RNA-binding proteins and the control of protein synthesis and cell growth. Cold Spring Harb Symp Quant Biol 2001;66:485-497.

[136] Schaffert D, Kiss M, Rodl W, Shir A, Levitzki A, Ogris M, et al. Poly(I:C)-mediated tumor growth suppression in EGF-receptor overexpressing tumors using EGF-polyethylene glycol-linear polyethylenimine as carrier. Pharm Res 2011 Apr;28(4): 731-741.

[137] Li Z, Zhao R, Wu X, Sun Y, Yao M, Li J, et al. Identification and characterization of a novel peptide ligand of epidermal growth factor receptor for targeted delivery of therapeutics. FASEB J 2005 Dec;19(14):1978-1985.

[138] Mohammadi Z, Dorkoosh FA, Hosseinkhani S, Gilani K, Amini T, Najafabadi AR, et al. In vivo transfection study of chitosan-DNA-FAP-B nanoparticles as a new non viral vector for gene delivery to the lung. Int J Pharm 2011 Dec 12;421(1):183-188.

[139] Ke W, Shao K, Huang R, Han L, Liu Y, Li J, et al. Gene delivery targeted to the brain using an Angiopep-conjugated polyethyleneglycol-modified polyamidoamine dendrimer. Biomaterials 2009 Dec;30(36):6976-6985.

[140] Huang S, Li J, Han L, Liu S, Ma H, Huang R, et al. Dual targeting effect of Angiopep-2-modified, DNA-loaded nanoparticles for glioma. Biomaterials 2011 Oct;32(28): 6832-6838.

[141] Nilsson B, Moks T, Jansson B, Abrahmsen L, Elmblad A, Holmgren E, et al. A synthetic IgG-binding domain based on staphylococcal protein A. Protein Eng 1987 Feb-Mar;1(2):107-113.

[142] Nord K, Gunneriusson E, Ringdahl J, Stahl S, Uhlen M, Nygren PA. Binding proteins selected from combinatorial libraries of an alpha-helical bacterial receptor domain. Nat Biotechnol 1997 Aug;15(8):772-777.

[143] Orlova A, Magnusson M, Eriksson TL, Nilsson M, Larsson B, Hoiden-Guthenberg I, et al. Tumor imaging using a picomolar affinity HER2 binding affibody molecule. Cancer Res 2006 Apr 15;66(8):4339-4348.

[144] Friedman M, Orlova A, Johansson E, Eriksson TL, Hoiden-Guthenberg I, Tolmachev V, et al. Directed evolution to low nanomolar affinity of a tumor-targeting epidermal growth factor receptor-binding affibody molecule. J Mol Biol 2008 Mar 7;376(5): 1388-1402.

[145] Li J, Lundberg E, Vernet E, Larsson B, Hoiden-Guthenberg I, Graslund T. Selection of affibody molecules to the ligand-binding site of the insulin-like growth factor-1 receptor. Biotechnol Appl Biochem 2010 Feb 25;55(2):99-109.

[146] Lindborg M, Cortez E, Hoiden-Guthenberg I, Gunneriusson E, von Hage E, Syud F, et al. Engineered high-affinity affibody molecules targeting platelet-derived growth factor receptor beta in vivo. J Mol Biol 2011 Mar 25;407(2):298-315.

[147] Wikman M, Steffen AC, Gunneriusson E, Tolmachev V, Adams GP, Carlsson J, et al. Selection and characterization of HER2/neu-binding affibody ligands. Protein Eng Des Sel 2004 May;17(5):455-462.

[148] Friedman M, Nordberg E, Hoiden-Guthenberg I, Brismar H, Adams GP, Nilsson FY, et al. Phage display selection of Affibody molecules with specific binding to the extracellular domain of the epidermal growth factor receptor. Protein Eng Des Sel 2007 Apr;20(4):189-199.

[149] Gopal V, Guruprasad K. Structure prediction and validation of an affibody engineered for cell-specific nucleic acid targeting. Syst Synth Biol 2010 Dec;4(4):293-297.

[150] Govindarajan S, Sivakumar J, Garimidi P, Rangaraj N, Kumar JM, Rao NM, et al. Targeting human epidermal growth factor receptor 2 by a cell-penetrating peptide-affibody bioconjugate. Biomaterials 2012 Mar;33(8):2570-2582.

[151] Beuttler J, Rothdiener M, Muller D, Frejd FY, Kontermann RE. Targeting of epidermal growth factor receptor (EGFR)-expressing tumor cells with sterically stabilized affibody liposomes (SAL). Bioconjug Chem 2009 Jun;20(6):1201-1208.

[152] Canine BF, Wang Y, Hatefi A. Biosynthesis and characterization of a novel genetically engineered polymer for targeted gene transfer to cancer cells. J Control Release 2009 Sep 15;138(3):188-196.

[153] Midoux P, Kichler A, Boutin V, Maurizot JC, Monsigny M. Membrane permeabilization and efficient gene transfer by a peptide containing several histidines. Bioconjug Chem 1998 Mar-Apr;9(2):260-267.

[154] Siomi H, Dreyfuss G. A nuclear localization domain in the hnRNP A1 protein. J Cell Biol 1995 May;129(3):551-560.

[155] Dufes C, Keith WN, Bilsland A, Proutski I, Uchegbu IF, Schatzlein AG. Synthetic anticancer gene medicine exploits intrinsic antitumor activity of cationic vector to cure established tumors. Cancer Res 2005 Sep 15;65(18):8079-8084.

[156] Chen L, Zheng J, Zhang Y, Yang L, Wang J, Ni J, et al. Tumor-specific expression of microRNA-26a suppresses human hepatocellular carcinoma growth via cyclin-dependent and -independent pathways. Mol Ther 2011 Aug;19(8):1521-1528.

[157] Mineo R, Fichera E, Liang SJ, Fujita-Yamaguchi Y. Promoter usage for insulin-like growth factor-II in cancerous and benign human breast, prostate, and bladder tissues, and confirmation of a 10th exon. Biochem Biophys Res Commun 2000 Feb 24;268(3):886-892.

[158] Ayesh B, Matouk I, Ohana P, Sughayer MA, Birman T, Ayesh S, et al. Inhibition of tumor growth by DT-A expressed under the control of IGF2 P3 and P4 promoter sequences. Mol Ther 2003 Apr;7(4):535-541.

[159] Amit D, Tamir S, Birman T, Gofrit ON, Hochberg A. Development of targeted therapy for bladder cancer mediated by a double promoter plasmid expressing diphtheria toxin under the control of IGF2-P3 and IGF2-P4 regulatory sequences. Int J Clin Exp Med 2011;4(2):91-102.

[160] Amit D, Matouk IJ, Lavon I, Birman T, Galula J, Abu-Lail R, et al. Transcriptional targeting of glioblastoma by diphtheria toxin-A driven by both H19 and IGF2-P4 promoters. Int J Clin Exp Med 2012;5(2):124-135.

[161] Hauschka PV, Wians FH,Jr. Osteocalcin-hydroxyapatite interaction in the extracellular organic matrix of bone. Anat Rec 1989 Jun;224(2):180-188.

[162] Ducy P, Desbois C, Boyce B, Pinero G, Story B, Dunstan C, et al. Increased bone formation in osteocalcin-deficient mice. Nature 1996 Aug 1;382(6590):448-452.

[163] Boskey AL, Gadaleta S, Gundberg C, Doty SB, Ducy P, Karsenty G. Fourier transform infrared microspectroscopic analysis of bones of osteocalcin-deficient mice provides insight into the function of osteocalcin. Bone 1998 Sep;23(3):187-196.

[164] Coleman RE, Mashiter G, Fogelman I, Whitaker KD, Caleffi M, Moss DW, et al. Osteocalcin: a potential marker of metastatic bone disease and response to treatment. Eur J Cancer Clin Oncol 1988 Jul;24(7):1211-1217.

[165] Koeneman KS, Yeung F, Chung LW. Osteomimetic properties of prostate cancer cells: a hypothesis supporting the predilection of prostate cancer metastasis and growth in the bone environment. Prostate 1999 Jun 1;39(4):246-261.

[166] Jung C, Ou YC, Yeung F, Frierson HF,Jr, Kao C. Osteocalcin is incompletely spliced in non-osseous tissues. Gene 2001 Jun 27;271(2):143-150.

[167] McCarthy HO, Coulter JA, Worthington J, Robson T, Hirst DG. Human osteocalcin: a strong promoter for nitric oxide synthase gene therapy, with specificity for hormone refractory prostate cancer. J Gene Med 2007 Jun;9(6):511-520.

[168] Coulter JA, Page NL, Worthington J, Robson T, Hirst DG, McCarthy HO. Transcriptional regulation of inducible nitric oxide synthase gene therapy: targeting early stage and advanced prostate cancer. J Gene Med 2010 Sep;12(9):755-765.

[169] Johnson NA, Chen BH, Sung SY, Liao CH, Hsiao WC, W K Chung L, et al. A novel targeting modality for renal cell carcinoma: human osteocalcin promoter-mediated gene therapy synergistically induced by vitamin C and vitamin D(3). J Gene Med 2010 Nov;12(11):892-903.

[170] Hatakeyama H, Akita H, Harashima H. A multifunctional envelope type nano device (MEND) for gene delivery to tumours based on the EPR effect: a strategy for overcoming the PEG dilemma. Adv Drug Deliv Rev 2011 Mar 18;63(3):152-160.

[171] Hatakeyama H, Ito E, Yamamoto M, Akita H, Hayashi Y, Kajimoto K, et al. A DNA microarray-based analysis of the host response to a nonviral gene carrier: a strategy for improving the immune response. Mol Ther 2011 Aug;19(8):1487-1498.

[172] Mishra S, Webster P, Davis ME. PEGylation significantly affects cellular uptake and intracellular trafficking of non-viral gene delivery particles. Eur J Cell Biol 2004 Apr; 83(3):97-111.

[173] Hatakeyama H, Akita H, Kogure K, Oishi M, Nagasaki Y, Kihira Y, et al. Development of a novel systemic gene delivery system for cancer therapy with a tumor-specific cleavable PEG-lipid. Gene Ther 2007 Jan;14(1):68-77.

[174] Kogure K, Moriguchi R, Sasaki K, Ueno M, Futaki S, Harashima H. Development of a non-viral multifunctional envelope-type nano device by a novel lipid film hydration method. J Control Release 2004 Aug 11;98(2):317-323.

[175] Masuda T, Akita H, Nishio T, Niikura K, Kogure K, Ijiro K, et al. Development of lipid particles targeted via sugar-lipid conjugates as novel nuclear gene delivery system. Biomaterials 2008 Feb;29(6):709-723.

[176] Akita H, Kudo A, Minoura A, Yamaguti M, Khalil IA, Moriguchi R, et al. Multi-layered nanoparticles for penetrating the endosome and nuclear membrane via a stepwise membrane fusion process. Biomaterials 2009 May;30(15):2940-2949.

[177] Hatakeyama H, Akita H, Ito E, Hayashi Y, Oishi M, Nagasaki Y, et al. Systemic delivery of siRNA to tumors using a lipid nanoparticle containing a tumor-specific cleavable PEG-lipid. Biomaterials 2011 Jun;32(18):4306-4316.

[178] Moriguchi R, Kogure K, Akita H, Futaki S, Miyagishi M, Taira K, et al. A multifunctional envelope-type nano device for novel gene delivery of siRNA plasmids. Int J Pharm 2005 Sep 14;301(1-2):277-285.

[179] Sakurai Y, Hatakeyama H, Sato Y, Akita H, Takayama K, Kobayashi S, et al. Endoso-
       mal escape and the knockdown efficiency of liposomal-siRNA by the fusogenic pep-
       tide shGALA. Biomaterials 2011 Aug;32(24):5733-5742.

[180] Hatakeyama H, Ito E, Akita H, Oishi M, Nagasaki Y, Futaki S, et al. A pH-sensitive
       fusogenic peptide facilitates endosomal escape and greatly enhances the gene silenc-
       ing of siRNA-containing nanoparticles in vitro and in vivo. J Control Release 2009
       Oct 15;139(2):127-132.

[181] Khalil IA, Kogure K, Futaki S, Hama S, Akita H, Ueno M, et al. Octaarginine-modi-
       fied multifunctional envelope-type nanoparticles for gene delivery. Gene Ther 2007
       Apr;14(8):682-689.

[182] Suzuki R, Yamada Y, Harashima H. Efficient cytoplasmic protein delivery by means
       of a multifunctional envelope-type nano device. Biol Pharm Bull 2007 Apr;30(4):
       758-762.

[183] Shaheen SM, Akita H, Nakamura T, Takayama S, Futaki S, Yamashita A, et al. KA-
       LA-modified multi-layered nanoparticles as gene carriers for MHC class-I mediated
       antigen presentation for a DNA vaccine. Biomaterials 2011 Sep;32(26):6342-6350.

Chapter 2

Gene Therapy Based on Fragment C of Tetanus Toxin in ALS: A Promising Neuroprotective Strategy for the Bench to the Bedside Approach

Ana C. Calvo, Pilar Zaragoza and Rosario Osta

Additional information is available at the end of the chapter

1. Introduction

Neurodegenerative diseases cover a wide range of neurogenetic disorders including Amyotrophic Lateral Sclerosis (ALS), Alzheimer's disease (AD), Huntington's disease (HD), the spinocerebellar ataxias, inherited prion diseases, the inherited neuropathies, and muscular dystrophies among others.

In particular, ALS belongs to the group of motor neuron diseases, involving the loss of cortex, brainstem, and spinal cord motor neurons that result in muscle paralysis [1]. Motor neurons, which are localized in the brain, brainstem and spinal cord, behave as a crucial links between the nervous system and the voluntary muscles of the body, as they let synaptic signals travel from upper motor neurons in the brain to lower motor neurons in the spinal cord and finally to muscles. In accordance with the revised El Escorial criteria [2], both the upper motor neurons and the lower motor neurons degenerate or die in ALS, and as a consequence the communication between neuron and muscle is lost, prompting the progressive muscle weakening and the appearance of fasciculations. In the later stages of the disease, patients become paralyzed although the disease usually does not impair a person's mind or intelligence.

Nowadays, the cause of ALS and its early manifestations still remain to be elucidated. The pathophysiological mechanisms that prompt the neurodegenerative process in both familial (FALS) and sporadic (SALS) ALS are unknown. However, there is growing evidence that the pathogenic process involved in ALS are multifactorial and include oxidative stress, glutamate excitotoxicity, mitochondrial dysfunction, axonal transport systems and dysfunction of glial cells, yielding the damage of critical proteins and organelles in the motor neuron triggering the neurodegeneration [3]. Due to the fact that FALS and SALS share clinical and pathological signs, the understanding of the pathophysiological process in FALS would provide a better understanding of the neurodegenerative mechanisms in SALS.

FALS follows a predominantly autosomal dominant pattern, while in SALS genetic factors that take place sporadically contribute to its pathogenesis. The majority of ALS cases are sporadic and 5-10% of cases correspond to FALS. Although the ages of onset of FALS, which follow a normal Gaussian distribution, correspond to a decade earlier than for SALS cases which have an age dependent incidence, males and females are affected equally in FALS [4].

The most significant candidate genes for SALS include *VEGF* (vascular endothelial growth factor), *angiogenin (ALS9), paraoxonoase, neurofilaments, peripherin* and *SMN* (spinal muscular atrophy). Although *ALS9, paraoxonase, neurofilaments, peripherin* and *SMN* mutations have been found in ALS patients, except for *VEGF* mutations, these genes may play a small role in the pathogenesis of ALS and previous studies are conflicting [5].

Regarding FALS candidate genes, the mutations in the copper/zinc superoxide-dismutase-1 gene (*SOD1*), Tar DNA-binding protein gene (*TARDBP*) and in the most recent discovered DNA/RNA-binding protein called *FUS* (fused in sarcoma) or *TLS* (translocation in liposarcoma) produce the typical adult onset ALS phenotype. Other candidate genes that have been described in genome association studies of FALS include *dynactin, senataxin (ALS4)* and *VAPB (ALS8)* (VAMP/synaptobrevin-associated membrane protein B gene) [5,6].

The pathophysiology of *SOD1* mutations is probably the most studied one. Many hypotheses have been suggested and reinforced in transgenic mouse models that overexpress the mutated *SOD1* gene and therefore develop an ALS-like syndrome. Among the proposed mechanisms that support these hypotheses are the toxic gain of function of the mutated SOD1 enzyme, which mainly increases the production of hydroxyl and free radicals, yielding improper binding metal properties, oxidative stress and inflammation induced by upregulation of proinflammatory cytokines [7,8]. Alternative hypothesis also suggested a conformational instability and misfolding of the SOD1 peptide, forming intracellular aggregates which have been reported in motor neuron and glial cells [9].

Neurotrophic factors have been initially identified as potential therapeutic agents in the treatment of ALS, opening the door to a new tool for the treatment of motor neuron diseases [10]. Based on previous studies ciliary and glial derived neurotrophic factors, insulin-like growth factor (IGF-1) and erythropoietin improved motor behaviour and reduce motor neuron loss, astrocyte and microglia activation in preclinical animal models [11], albeit clinical trials in ALS patients showed lack of therapeutic efficacy [12].

The failure of standard treatments in ALS could rely on the inappropriate route of administration and/or the poor bioavailability of molecules to the target cell [13]. The subcutaneous and intrathecal delivery of neurotrophic factors can cause adverse side effects such as weight loss, fever, cough, fatigue and behavioral changes [14], whereas viral gene therapy based on the use of an adeno-associated virus or lentivirus vectors is more efficient than the neurotrophic factor delivery but can induce several inherent hazards [15].

An alternative strategy that effectively reaches motor neurons, can exert neuroprotective properties and does not show such adverse side effects implies the use of the nontoxic fragment C

(TTC) of tetanus toxin. Tetanus toxin is a neurotoxin produced by *Clostridium tetani*, an anaerobic bacterium whose spores are commonly found in soil and animal waste. This toxin affects the nervous system and causes generalized muscle contractions, called titanic spasms [16, 17].

Tetanus toxin is a single peptide of approximately 150 kDa, which consists of 1315 amino-acid residues. The toxin forms a two-chain activated molecule composed of a heavy chain (HC) and a light chain (LC) linked by a disulfide bond. The catalytic domain of the toxin resides in the LC, while the translocation and receptor-binding domains are present in HC [18–21] (Figure 1). Tetanus and botulinum toxins are zinc metalloproteases that cleave SNARE (soluble NSF attachment receptor) proteins, which interfere with the fusion of synaptic vesicles to the plasma membrane and ultimately blocks neurotransmitter release in nerve cells [22].

The nature of the action of tetanus toxin has been widely described in different animal models [23–28], exploring its effect not only in the spinal cord but also in the cerebral cortex [29]. One of the unique characteristics of tetanus toxin is that it can be transported retrogradely to the central nervous system and shows remarkable affinity and specificity to neuronal terminals. The ganglioside-recognition domain in the C-terminal region of HC allows the toxin to be internalized into the neuron at the neuromuscular junction where it enters the axonal retrograde transport pathway and is subsequently transported to the neuronal soma in the CNS [30,31]. Once the toxin reaches the cytoplasm, it specifically cleaves neuronal proteins integral to vesicular trafficking and neurotransmitter release. In particular, the synaptic vesicle protein synaptobrevin (VAMP) is the target of tetanus toxin. This protein belongs to a family of proteins that facilitate exocytosis in neurons known as SNARE proteins. The other members of this family are syntaxin and SNAP-25, which are the main molecular targets of botulinum toxin. SNARE proteins are formed by coiled-coil interactions of the alpha-helices of its members, which is required for membrane fusion [32–35].

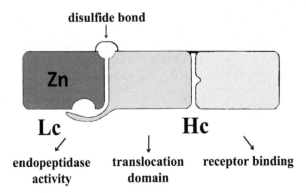

Figure 1. Diagram of the tetanus toxin molecule. The targeting and the translocation domains are located in the heavy-chain (HC), whereas the catalytic domain is located in the light-chain (LC) of the molecule. Its proteolytic activity is Zn^{2+}-dependent, and heavy-metal chelators generate inactive apo-neurotoxins. TTC is approximately 50 KDa and resides in the HC of the toxin. The ganglioside-recognition domain in TTC allows the toxin to be internalized into the neuron [35].

From the gene therapy point of view, the most interesting part of the toxin that must be out-standing is TTC. This fragment of the toxin is located in the HC of tetanus toxin molecule and it plays an important role in the neuronal internalization (Figure 1). In fact, TTC main-tains transport properties of the native tetanus toxin without causing toxic effects, in such a way that in the absence of TTC, the toxin retains little ability to paralyze neuromuscular transmission [35,36].

The trans-synaptic transport of TTC was intensively studied in one of the best-characterized systems, the primary visual pathway [37, 38], confirming its capacity as a carrier once it was injected intramuscularly [39-41]. Furthermore, the possibility of constructing recombinant molecules with TTC has opened the door to an interesting research field, the discovery of neuro-anatomical tracers, whose main purpose is to map synaptic connections between neu-ronal cells.

One of the most well-known recombinant proteins that have been used for this purpose is the protein encoded by *lacZ*-TTC. This protein has been tested *in vitro* and *in vivo* to deter-mine its activity in the hypoglossal system, and the detection of the labeled motor neurons was dependent on time post-injection [40-42]. Since neuronal integrity is crucial for TTC in-ternalization, the transneuronal molecular pathway at neuromuscular junctions was inten-sively studied using this recombinant protein [43]. The protein was detected not only in the neuromuscular junction postsynaptic side but also the soma of the motor neuron, away from the active zones in large uncoated vesicles.

The advances in the understanding of these recombinant proteins have paved the way for new therapeutic approaches using TTC as a carrier of molecules to ameliorate the disease process of motor neuron diseases, neuropathies and pain. As an example, several proteins conjugated to TTC that have been used to study neuronal internalization *in vitro* and *in vivo* are horseradish peroxidise (HPRT), glucose oxidase (GO), green fluorescent protein (GFP), β-Nacetylhexosaminidase-A (HEXA), superoxide dismutase 1 (SOD1), survival motor neuron 1 (SMN1), cardiotrophin-1 (CT1), B-cell lymphomaextra large (Bcl-xL), IGF-1, glial derived neurotrophic factor (GDNF) and brain derived neurotrophic factor (BDNF) [17]. More re-cently, a novel multi-component nanoparticle system using polyethylene imine (PEI) has been evaluated to elicit the expression of BDNF in neuronal cell lines [44].

Apart from the carrier properties of TTC, the neuroprotective nature of TTC was one of the best kept properties to discover.

The neurotrophin family has been shown to regulate survival, development and functional aspects of neurons in the central and peripheral nervous systems through the activation of one or more of the three members of the receptor tyrosine kinases (TrkA, TrkB, and TrkC) in cooperation with p^{75NTR} [45-48]. Nerve growth factor (NGF) can bind to the TrkA receptor or a complex of TrkA and p^{75NTR} [45], BDNF and neurotrophin-4/5 can bind to TrkB, and neuro-trophin-3 binds to TrkC. Interestingly, the retrograde pathway of TTC is shared by $p75^{NTR}$, TrkB and BDNF, which is strongly dependent on the activities of the small GTPases Rab5 and Rab7 [49], therefore TTC alone might have a neuroprotective role and therefore it can be a valuable non-viral therapeutic agent in ALS.

2. Neuroprotective nature of TTC

Many authors have suggested that the trans-synaptic transcytosis pathway used by tetanus toxin was most likely "designed" for the trafficking of trophic factors through a chain of connected neurons [50]. Furthermore, two trophic factors, GDNF and BDNF, have been reported to possess similar trans-synaptic transcytotic properties to those of tetanus toxin [51].

Tetanus toxin can induce an increase in serotonin synthesis in the central nervous system, suggesting that the toxin-affected serotonergic innervation in the perinatal rat brain can trigger the translocation of calcium phosphatidylserine-dependent protein kinase C (PKC) [52]. In particular, tetanus toxin is able to alter a component involving inositol phospholipid hydrolysis, which is associated with PKC activity translocation [53,54]. In addition to this translocation, an enhancement of the tyrosine phosphorylation of the tyrosine receptor TrkA, phospholipase C (PLCγ-1) and ERK-1/2 can be also observed [55]. Due to the fact that TTC can stimulate the PLC-mediated hydrolysis of phosphoinositides in rat brain neurons, TTC seems to modulate some signaling pathways involving the transport of serotonin [56].

Moreover, the activation of intracellular pathways related to the PLCγ-1 phosphorylation and activation of PKC isoforms and the kinases Akt (at Ser 473 and Thr 308) and ERK-1/2 (at Thr 202/Tyr 204) is induced by TTC in rat brain synaptosomes and cultured cortical neurons. This signal pathway activation is dependent on time and concentration, therefore TTC can exert neuroprotective effects, activating TrkA and TrkB receptors in a similar manner as do NGF and BDNF or neurotrophin-4/5 [57,58].

The neuroprotective role of TTC is also supported by the fact that it can also protect cerebellar granular cells against potassium deprivation-induced apoptotic death [59] and act as a neuroprotector in a model of 1-methyl-4-phenylpyridinium (MPP+)-triggered apoptosis, enhancing the survival pathways in rats with a dopaminergic lesion and improving different motor behaviors. Particularly, TTC is able to induce Ser 112 and Ser 136 BAD phosphorylation, activate the transcription factor NF-κB, which prevents neuronal death, and induce a decrease in the release of cytochrome c and, consequently, a reduction in the activation of procaspase-3 and chromatin condensation [60,61].

More recently, the nature of TTC described by Longstreth and colleagues [62] and Larsen and colleagues [63], based on its stability to reach motor neurons specifically through the retrograde axonal transport system, has been reinforced as a potential neuroprotective agent in previous *in vivo* studies of gene and protein expression after injection of plasmid-DNA in transgenic SOD1^{G93A} mice, which carries the mutation G93A in human superoxide dismutase 1 (SOD1) [64]. These studies suggested that intramuscular naked-DNA TTC gene therapy administered into neurodegenerative mouse model delayed the onset of symptoms (by approximately 5 days), prolonged survival (by approximately 13 days) and improved the motor function activity in TTC-treated mice throughout disease progression, by increasing numbers of surviving motor neurons (Figure 2).

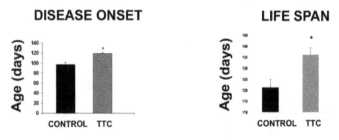

	ONSET	END POINT
CONTROL	97,1 ± 4,7	121,3 ± 3,6
TTC	118,7 ± 1,9	136,0 ± 3,2

DISEASE ONSET   **LIFE SPAN**

Figure 2. Functional and survival effect under TTC treatment. Intramuscular injection of TTC-encoding plasmid in SOD1^{G93A} mice (grey bars) delays significantly disease onset and mortality compared to the control group (*p<0,05, error barrs indicate SEM) (Reprinted from Orphanet J. Rare Dis., 6: 10, Calvo AC, Moreno-Igoa M, Mancuso R. et al. Lack of a synergistic effect of a non-viral ALS gene therapy based on BDNF and a TTC fusion molecule, Copyright (2011), [65] with permission from BioMed Central).

Apart from functional and survival results obtained *in vivo* in transgenic SOD1^{G93A} mice, the electrophysiological studies showed that, from three to four months of age, TTC treatment played a partial protective effect as demonstrated by the lower decline in amplitudes of the M waves, improvement in motor behavioral tests, and increased survival of motor neurons in the TTC-treated animals' lumbar spinal cord [64] (Figure 3).

Interestingly, TTC administration can also affect antiapoptic pathways by means of calcium-related mechanisms [64]. The positive effects on motor neuron preservation, animal motor function, and survival were confirmed with studies of anti-apoptotic effects and survival signals in the spinal cords of treated animals. Transcriptional caspase-1 and caspase-3 levels were downregulated in the spinal cord of TTC-treated animals as well as significant variations in calcium-related gene expression were found [64]. Furthermore, a downregulation of the caspase-3 activation protein levels in the spinal cord of TTC-treated animals indicated that TTC might act through an anti-apoptotic pathway. Actually, Bax, Bcl2, phospho-Akt and phospho-ERK 1/2 protein expression levels in TTC-treated animals were statistically significant and close to those of wild-type animals, suggesting a decrease of apoptosis and a lower degree of motor neuron neurodegeneration due to TTC treatment [64].

Taking all these results obtained *in vitro* and *in vivo* as a whole, non-viral gene therapy treatment based on TTC could be a safe and promising neuroprotective strategy for neurodegenerative diseases, especially in ALS. However, the next question to be tackled is whether a recombinant molecule of TTC may have a synergistic effect and enhance the neuroprotective properties of TTC alone.

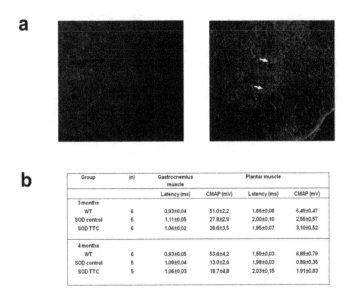

a

b

Group	(n)	Gastrocnemius muscle		Plantar muscle	
		Latency (ms)	CMAP (mV)	Latency (ms)	CMAP (mV)
3 months					
WT	6	0,93±0,04	51,0±2,2	1,66±0,08	6,49±0,47
SOD control	6	1,11±0,05	27,8±2,9	2,00±0,10	2,55±0,57
SOD TTC	6	1,04±0,02	28,6±3,5	1,95±0,07	3,10±0,52
4 months					
WT	6	0,93±0,05	53,6±4,2	1,59±0,03	6,89±0,79
SOD control	5	1,09±0,04	13,0±2,6	1,98±0,03	0,89±0,35
SOD TTC	5	1,06±0,03	18,7±4,8	2,03±0,15	1,91±0,83

Figure 3. Motor neuron survival and neurophysiological study in gastrocnemius and plantar muscles in SOD1^{G93A} mice. (a) Presence of TTC in the grey matter of the ventral horn of (a) positive control (SOD1^{G93A} transgenic mice injected with empty plasmid) and (b) SOD1^{G93A}-TTC treated mice. Arrows point to some of the neurons positively stained for TTC. Bar = 200 μm. (b) Electrophysiological study of compound muscle action potential (CMAP) in gastrocnemius and plantar muscles in wild-type mice (WT), control SOD1^{G93A} mice, and SOD1^{G93A} mice treated with naked DNA encoding for TTC. Values are the mean ± SEM. CMAP, compound muscle action potential; n, number of mice. *P < 0.05 vs. WT group at the same age (Reprinted from Orphanet J. Rare Dis., 6: 10, Calvo AC, Moreno-Igoa M, Mancuso R. et al. Lack of a synergistic effect of a non-viral ALS gene therapy based on BDNF and a TTC fusion molecule, Copyright (2011), [65] with permission from BioMed Central).

3. Neuroprotective properties of recombinant molecules of TTC in a mouse model of ALS

It has been very well described the specificity of a trophic factor for motoneurons and precisely this specificity could be increased by genetically fusing it to TTC, while the trophic factor could contribute to enhance the benefits observed for TTC. Therefore the next inevitable approach is to test naked-DNA gene delivery to encode for a chimeric molecule, to study the potential synergistic effect.

As previously mentioned, BDNF belongs to the family of neurotrophins and binds specifically to TrkB receptors to activate the intracellular signaling pathways that promote neuronal survival and the differentiation of neurons. The neurotrophic effects of BDNF on motoneuronal degeneration have been widely studied *in vitro* and *in vivo* [66,67]. This neurotrophin has also been proposed as a potential therapeutic agent for the treatment of human ALS [68], although no successful results have been achieved. This failure in the clinical application of BDNF may be due to the low efficacy of targeting the neurotrophic factor to motoneurons. Alternatively, TTC possesses a high affinity for motoneurons [40], and the fusion of BDNF to the TTC protein might increase its accessibility. A previous study reported that some neurotrophic factors, in particular BDNF, facilitate the internalization of TTC recombinant molecules in motor nerve terminals [69]. In addition, TTC and the recombinant protein BDNF-TTC can inhibit apoptosis in cultured neurons, with the quimeric molecule being more effective than TTC alone [70]. Interestingly, BDNF may cause a relocalization of membrane domains containing TTC receptors by activating Trk receptors, thereby facilitating the neuronal internalization of TTC. This observation is supported by other authors who state that TTC activates intracellular pathways involving Trk receptors [58]. Therefore, the hypothesis of a synergistic positive effect based on the fusion of the mature form of BDNF genes to TTC in a mouse model of ALS needs to be pointed out for the bench to the bedside approach.

Similarly to the results observed in transgenic SOD1^{G93A} mice [64], an amelioration of the decline in hindlimb muscle innervation was observed in the animals that were injected with either naked DNA encoding TTC or naked DNA encoding the recombinant molecule TTC and BDNF (BDNF-TTC) [65] (Figures 4,5), in addition to a significant delay in the onset of symptoms and functional deficits (Figure 6), an improvement in the spinal motor neuron survival (Figure 7) (down-regulation of caspase-1 and caspase-3 levels and a significant phosphorylation of serine/threonine protein kinase Akt) (Figure 8) and a prolonged lifespan under both treatments [64,65].

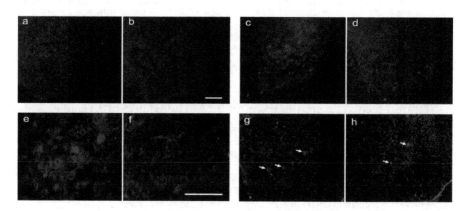

Figure 4. Motoneuronal preservation in transgenic SOD1^{G93A} mice under TTC, BDNF and BDNF-TTC treatments. Immunohistochemical labeling for BDNF expression in the grey matter of the ventral horn of (a) positive control (SOD1^{G93A} transgenic mice injected with empty plasmid), (b) SOD1^{G93A}-BDNF and (c) L2 and (d) L4 spinal segments of SOD1^{G93A}-BDNF-TTC mice. (e, f) Detail of BDNF immunolabeling of the sections shown in c and d, at higher magnification. Presence of TTC in the grey matter of the ventral horn of (g) SOD1^{G93A}-BDNF-TTC and (h) SOD1^{G93A}-TTC treated mice. Arrows point to some of the neurons positively stained for TTC. Bar = 200 μm in a, b, c, d, g and h; bar = 100 μm in e and f (Reprinted from Orphanet J. Rare Dis., 6: 10, Calvo AC, Moreno-Igoa M, Mancuso R. et al. Lack of a synergistic effect of a non-viral ALS gene therapy based on BDNF and a TTC fusion molecule, Copyright (2011), [65] with permission from BioMed Central).

a

Group	(n)	Gastrocnemius muscle		Plantar muscle	
		Latency (ms)	CMAP (mV)	Latency (ms)	CMAP (mV)
3 months					
WT	(6)	0.93 ± 0.04	51.9 ± 2.2	1.66 ± 0.08	6.49 ± 0.47
SOD control	(6)	1.11 ± 0.05	27.8 ± 2.9*	2.00 ± 0.10	2.55 ± 0.57*
SOD BDNF	(7)	1.12 ± 0.05	32.1 ± 5.0	1.89 ± 0.08	2.69 ± 0.44*
SOD TTC	(6)	1.04 ± 0.02	28.6 ± 3.5	1.95 ± 0.07	3.10 ± 0.52*
SOD BDNF-TTC	(8)	1.10 ± 0.05	32.1 ± 7.4	2.01 ± 0.11	2.64 ± 0.47*
4 months					
WT	(6)	0.93 ± 0.05	53.6 ± 4.2	1.59 ± 0.03	6.89 ± 0.79
SOD control	(5)	1.09 ± 0.04	13.0 ± 2.6*	1.98 ± 0.03	0.89 ± 0.35*
SOD BDNF	(5)	1.10 ± 0.06	18.1 ± 3.1*	1.88 ± 0.04	1.52 ± 0.41*
SOD TTC	(5)	1.06 ± 0.03	18.7 ± 4.8*	2.03 ± 0.15*	1.91 ± 0.83*
SOD BDNF-TTC	(5)	1.11 ± 0.07	20.9 ± 9.3*	2.02 ± 0.16*	1.68 ± 0.71*

b

Figure 5. Neurophysiological study in gastrocnemius and plantar muscles. (a) Results of wild-type mice (WT), control SOD1[G93A] mice, and SOD1[G93A] mice treated with naked DNA encoding for BDNF, TTC, and BDNF-TTC are shown. Values are the mean ± SEM. CMAP, compound muscle action potential; n, number of mice. *$p < 0.05$ vs. WT group at the same age. (b) Histogram representation of the decrement in the amplitude of the compound muscle action potential. CMAP was compared at 4 months with respect to values at 3 months of age in SOD1[G93A] mice, untreated and treated with naked DNA encoding for BDNF, TTC or BDNF-TTC. For each group, the left bar corresponds to the gastrocnemius muscle and the right bar to the plantar muscle (Reprinted from Orphanet J. Rare Dis., 6: 10, Calvo AC, Moreno-Igoa M, Mancuso R. et al. Lack of a synergistic effect of a non-viral ALS gene therapy based on BDNF and a TTC fusion molecule, Copyright (2011), [65] with permission from BioMed Central).

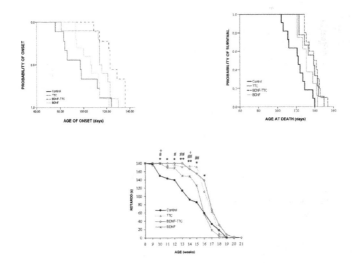

Figure 6. Improvement in disease clinical outcomes in transgenic SOD1[G93A] mice under TTC, BDNF and BDNF-TTC treatments. Cumulative probability of the onset of disease symptoms (hanging-wire test) and survival in SOD1[G93A] mice injected

at 60 days of age with TTC, BDNF-TTC, BDNF or empty (positive control) plasmids. Strength and motor function were tested using the rotarod at 15 rpm. Mice were given up to 180 s for the test performance and the time at which mice fell was recorded (*, #, +, P < 0.05; **, ##, P < 0.01; error bars indicate SEM); * for BDNF-TTC vs. positive control comparisons; # for TTC vs. control comparisons; + for BDNF vs. positive control comparisons (Reprinted from Orphanet J. Rare Dis., 6: 10, Calvo AC, Moreno-Igoa M, Mancuso R. et al. Lack of a synergistic effect of a non-viral ALS gene therapy based on BDNF and a TTC fusion molecule, Copyright (2011), [65] with permission from BioMed Central).

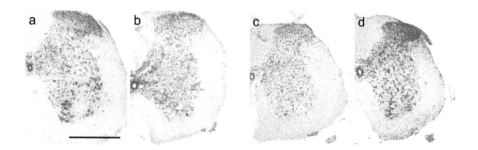

Figure 7. Spinal motor neuron survival of transgenic SOD1^{G93A} mice under TTC, BDNF and BDNF-TTC treatments. Representative micrographs showing cross-sections of lumbar spinal cords stained with cresyl violet from wild-type, (a) SOD1^{G93A} control (positive control), (b) BDNF-treated, (c) and BDNF-TTC-treated, (d) mice at 16 weeks of age. Bar = 500 µm (Reprinted from Orphanet J. Rare Dis., 6: 10, Calvo AC, Moreno-Igoa M, Mancuso R. et al. Lack of a synergistic effect of a non-viral ALS gene therapy based on BDNF and a TTC fusion molecule, Copyright (2011), [65] with permission from BioMed Central).

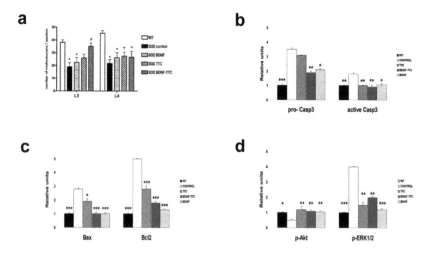

Figure 8. Apoptotic and survival pathways under TTC, BDNF and BDNF-TTC treatments. (a) Histogram representation of the average number of stained motoneurons per section in L2 and L4 spinal cord segments of wild-type littermates, control SOD1^{G93A} and treated mice (n = 4-5 mice per group). * p < 0.05 vs. wild type; # p < 0.05 vs. SOD1^{G93A} control mice. (b) Fold-changes in the expression of pro-Casp3 and active Casp3 proteins, (c) Bax and Bcl2 proteins and (d) phosphorylated states of Akt and ERK1/2 proteins in spinal cord lysates of control SOD1^{G93A} animals (white) and ani-

mals treated with TTC (grey), BDNF-TTC (blue, BTTC) and BDNF (soft blue). Western blot quantities are shown as the
ratios to b-tubulin and then related to age-matched wild-type (black) mice data (*P < 0.05 and **P < 0.01 vs. control
SOD1^{G93A} mice; ***p < 0.001; error bars indicate SEM) (Reprinted from Orphanet J. Rare Dis., 6: 10, Calvo AC, Moreno-
Igoa M, Mancuso R. et al. Lack of a synergistic effect of a non-viral ALS gene therapy based on BDNF and a TTC fusion
molecule, Copyright (2011), [65] with permission from BioMed Central).

Additionally, GDNF is another candidate neurotrophic factor for ALS therapy. This factor
has been described to show potent trophic effects on proliferation, differentiation and survival of motor neurons *in vitro* and *in vivo* [63,71-76]. Furthermore, after the retrograde
transport of GDNF to the cell bodies, a fraction of this trophic factor avoided degradation
and was sorted to dendrites [51], similar to the known movement of the TTC [39]. It was also
suggested that the transsynaptic and transcytotic pathway used by GDNF was similar to
that of TTC, but not identical, and that GDNF protein degradation was lower than that of
TTC protein. Furthermore, the combination of TTC and GDNF has been evaluated in a neonatal rat axotomy model [63] and in the ALS mouse model [77]. The combination of TTC
with insulin growth factor (IGF-1) has also been assayed in transgenic SOD1^{G93A} mice [78],
although the effect of TTC alone has not been compared in any of these studies. When the
effect of TTC was compared to the recombinant molecule *in vitro*, a significant increase in
the survival capacity of neuronal cells was found [77]. However *in vivo*, no significant differences were observed, which is probably due to the possibility that the recombinant molecule
might follow a GDNF route and not the TTC route under axotomy conditions [63].

When focusing the study *in vivo* in a mouse model of ALS, the recombinant molecule TTC
and GDNF (GDNF-TTC), GDNF and TTC treatments prompted a delay in disease onset, an
improvement in motor function and a longer lifespan in transgenic SOD1^{G93A} mice, comparing to empty-plasmid injected control mice [79] (Figure 9).

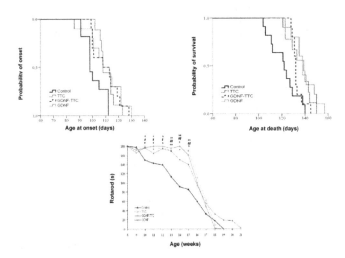

Figure 9. Improvement in disease clinical outcomes in transgenic SOD1^{G93A} mice under TTC, GDNF and GDNF-TTC
treatments. Cumulative probability of the onset of disease symptoms (hanging-wire test) and survival in SOD1^{G93A}
mice injected at 60 days of age with TTC, GDNF-TTC, GDNF or empty (positive control) plasmids. Strength and motor

function were tested using the rotarod at 15 rpm. Mice were given up to 180 s for the test performance and the time at which mice fell was recorded (*, #, +, P < 0.05; **, ##, P < 0.01; error bars indicate SEM); *GDNF-TTC vs. control comparisons; # TTC vs. control comparisons; + GDNF vs. control comparisons (*,#, +, P<0.05; **, ##, P<0.01; error bars indicate SEM) (Reprinted from Restor. Neurol. Neurosci, 30, Moreno-Igoa M, Calvo AC, Ciriza J. et al. Non-viral gene delivery of the GDNF, either alone or fused to the C-fragment of tetanus toxin protein, prolongs survival in a mouse ALS model, p. 69-80, Copyright (2012), [79] with permission from IOS Press).

Moreover, the recombinant molecule GDNF-TTC and full-length GDNF inhibited apoptotic pathways in spinal cords of SOD1^{G93A} mice by reducing the activation of caspase-3, as well as Bax and Bcl2 protein levels reached a profile expression similar than the one observed in wild type mice, highlighting the fact that treated mice biochemically resemble non-transgenic mice (Figure 10). In addition, all treatment molecules activated the PI3K survival pathway by phosphorylating Akt and ERK1/2, resembling again the wild type levels [79] (Figure 10).

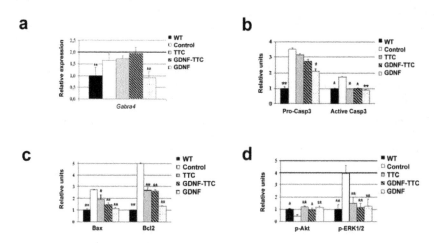

Figure 10. Apoptotic and survival pathways under TTC, GDNF and GDNF-TTC treatments. (a) Fold-changes in the expression of GABA(A) receptor subunit-4 (*Gabra4*) mRNA levels in total spinal cord of wild type, control transgenic mice and treated transgenic mice (n=5 per group). (*P<0.05, **P<0.01; error bars indicate SEM). Fold changes in the expression of (b) pro-Casp3 and active Casp3 proteins, (c) Bax and Bcl2 proteins, and (d) phosphorylated states of Akt and ERK1/2 proteins. Western blots from spinal cord lysates of control animals (white) and treated with TTC (gray), GDNFTTC (hatched-columns) and GDNF (dotted-columns). Western blot quantities are shown as the ratio to β-tubulin and then related to age-matched wild type (black) mice data (Reprinted from Restor. Neurol. Neurosci, 30, Moreno-Igoa M, Calvo AC, Ciriza J. et al. Non-viral gene delivery of the GDNF, either alone or fused to the C-fragment of tetanus toxin protein, prolongs survival in a mouse ALS model, p. 69-80, Copyright (2012), [79] with permission from IOS Press).

Summarizing, albeit a significant improvement in behavioral assays together with an activation of anti-apoptotic and survival pathways under BDNF and GDNF treatments was observed in transgenic SOD1^{G93A} mice, no synergistic effect was found neither using the BDNF-TTC nor GDNF-TTC recombinant molecules. Interestingly, recombinant plasmids BDNF-TTC and GDNF-TTC were detected in skeletal muscle and the corresponding recombinant protein reached the spinal cord tissue of transgenic SOD1^{G93A} mice (Figure 11), reinforcing the carrier properties of TTC.

As a final point, the active state of the neurotrophic factors BDNF and GDNF in the recombinant molecule could suggest that either BDNF or GDNF could exert an autocrine and neuroprotective role together with TTC to a similar extent as TTC alone; however this effect could
not be sufficient enough to prompt a synergistic effect. As a consequence, the recombinant
molecules could mainly use the same pathway that mimics a neurotrophic secretion route,
prompting survival signals in the spinal cord of transgenic SOD1^{G93A} mice [65,79]. Despite
all these contributions to the understanding of the neuroprotective properties of recombinant molecules, it is undoubtedly that TTC has open the door to an alternative therapeutic
strategy for more neurodegenerative diseases although its molecular pathways is not yet
well characterized.

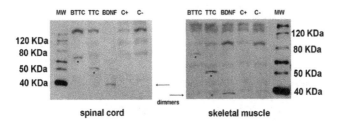

Figure 11. TTC and BDNF detection in skeletal muscle and spinal cord of ALS transgenic SOD1^{G93A} mice. Western blot
detection of TTC in spinal cord and skeletal muscle tissues of wild-type (C-, negative control), SOD1^{G93A} transgenic mice
injected with empty plasmid (C+, positive control), TTC- and BDNFTTC (BTTC)-treated mice. In TTC and BDNF-TTC treated groups, the detected band was approximately of 50 and ~ 70 KDa respectively (*), using both anti-TTC and anti-
BDNF antibodies. In the BDNF group, the dimeric conformation, indicated by arrows, was observed at approximately
40 KDa (Reprinted from Orphanet J. Rare Dis., 6: 10, Calvo AC, Moreno-Igoa M, Mancuso R. et al. Lack of a synergistic
effect of a non-viral ALS gene therapy based on BDNF and a TTC fusion molecule, Copyright (2011), [65] with permission from BioMed Central).

4. Conclusions

At present, gene and stem cell therapies are holding the hope for an efficient treatment in
ALS. Regarding gene therapy, the possibility of delivering therapeutic molecules to damaged tissues crossing the blood-brain barrier has made possible the study of viral (adenovirus, adeno-associated and lentivirus) and non-viral (fragment C of tetanus toxin) vectors,
which are retrogradely transported to motor neurons, in preclinical animal models showing
promising neuroprotective effects.

Although therapeutic strategies, which tend to stop or slow down the progression of ALS,
are one of the main goals in this field of research, the new property of TTC has opened the
door to new non-viral therapeutic strategies in this disease. The fact that TTC as well as the
recombinant molecules BDNF-TTC and GDNF-TTC can be transported through motoneurons to induce a later onset of symptoms, improve motoneuron survival and extend the survival of SOD1^{G93A} mice support the fact that the naked DNA-mediated intramuscular

delivery of TTC and fusion molecules can promote neuroprotective effects in the SOD1^{G93A} murine model of ALS. The active states of BDNF and GDNF in the recombinant molecules also confirm that these neurotrophic factors could exert an autocrine and neuroprotective role together with TTC to a similar extent as TTC alone, but this effect was not sufficient to enhance the survival signals observed under TTC treatment alone.

Definitively, the neuroprotective role of fragment C has shed light on the understanding of the disease neurodegeneration processes and the study of this promising property of TTC can be extended to other neurodegenerative diseases, such as Parkinson's disease, Alzheimer's disease and Spinal Muscular Atrophy (SMN). Essentially, a better understanding of these neurodegenerative diseases will facilitate the translation from animal model to patients to find a definitive therapeutic approach.

Acknowledgements

This work was supported by from Caja Navarra: "Tú eliges, tú decides"; PI10/0178 from the Fondo de Investigación Sanitaria of Spain; ALS association Nº S54406 and Ministerio de Ciencia e Innovacion INNPACTO IPT-2011-1091-900000.

Author details

Ana C. Calvo, Pilar Zaragoza and Rosario Osta*

*Address all correspondence to: osta@unizar.es

Laboratory of Genetics and Biochemistry (LAGENBIO-I3A), Aragon's Institute of Health Sciences (IACS), Faculty of Veterinary School, University of Zaragoza, Spain

References

[1] Jiasheng Zhang EJH. Dynamic expression of neurotrophic factor receptors in postnatal spinal motoneurons and in mouse model of ALS. J Neurobiol 2006;66: 882–895.

[2] Brooks BR, Miller RG, Swash M, Munsat TL. El Escorial revisited: revised criteria for the diagnosis of amyotrophic lateral sclerosis. Amyotroph. Lateral Scler. Other Motor Neuron Disord. 2000;1: 293-299.

[3] Vucic S, Kiernan MC. Pathophysiology of neurodegeneration in familial amyotrophic lateral sclerosis. Curr. Mol. Medicine 2009;9: 255-272.

[4] Wijesekera LC, Leigh PN. Amyotrophic lateral sclerosis. Orphanet Journal of Rare Diseases 2009; 4:3, doi:10.1186/1750-1172-1184-1183.

[5] Sreedharan J, Shaw C. The genetics of Amyotrophic Lateral Sclerosis. ACNR 2009;9: 10-16.

[6] Van Blitterswijk M, van Es MA, Koppers M, van Rheenen W et al. VAPB and C9orf72 mutations in 1 familial amyotrophic lateral sclerosis patient. Neurobiol. Aging, 2012;Aug 7.

[7] Cluskey S, Ramsden DB. Mechanism of neurodegeneration in amyotrophic lateral sclerosis. J. Clin. Pathol. 2001;54(6):386-92.

[8] Hensley K, Mhatre M, Mou S, Pye QN. et al. On the relation of oxidative stress to neuroinflammation: lessons learned from the G93A-SOD1 mouse model of amyotrophic lateral sclerosis. Antioxid. Redox. Signal. 2006;8: 2075-2087.

[9] Bruijn LI, Houseweart MK, Kato S, Anderson KL. et al. Aggregation and motor neuron toxicity of an ALS-linked SOD1 mutant independent from wild-type SOD1. Science 1998;281: 1851-1854.

[10] Jiasheng Zhang EJH. Dynamic expression of neurotrophic factor receptors in postnatal spinal motoneurons and in mouse model of ALS. J Neurobiol 2006;66: 882–895.

[11] Goodall EF, Morrison KE. Amyotrophic lateral sclerosis (motor neuron disease): proposed mechanisms and pathways to treatment. Expert Rev. Mol. Med. 2006;8: 1-22.

[12] Kalra S, Genge A, Arnold DL. A prospective, randomized, placebo-controlled evaluation of corticoneuronal response to intrathecal BDNF therapy in ALS using magnetic resonance spectroscopy: feasibility and results. Amyotroph. Lateral Scler. Other Motor Neuron Disord. 2003;4: 22-26.

[13] Thorne RG; Frey WH. Delivery of neurotrophic factors to the central nervous system: pharmacokinetic considerations. Clin Pharmacokinet 2001;40: 907–946.

[14] Borasio GD, Robberecht W, Leigh PN. et al. A placebo-controlled trial of insulin-like growth factor-I in amyotrophic lateral sclerosis. European ALS/IGF-I Study Group. Neurology 1998;51: 583–586.

[15] Check, E. Harmful potential of viral vectors fuels doubts over gene therapy. Nature 2003;423: 573–574.

[16] Farrar JJ, Yen L.M, Cook T, Fairweather N. et al. Tetanus. J. Neurol. Neurosurg. Psychiatr. 2000;69: 292–301.

[17] Toivonen JM, Oliván S, Osta R. Tetanus toxin-C fragment: the curier and the cure?. Toxins 2010;2: 2622-2644. doi:10.3390/toxins2112622.

[18] Johnson EA. Clostridial toxins as therapeutic agents: Benefits of nature's most toxic proteins. Ann. Rev. Microbiol. 1999;53: 551-575.

[19] Pellizari R, Rossetto O, Schiavo G, Montecucco C. Tetanus and botulinum neurotoxins: mechanism of action and therapeutic uses. Phil. Trans. R. Soc. Lond. B 1999;354: 259-268.

[20] Montal M. Botulinum neurotoxin. Annu. Rev. Biochem. 2010;79: 591-617.

[21] Habermann E, Dreyer F. Clostridial neurotoxins: handling and action at the cellular and molecular level. Curr. Top Microbiol. Immunol. 1986;129: 93-179.

[22] Chen S, Karalewitz APA, Barbieri JT. Insights into the different catalytic activities of Clostridium neurotoxins. Biochemistry 2012;Apr 24, Epub ahead of print.

[23] Firor WM, Lamont A. The apparent alteration of tetanus toxin within the spinal cord of dogs. Ann. Surgery 1938;108: 941-957.

[24] Martini E, Torda C, Zironi A. The effect of tetanus toxin on the choline esterase activity of the muscles of rats. J. Physiol. 1939; 96: 168-171.

[25] Harvey AM. The peripheral action of tetanus toxin. J. Physiol. 1939;96: 348-365.

[26] Manwaring WH. Types of tetanus toxin. Cal West Med. 1943;59: 306-307.

[27] Ipsen, J. The effect of environmental temperature on the reaction of mice to tetanus toxin. J. Immunol. 1951;66: 687-694.

[28] Wright, E.A. The effect of the injection of tetanus toxin into the central nervous system of rabbits. J. Immunol. 1953;71: 41-44.

[29] Roaf, M.D.; Sherrington, C.S. Experiments in examination of the locked jaw induced by tetanus toxin. J Physiol. 1906;34: 315-31.

[30] Lalli G, Gschmeissner S, Schiavo G. Myosin Va and microtubule-based motors are required for fast axonal retrograde transport of tetanus toxin in motor neurons. J. Cell Sci. 2003;116: 4639–4650

[31] Price DL, Griffin J, Young A, Peck K. et al. Tetanus toxin: Direct evidence for retrograde intraaxonal transport. Science 1975;188: 945–947.

[32] Mochida S. Protein-protein interactions in neurotransmitter release. Neurosci. Res. 2000;36: 175-182.

[33] Humeau Y, Doussau F, Grant NJ, Poulain B. How botulinum and tetanus neurotoxins block neurotransmitter release. Biochimie 2000;82:427-446.

[34] Ungar D, Hughson FM. SNARE protein structure and function. Annu. Rev. Cell Dev. Biol. 2003;19: 493–517.

[35] Calvo AC, Oliván S, Manzano R. et al. Fragment C of tetanus toxin: new insights into its neuronal signalling pathway. Int. J. Mol. Sci. 2012;13(6): 6883-6901. doi:10.3390/ijms13066883 (accessed 7 June 2012).

[36] Simpson LL, Hoch DH. Neuropharmacological characterization of fragment B from tetanus toxin. J. Pharmacol. Exp. Ther. 1985;232: 223-227.

[37] Evinger C, Erichsen JT. Transsynaptic retrograde transport of fragment C of tetanus toxin demonstrated by immunohistochemical localization. Brain Res. 1986;380: 383-388.

[38] Manning KA, Erichsen JT, Evinger C. Retrograde transneuronal transport properties of fragment C of tetanus toxin. Neuroscience 1990;34: 251-263.

[39] Fishman PS, Carrigan DR. Retrograde transneuronal transfer of the fragment C of tetanus toxin. Brain Res. 1987;406: 275-279.

[40] Coen L, Osta R, Maury M, Brulet P. Construction of recombinant proteins that migrate retrogradely and transynaptically into the central nervous system. Proc Natl Acad Sci USA 1997;94: 9400–9405.

[41] Miana-Mena FJ, Munoz MJ, Roux S. et al. A non-viral vector for targeting gene therapy to motoneurons in the CNS. Neurodegener Dis. 2004;1: 101–108.

[42] Miana-Mena FJ, Muñoz MJ, Ciriza J. et al. Fragment C tetanus toxin: A putative activity-dependent neuroanatomical tracer. Acta Neurobiol. Exp. 2003;63: 211-218.

[43] Miana-Mena FJ, Roux S, Benichou JC. et al. Neuronal activity-dependent membrane traffic at the neuromuscular junction. Proc. Nat. Acad. Sci. 2002;99: 3234-3239.

[44] Oliveira H, Fernandez R, Pires LR. et al. Targeted gene delivery into peripheral sensorial neurons mediated by self-assembled vectors composed of poly (ethylene imine) and tetanus toxin fragment C. J. Control Release 2010;143: 350-358.

[45] Skeldal S, Matusica D, Nykjaer A, Coulson EJ. Proteolytic processing of the p75 neurotrophin receptor: A prerequisite for signalling? Neuronal life, growth and death signaling are crucially regulated by intra-membrane proteolysis and trafficking of p75(NTR). Bioessays 2011;33: 614–625.

[46] Skaper SD. The biology of neurotrophins, signalling pathways, and functional peptide mimetics of neurotrophins and their receptors. CNS Neurol. Disord. Drug Targets 2008;7: 46–62.

[47] Deinhardt K, Berninghausen O, Willison HJ. et al. Tetanus toxin is internalized by a sequential clathrin-dependent mechanism initiated within lipid microdomains and independent of epsin (eosin?) 1. J. Cell Biol. 2006;174: 459–471.

[48] Deinhardt K, Reversi A, Berninghausen O. et al. Neurotrophins redirect p[75NTR] from a clathrin-independent to a clathrin-dependent endocytic pathway coupled to axonal transport. Traffic 2007;8: 1736–1749.

[49] Deinhardt K, Salinas K, Verastigui C, Watson R. et al. Rab5 and Rab7 control endocytic sorting along the axonal retrograde transport pathway. Neuron 2006;52: 293-305.

[50] Schwab M, Thoenen H. Selective trans-synaptic migration of tetanus toxin after retrograde axonal transport in peripheral sympathetic nerves: a comparison with nerve growth factor. Brain Res. 1977;122: 459–474.

[51] Rind HB, Butowt R, von Bartheld CS. Synaptic targeting of retrogradely transported trophic factors in motoneurons: comparison of glial cell line-derived neurotrophic

factor, brainderived neurotrophic factor, and cardiotrophin-1 with tetanus toxin. J Neurosci. 2005;25: 539–549.

[52] Aguilera J, Lopez LA, Yavin E. Tetanus toxin-induced protein kinase C activation and elevated serotonin levels in the perinatal rat brain. FEBS 1990;263: 61–65.

[53] Gil C, Ruiz-Meana M, Álava M. et al. Tetanus toxin enhances protein kinase C activity translocation and increases polyphosphoinositide hydrolysis in rat cerebral cortex preparations. J. Neurochem. 1998;70: 1636–1643.

[54] Inserte J, Najib A, Pelliccioni P. et al. Inhibition by tetanus toxin of sodium-dependent, high-affinity [3H]5-hydroxitryptamine uptake in rat synaptosomes. Biochem. Pharmacol. 1999;57: 111–120.

[55] Gil C, Chaib I, Pelliccioni P, Aguilera J. Activation of signal transduction pathways involving TrkA, PLCγ-1, PKC isoforms and ERK-1/2 by tetanus toxin. FEBS Lett. 2000;481: 177–182.

[56] Pelliccioni P, Gil C, Najib A. et al. Tetanus toxin modulates serotonin transport in rat-brain neuronal cultures. J. Mol. Neurosci. 2001;17: 303–310.

[57] Gil C, Chaib-Oukadour I, Blasi J, Aguilera J. HC fragment (C-terminal portion of the heavy chain) of tetanus toxin activates protein kinase C isoforms and phosphoproteins involved in signal transduction. Biochem. J. 2001;356: 97–103.

[58] Gil, C.; Chaib-Oukadour, I.; Aguilera, J. C-terminal fragment of tetanus toxin heavy chain activates Akt and MEK/ERK signalling pathways in a Trk receptor-dependent manner in cultured cortical neurons. Biochem. J. 2003;373: 613–620.

[59] Chaib-Oukadour I, Gil C, Aguilera J. The C-terminal domain of heavy chain of tetanus toxin rescues cerebellar granule neurons from apoptotic death: Involvement of phosphatidylinositol 3-kinase and mitogen-activated protein kinase pathways. J. Neurochem. 2004;90: 1227–1236.

[60] Mendieta L, Venegas B, Moreno N. et al. The carboxyl-terminal domain of the heavy chain of tetanus toxin prevents dopaminergic degeneration and improves motor behaviour in rats with striatal MPP+-lesions. Neurosci. Res. 2009;65: 98–106.

[61] Chaib-Oukadour I, Gil C, Rodríguez-Álvarez J. et al. Tetanus toxin HC fragment reduces neuronal MPP+ toxicity. Mol. Cell. Neurosci. 2009;41: 297–303.

[62] Longstreth WTJr, Meschke JS, Davidson SK. et al. Hypothesis: a motor neuron toxin produced by a clostridial species residing in gut causes ALS. Med Hypotheses 2005;64: 1153–1156.

[63] Larsen KE, Benn SC, Ay I. et al. A glial cell line-derived neurotrophic factor (GDNF): tetanus toxin fragment C protein conjugate improves delivery of GDNF to spinal cord motor neurons in mice. Brain Res. 2006;1120: 1–12.

[64]   Moreno-Igoa M, Calvo AC, Penas C. et al. Fragment C of tetanus toxin, more than a carrier. Novel perspectives in non-viral ALS gene therapy. Journal of Molecular Medicine 2010;88: 297-308.

[65]   Calvo AC, Moreno-Igoa M, Mancuso R. et al. Lack of a synergistic effect of a non-viral ALS gene therapy based on BDNF and a TTC fusion molecule. Orphanet J. Rare Dis. 2011;6: 10. http://www.ojrd.com/content/6/1/10.

[66]   Ikeda K, Klinkosz B, Greene T. et al. Effects of brain-derived neurotrophic factor on motor dysfunction in wobbler mouse motor neuron disease. Ann Neurol. 1995;37: 505-511.

[67]   Lohof AM, Ip NY, Poo MM. Potentiation of developing neuromuscular synapses by the neurotrophins NT-3 and BDNF. Nature 1993;363: 350-353.

[68]   A controlled trial of recombinant methionyl human BDNF in ALS: The BDNF Study Group (Phase III). Neurology 1999;52: 1427-1433.

[69]   Roux S, Saint Cloment C, Curie T. et al. Brain-derived neurotrophic factor facilitates in vivo internalization of tetanus neurotoxin C-terminal fragment fusion proteins in mature mouse motor nerve terminals. Eur. J. Neurosci. 2006;24: 1546-1554.

[70]   Ciriza J, Garcia-Ojeda M, Martín-Burriel I. et al. Antiapoptotic activity maintenance of brain derived neurotrophic factorand the C fragment of the tetanus toxin genetic fusion protein. Cent Eur J Biol 2008;3: 105-112.

[71]   Henderson CE, Phillips HS, Pollock RA. et al. GDNF: a potent survival factor for mo-toneurons present in peripheral nerve and muscle. Science 1994;266: 1062-1064.

[72]   Oppenheim RW, Houenou LJ, Johnson JE. et al. Developing motor neurons rescued from programmed and axotomy-induced cell death by GDNF. Nature 1995;373: 344-346.

[73]   Mohajeri MH, Figlewicz DA, Bohn MC. Intramuscular grafts of myoblasts genetical-ly modified to secrete glial cell line-derived neurotrophic factor prevent motoneuron loss and disease progression in a mouse model of familial amyotrophic lateral sclero-sis. Hum. Gene Ther. 1999;10: 1853-1866.

[74]   Acsadi G, Anguelov RA, Yang H, et al. Increased survival and function of SOD1 mice after glial cell-derived neurotrophic factor gene therapy. Hum. Gene Ther. 2002;13: 1047-1059.

[75]   Wang LJ, Lu YY, Muramatsu S. et al. Neuroprotective effects of glial cell line-derived neurotrophic factor mediated by an adenoassociated virus vector in a transgenic ani-mal model of amyotrophic lateral sclerosis. J Neurosci. 2002;22: 6920-6928.

[76]   Manabe Y, Nagano I, Gazi MS. et al. Glial cell line-derived neurotrophic factor pro-tein prevents motor neuron loss of transgenic model mice for amyotrophic lateral sclerosis. Neurol. Res. 2003;25; 195-200.

[77] Ciriza J, Moreno-Igoa M, Calvo AC. et al. A genetic fusion GDNF-C fragment of teta-
      nus toxin prolongs survival in a symptomatic mouse ALS model. Restorative Neurol-
      ogy and Neuroscience 2008;26: 459-465.

[78] Chian RJ, Li J, Ay I. et al. IGF-1: Tetanus toxin fragment C fusion protein improves
      delivery of IGF-1 to spinal cord but fails to prolong survival of ALS mice. Brain Re-
      search 2009;1287: 1-19.

[79] Moreno-Igoa M, Calvo AC, Ciriza J. et al. Non-viral gene delivery of the GDNF, ei-
      ther alone or fused to the C-fragment of tetanus toxin protein, prolongs survival in a
      mouse ALS model. Restor. Neurol. Neurosci. 2012;30: 69-80.

Chapter 3

Mesenchymal Stem Cells as Gene Delivery Vehicles

Christopher D. Porada and Graça Almeida-Porada

Additional information is available at the end of the chapter

1. Introduction

Mesenchymal stem cells (MSCs) possess a battery of unique properties which make them ideally suited not only for cellular therapies/regenerative medicine, but also as vehicles for gene delivery in a wide array of clinical settings. These include: 1) widespread distribution throughout the body; 2) ease of isolation and ability to be extensively expanded in culture without loss of potential; 3) the ability to differentiate into a wide array of functional cell types in vitro and in vivo; 4) they exert pronounced anti-inflammatory and immunomodulatory effects upon transplantation; and 5) the ability to home to damaged tissues, solid tumors, and metastases following in vivo administration.

In this Chapter, we will summarize the latest research in the use of MSC in regenerative medicine, focusing predominantly on their use as vehicles for transferring exogenous genes. To highlight the immense potential these cells possess for gene therapy applications, we will attempt to paint as broad a canvas as possible, starting with a discussion about the basic biology of MSC, and their unique properties which combine to make MSC one of the most promising stem cell populations for use in gene therapy studies and trials. We will reveal the versatility of MSC as gene delivery vehicles by summarizing some of the most recent studies showing the ease with which MSC can be modified with a wide range of both viral and non-viral vector systems, and highlighting some of the advantages to delivering transgenes within a cellular vehicle, as opposed to administering vectors directly into the body. We will then discuss the engineering of MSC to enhance their natural abilities to mediate repair within various tissues; one of the most popular uses of MSC to-date in the gene therapy arena. We will discuss our recent work, and that of others, using MSC to deliver coagulation factors to treat the hemophilias, with hemophilia A serving as a paradigm for how MSC could be used to deliver a therapeutic transgene, and thereby correct essentially any inherited disease. The Chapter will conclude with a discussion of MSC's ability to selectively migrate to forming solid tumors following intravenous administration, and to actively seek out metastases at sites far removed from the primary site of the tumor. We will summarize exciting recent work showing that it is possible to exploit this property to achieve sustained, high-level expression of pro-apoptotic gene products within the tumor, obtaining greatly improved anti-tumor effects, while essentially eliminating the systemic toxicities that plague current radiation/chemotherapy-based treatments.

2. Isolation and characterization of MSC

More than 30 years ago, Friedenstein pioneered the concept that the marrow microenvironment resided within the so-called stromal cells of the marrow, by demonstrating that fibroblastoid cells obtained from the bone marrow were capable of transferring the hematopoietic microenvironment to ectopic sites [1, 2]. Years later, scientists began to explore the full potential of these microenvironmental cells, and results of these studies led to the realization that this population harbored cells with properties of true stem cells. These cells were officially termed mesenchymal stem cells (MSC) [3]. MSC are now recognized to be a key part of the microenvironment/niche that supports the hematopoietic stem cell and drives the process of hematopoiesis, yet despite serving this vital function, MSC only comprise ~0.001-0.01% of cells within the marrow [4], making methods for isolating/enriching and for expanding these cells essential to their study and their ultimate clinical use. The most straightforward method for obtaining MSC is to exploit their propensity to adhere to plastic and their ability to be passaged with trypsin (contaminating hematopoietic cells do not passage with trypsin) to rapidly obtain a relatively morphologically homogeneous population of fibroblastic cells from a bulk mononuclear cell preparation [5-7]. Unfortunately, true MSC (defined by function) account for only a small percentage of the highly heterogeneous resultant population, making results obtained with cells prepared in this fashion difficult to interpret, and inconsistent from experiment-to-experiment and from group-to-group. The identification of antigens that are unique to MSC would eliminate this problem. Human MSC do not express markers which have been associated with other stem cell populations (like hematopoietic stem cells) such as CD34, CD133, or c-kit, nor hematopoietic markers such as CD45, CD14, and CD19. Moreover, no marker has been identified to date that specifically identifies MSC. Nevertheless, several surface antigens have proven useful for obtaining highly enriched MSC populations. The first of these markers to be identified was Stro-1, an antibody that reacts with non-hematopoietic bone marrow stromal precursor cells [8]. Although the antigen recognized by this antibody has not yet been identified, we and others have found that by tri-labeling bone marrow cells with Stro-1, anti-CD45, and anti-GlyA, and selecting the Stro-1+CD45-GlyA- cells, it is possible to consistently obtain a homogeneous population that is highly enriched for MSC [9-15]. In addition to Stro-1, antibodies such as SB-10, SH2, SH3, and SH4 have been developed over the years and numerous surface antigens such CD13, CD29, CD44, CD63, CD73, CD90, CD105, and CD166 have been used to attempt to identify and isolate MSC [16-18]. Unfortunately, all of these antigens appear to be expressed on a wide range of cell types within the body in addition to MSC. This lack of a unique marker suggests that to obtain a pure population of MSC that are functionally homogeneous, investigators will likely either have to await the development of novel antibodies that recognize as yet unidentified antigens that are unique to primitive MSC, or employ strategies in which multiple antibodies are combined to allow for positive selection of MSC and depletion of cells of other lineages that share expression of the antigens recognized by the MSC antibody in question, as we have done with Stro-1, CD45, and GlyA.

3. Sources of MSC

Although much of the work to date has focused on MSC isolated from adult bone marrow, we and others have isolated cells that appear phenotypically and functionally to be MSC, from numerous tissues including brain, liver, lung, fetal blood, umbilical cord blood, kidney, and even liposuction material [19-26]. The broad distribution of MSC throughout the body leads one to postulate that MSC may play a critical role in organ homeostasis by providing supportive factors and/or mediating maintenance/repair within their respective tissue. Importantly, although MSC from each of these tissues appear similar with respect to phenotype and overall differentiative potential, studies at the RNA and protein level have now revealed that subtle differences exist between MSC from these various tissues, with MSC from each tissue possessing a molecular fingerprint indicative of their tissue of origin [21, 22, 27-31]. Using a non-injury fetal sheep transplantation model, we showed that these differences result in a bias for human MSC to home to and give rise to cells of their tissue of origin in vivo [32, 33]. This suggests that, to use MSC as therapeutics or as gene delivery vehicles, the ideal source of MSC may differ depending on the specific disease to be treated and the desired target organ.

Despite the apparent presence of MSC within many of the major organs of the body, the relatively non-invasive fashion with which adipose tissue or bone marrow can be obtained, and the fact that both these tissues could readily be obtained autologously, combine to suggest that these two tissues will likely be the predominant source of MSC employed in clinical applications in the foreseeable future. However, additional experiments will need to be performed to rigorously assess the inherent safety of adipose tissue-derived MSC before these cells will see widespread clinical use, since several recent studies have suggested that they may be inherently less genetically stable than MSC isolated from bone marrow [34], exhibiting aneuploidy [35, 36] and undergoing transformation [37, 38] upon prolonged propagation in vitro. However, another recent study provided evidence that, even if genomic instability is intentionally induced with genotoxic agents, adipose tissue-derived MSC respond to this insult by undergoing terminal adipogenic differentiation rather than transformation [39]. The dramatically conflicting nature of the results from these different studies could, perhaps, be due to differing methods employed for isolating and culturing MSC, differing levels of contaminating non-MSC cells in the cultures, as well as the duration of the culture (i.e., the number of times the cells have been passaged). Bearing this possible instability in mind, the recommendation has been put forward to only make clinical use of cells that have been passaged fewer than 25 times in culture, regardless of the source of MSC [40].

4. MSC as vehicles for delivering therapeutic genes

While MSC possess tremendous therapeutic potential by virtue of their ability to lodge/engraft within multiple tissues in the body and both give rise to tissue-specific cells and release trophic factors that trigger the tissue's own endogenous repair pathways [41-59], gene therapists have realized that these properties are just the beginning of the therapeutic applications for MSC [24, 60, 61]. By using gene therapy to engineer MSC to either augment their own natural production of specific desired proteins or to enable them to express proteins outside of their native repertoire, it is possible to greatly broaden the spectrum of diseases for which MSC could provide therapeutic benefit. Unlike hematopoietic stem cells which are notoriously difficult to modify with most viral vectors while preserving their in vivo potential, MSC can be readily transduced with all of the major clinically prevalent viral vector systems including those based upon adenovirus [62-64], the murine retroviruses [64-68], lentiviruses [69-74], and AAV [75, 76], and efficiently produce a wide range of cytoplasmic, membrane-bound, and secreted protein products. This ease of transduction coupled with the ability to subsequently select and expand only the gene-modified cells in vitro to generate adequate numbers for transplantation combine to make MSC one of the most promising stem cell populations for use in gene therapy studies and trials.

To date, the majority of studies using gene-modified MSC have been undertaken with the purpose of enhancing the natural abilities of MSC to mediate repair within various tissues. Using the heart as an example, once investigators discovered the identity of some of the key trophic factors responsible for MSC's beneficial effect on the injured myocardium, they undertook studies using MSC engineered to overexpress a number of these factors [69, 77-86]. As anticipated, the "gene-enhanced" MSC were substantially more effective than their unmodified counterparts, producing greatly enhanced therapeutic effects. Similar studies have also been performed to repair the damaged/diseased CNS using MSC engineered to produce neurotrophic factors [87-94], to repair the injured liver using MSC expressing proteins involved in hepatocyte differentiation and/or proliferation [95, 96], to repair ischemia/reperfusion injury [97-102], and to repair the kidney [103-105]. In each case thus far, MSC engineered to express higher levels of proteins known to be beneficial for the tissue in question and/or to promote survival have produced markedly better results than unmodified MSC.

Despite the many advantages of using MSC as gene delivery vehicles, however, relatively few studies have thus far explored this potential for the treatment of genetic diseases. One disease for which we and others are actively investigating MSC for delivery of a therapeutic gene is hemophilia A [106-112].

5. Hemophilia A as a paradigm for the use of gene-modified msc to correct genetic diseases

Hemophilia A represents the most common inheritable deficiency of the coagulation proteins [113]. The severity of hemophilia A is traditionally based on plasma levels of FVIII, with persons exhibiting less than 1% normal factor (<0.01 IU/mL) being considered to have severe hemophilia, persons with 1-5% normal factor moderately severe, and persons with 5%-40% of the normal FVIII levels mild [114-116]. Up to 70% of hemophilia A patients present with the severe form of the disease, and suffer from frequent hemorrhaging, leading to chronic debilitating arthropathy, hematomas of subcutaneous connective tissue/muscle, and internal bleeding. Over time, the collective complications of recurrent hemorrhaging result in chronic pain, absences from school and work, and permanent disability [114]. Current state-of-the-art treatment consists of frequent prophylactic infusions of plasma-derived or recombinant FVIII protein to maintain hemostasis, and has greatly increased life expectancy and quality of life for many hemophilia A patients.

This treatment approach is, however, far from ideal, due to the need for lifelong intravenous infusions and the high treatment cost. Moreover, this treatment is unavailable to a large percentage of the world's hemophiliacs, placing these patients at great risk of severe, permanent disabilities and life-threatening bleeds. Furthermore, even among the patients who are fortunate enough to have access to, and the financial means to afford, prophylactic FVIII infusions, approximately 30% will form FVIII inhibitors [117]. The formation of these inhibitors greatly reduces the efficacy of subsequent FVIII infusions, and can ultimately lead to treatment failure, placing the patient at risk of life-threatening hemorrhage. There is thus a significant need to develop novel, longer-lasting hemophilia A therapies.

In the past three decades, the remarkable progress in the understanding of the molecular basis of the disease, the identification and characterization of FVIII gene, structure, and biology has heightened the interest and feasibility of treating hemophilia A with gene therapy. In contrast to current protein-based therapeutics, lifelong improvement or permanent cure of hemophilia A is theoretically possible after only a single gene therapy treatment; indeed, several aspects of hemophilia A make it ideally suited for correction by gene therapy [118-126]. First, in contrast to many other genetic diseases, the missing protein (coagulation FVIII) does not need to be expressed in either a cell- or tissue-specific fashion to mediate correction. Although the liver is thought to be the primary natural site of synthesis of FVIII, expression of this factor in other tissues exerts no deleterious effects. As long as the protein is expressed in cells which have ready access to the circulation, it can be secreted into the bloodstream and exert its appropriate clotting activity. Second, even modest levels (3-5%) of FVIII-expressing cells would be expected to convert severe hemophilia A to a moderate/mild phenotype, reducing or eliminating episodes of spontaneous bleeding and greatly improving quality of life. Thus, even with the low levels of transduction that are routinely obtained with many of the current viral-based gene delivery systems, a marked clinical improvement would be anticipated in patients with hemophilia A. Conversely, even supraphysiologic levels of FVIII as high as 150% of normal are predicted to be well tolerated, making the therapeutic window extremely wide [116]. Based on this knowledge, the American Society of Gene and Cell Therapy (www.ASGCT.org) recently provided NIH director, Dr. Francis Collins, with a roadmap of disease indications that it feels will be viable gene therapy products within the next 5-7 years. The hemophilias were identified as belonging to the most promising, "Target 10", group of diseases.

6. Mesenchymal Stem Cells (MSC) as hemophilia A therapeutics

As discussed in the preceding section, the liver is thought to be the primary site of FVIII syn-thesis within the body. We and others have devoted a great deal of energy to demonstrating the ability of MSC from various sources to serve as therapeutics for liver disease [11, 13, 14, 33, 96, 127-152]. It is now clear that, not only do MSC have the ability to generate, in vitro and in vivo, cells which are indistinguishable from native hepatocytes, but transplantation of MSC in a range of model systems can result in fairly robust formation of hepatocytes which repair a variety of inborn genetic defects, toxin-induced injuries, and even fibrosis. The fetal sheep model provides a unique system in which to explore the full differentiative potential of various stem cell populations, since the continuous need for new cells within all of the organs during fetal development provides a permissive milieu in which gene-modi-fied donor cells can engraft, proliferate, and differentiate. Furthermore, by performing the transplant at a stage in gestation when the fetus is considered to be largely immuno-naïve, it is possible to engraft human cells at significant levels, which persist for the lifespan of the animal due to induction of donor-specific tolerance [130-132]. Indeed, in ongoing studies, we have found that, after transplantation into fetal sheep, human MSC engraft at levels of up to 12% within the recipient liver [11, 131, 132, 153-158], and contribute to both the paren-chyma and the perivascular zones of the engrafted organs, placing them ideally for deliver-ing FVIII into the circulation. Since FVIII levels of 3-5% of normal would convert a patient with severe hemophilia A to a moderate or mild phenotype, these levels of engraftment should be highly therapeutic. These collective results thus suggest that MSC may represent an ideal cell type for treating hemophilia A.

However, although MSC engrafted (following transplantation in utero) at significant levels within organs that are natural sites of FVIII synthesis, only a small percent expressed endog-enous FVIII, suggesting that simply transplanting "healthy" MSC will not likely provide an effective means of treating/curing hemophilia A. By using gene therapy to engineer MSC to express FVIII, however, it is highly probable that the levels of engrafted MSC we have thus far achieved in utero would provide marked therapeutic benefit in hemophilia A. By trans-ducing the MSC in vitro, rather than performing gene therapy by injecting the vector direct-ly, as is the current practice in clinical gene therapy trials, there is no risk of off-target transduction, and the vector being employed simply needs a strong constitutively active promoter to ensure that all cells derived from the transplanted MSC continue to express FVIII and mediate a therapeutic effect. Importantly, the only documented cases of retroviral-induced insertional mutagenesis have been observed following genetic modification of hem-atopoietic stem cells [159-161]; there is no evidence that MSC transform or progress to clonal dominance following transduction, suggesting they represent safe cellular vehicles for deliv-ering FVIII (or other transgenes).

Importantly, critical proof-of-principle studies have already shown that MSC can be trans-duced with FVIII-expressing viral vectors and secrete high levels of FVIII protein in vitro and following transplantation in vivo [106-109]. FVIII purified from the conditioned medi-um of the transduced MSC was proven to have a specific activity, relative electrophoretic mobility, and proteolytic activation pattern that was virtually identical to that of FVIII produced by other commercial cell lines [109]. Given the widespread distribution and engraftment of MSC following their systemic infusion, the ability of MSC to give rise, in vivo, to cells of numerous tissue types, and their ability to efficiently process and secrete high amounts of biologically active FVIII, they are, not surprisingly, being viewed as ideal vehicles for delivering a FVIII transgene throughout the body and thus providing long-term/permanent correction of hemophilia A [106-109, 162].

In addition to their widespread engraftment and their ability to serve as delivery vehicles for the FVIII gene, the rather unique immunological properties of MSC may further increase their utility for treating hemophilia A. MSC do not normally express MHC class II or the co-stimulatory molecules CD80 and CD82, unless they are stimulated with IFN-γ, and are thus viewed as being relatively hypo-immunogenic. As such, they do not provoke the proliferation of allogeneic lymphocytes or serve as very effective targets for lysis by cytotoxic T cells or NK cells. In fact, a large body of evidence is now accumulating that MSC can be readily transplanted across allogeneic barriers without eliciting an immune response [163, 164]. Thus, if one wished to use MSC to treat hemophilia A, off-the-shelf MSC from an unrelated donor could theoretically be used, greatly increasing the feasibility of obtaining and using these stem cells for therapy.

Perhaps even more important from the standpoint of their potential use as hemophilia A therapeutics, more recent studies have provided evidence that MSC also appear to have the ability to exert both immunosuppressive and anti-inflammatory properties both in vitro and in vivo. These properties appear to result from MSC's ability to intervene, at multiple levels, with the generation and propagation of an immune response. To name just a few examples, MSC have been demonstrated to interfere with the generation and maturation of cytotoxic and helper T cells [165-174], dendritic cells [175-178], and B cells [179]. In addition to actively shutting down the generation of immune effector cells, MSC also have the ability to induce the formation of potent Tregs, although the mechanism by which this comes about is still the subject of active research [40, 180-182]. MSC are also known to express a battery of factors [40, 168-170, 180, 183-187] that reduce local inflammation, blunt immune response, and counteract the chemotactic signals responsible for recruiting immune cells to sites of injury/inflammation. One could thus envision these immune-dampening properties enabling the delivery of FVIII without eliciting an immune response and subsequent inhibitor formation, thus overcoming one of the major hurdles that plague current treatment/management of hemophilia A. As will be discussed in the next section, however, our postnatal studies in the hemophilic sheep suggest that further work will be required to discover how to obtain these potential immune benefits in the context of the ongoing injury/inflammation present in animals/patients with clinically advanced hemophilia A.

In addition to the aforementioned properties, preclinical animal studies examining the potential of MSC isolated from adult tissues have also highlighted another interesting and clinically valuable characteristic of MSC; their ability to selectively navigate to sites of injury and/or inflammation within the body. Once reaching these specific sites, the MSC then mediate repair both by engrafting and generating tissue-specific cells within the injured tissue

[188-190], and by releasing trophic factors that blunt the inflammatory response and often promote healing by activating the tissue's own endogenous repair mechanisms. While the mechanisms responsible for this trafficking to sites of injury are still being elucidated [191-193], this observation raises the exciting possibility that, following systemic infusion, FVIII-expressing MSC could efficiently migrate to sites of active bleeding/injury, thereby releasing FVIII locally and focusing the therapy where it is most needed. As will be discussed in the following section, over the past 2-3 years, we have begun exploring whether it is possible to exploit these many advantages of MSC as a cellular vehicle for delivering a FVIII gene by testing the ability of FVIII-expressing MSC to correct hemophilia A in a new large animal model; sheep.

7. Establishment of a new preclinical model of hemophilia A and success with MSC-based treatment

A number of animal models have been developed to evaluate new methods of not only treatment of coagulation disorders, but also the prevention and treatment of inhibitor formation. Transient hemophilic rabbit models induced by infusion of plasma containing inhibitors have been used to evaluate the effect of different bypass products to factor VIII [194], but these models, while valuable for inhibitor studies, do not accurately recapitulate the human disease, precluding their use for gene therapy studies. Fortunately, dog models of hemophilia A with congenital deficiency [195, 196] and mouse models obtained by gene targeting and knockout technology [197] are available to study FVIII function and gene therapy approaches for treating hemophilia A. Therapeutic benefit has been obtained in numerous studies using a variety of vector systems in the murine model [121, 122, 198-204], and phenotypic correction of hemophilia A in the dog has been achieved, but has proven to be far more difficult than in mice [205, 206]. Despite promising results in both canine and murine models, however, no clinical gene therapy trial has shown phenotypic/clinical improvement of hemophilia A in human patients. This is in marked contrast to the recent clinical successes with gene therapy for hemophilia B [207]. The reasons for the disparity in the efficacy of gene therapy for treating hemophilia A versus B is not presently clear. Nonetheless, based on the disappointing results to-date, there are currently no active hemophilia A clinical gene therapy trials, even though hemophilia A accounts for roughly 80% of all cases of hemophilia.

The difficulties seen thus far translating success in animal models into therapeutic benefit in human patients underscores the importance of preclinical animal models that both precisely mimic the disease process of hemophilia A, and closely parallel normal human immunology and physiology. To this end, between 1979 and 1982, a number of male offspring of a single white alpine ewe at the Swiss Federal Institute of Technology all died several hours postpartum due to severe bleeding from the umbilical cord [208-210]. Daughters and granddaughters of this ewe also gave birth to lambs exhibiting the same pathology. Investigation of the affected animals showed extensive subcutaneous and intramuscular hematomas. Spontaneous hemarthroses were also frequent, leading to reduced locomotion and symp toms of pain in standing up, restricting nursing activity. Stronger injuries that arose when animals were not placed in carefully controlled isolation resulted in heavy bleeding and intensive pain. Laboratory tests showed increased PTT, and FVIII levels (as assessed by aPTT) of about 1% of control animals. Replacement therapy with human FVIII (hFVIII) concentrate or fresh sheep plasma resulted in remission of disease and rapid clinical improvement.

Unfortunately, due to the expense and effort of maintaining these sheep, the Swiss investigators allowed the line to die out, saving only a few straws of semen prior to allowing this valuable resource to pass into extinction. We recently used a variety of reproductive technologies to successfully re-establish this line of hemophilia A sheep, and fully characterized both the clinical parameters and the precise molecular basis for their disease [211-216]. In similarity to mutations seen in many human patients [217], these animals possess a premature stop codon with a frameshift mutation. This is the only animal model of hemophilia A with this clinically relevant mutation-type, providing a unique opportunity to study therapies in this context. All ten animals to-date have exhibited bleeding from the umbilical cord, prolonged tail and "cuticle" bleeding time, and multiple episodes of severe spontaneous bleeding including hemarthroses, muscle hematomas, and hematuria, all of which have responded to human FVIII. Just like human patients with severe hemophilia A, a hallmark symptom in these sheep is repeated spontaneous joint bleeds, which lead to chronic, debilitating arthropathies and reduced mobility. Importantly, chromogenic assays performed independently at the BloodCenter of Wisconsin and Emory University revealed undetectable FVIII activity in the circulation of these sheep, explaining their severe, life-threatening phenotype.

In addition to the value of another large animal model of hemophilia A and the uniqueness of the mutation, sheep possess many characteristics that make them an ideal preclinical model for gene therapy. The first of these is the size. Sheep are fairly close in size to humans, weighing roughly 8lbs at birth and 150-200lbs as adults, likely obviating the need for scale-up of cell/vector dose to move from experiments in sheep to trials in humans. This is in marked contrast to mice which are ~2800 times smaller than a typical human patient [218]. Secondly, sheep share many important physiological and developmental characteristics with humans; for example, the pattern of fetal to adult hemoglobin switching, and the naturally occurring changes in the primary sites of hematopoiesis from yolk sac to fetal liver and finally to the bone marrow near the end of gestation. Thirdly, sheep are outbred, and thus represent a wide spectrum of genetic determinants of the immune response, as do humans. As the immune response to both the vector and the vector–encoded FVIII are likely to play a key role in FVIII inhibitor formation (or lack thereof), this represents an advantage not found in most other models, with the possible exception of the dog, which could conceivably be outbred as well to achieve a broader genetic spectrum. In addition, the development of the sheep immune system has been investigated in detail [219-225], making sheep well suited for studying the immunological aspects of gene-based therapies for hemophilia A. Importantly, the large size of the sheep, their long life span (9-12 years), and their relative ease of maintenance and breeding make it possible to conduct long-term studies in relatively large numbers of animals to fully evaluate the efficacy and safety issues related to gene therapy. For these reasons, we feel that the sheep are a particularly relevant model in which to examine gene and cell-based therapies for hemophilia A. An additional unique advantage to using sheep to study hemophilia A treatment is that in sheep, like human, a large percentage of the vWF is found within platelets rather than free in plasma. This is in contrast to dog (in which vWF circulates free in plasma [226, 227]), and makes the sheep an ideal large animal model in which to explore the use of platelet-targeted gene therapy for hemophilia A [126, 228-230].

To experimentally test the ability of MSC to serve as FVIII delivery vehicles and thus treat hemophilia A, we recently tested a novel, non-ablative transplant-based gene therapy in 2 pediatric hemophilia A lambs [110-112]. During the first 3-5 months of life, both these animals had received frequent, on-demand infusions of human FVIII for multiple hematomas and chronic, progressive, debilitating hemarthroses of the leg joints which had resulted in severe defects in posture and gait, rendering them nearly immobile. In an ideal situation, one would use autologous cells to deliver a FVIII transgene, and thus avoid any complications due to MHC-mismatching. Unfortunately, the severe life-threatening phenotype of the hemophilia A sheep prevented us from collecting bone marrow aspirates to isolate autologous cells. We therefore elected to utilize cells from the ram that had sired the two hemophiliac lambs, hoping that, by using paternal (haploidentical) MSC, immunologic incompatibility between the donor and recipient should be minimized sufficiently to allow engraftment, especially given the large body of evidence now accumulating that MSC can be transplanted across allogeneic barriers without eliciting an immune response [163, 164].

Based on our prior work in the fetal sheep model, we knew that the intraperitoneal (IP) transplantation of MSC results in widespread engraftment throughout all of the major organs [11, 131, 157, 231-233] and durable expression of vector-encoded genes [232-234]. We further reasoned that using the IP route would also have the advantage of enabling the cells to enter the circulation in an almost time-release fashion, after being engulfed by the omentum and absorbed through the peritoneal lymphatics. Importantly, we also felt that the use of the IP route would enable us to avoid the lung-trapping which hinders the efficient trafficking of MSC to desired target organs following IV administration, and also poses clinical risks due to emboli formation [235, 236].

Following isolation, MSC were simultaneously transduced with 2 HIV-based lentivectors, the first of which encoded an expression/secretion optimized porcine FVIII (pFVIII) transgene [112]. We selected a pFVIII transgene for two reasons. First, we had not yet cloned the ovine FVIII cDNA and constructed a B domain-deleted cassette that would fit in a lentivector. Secondly, the pFVIII transgene had previously been shown, in human cells, to be expressed/secreted at 10-100 times higher levels than human FVIII [120, 121, 237]. We thus felt that these very high levels of expression/secretion might enable us to achieve a therapeutic benefit, even in the event we obtained very low levels of engraftment of the transduced paternal MSC. The second lentivector encoded eGFP to facilitate tracking and identification of donor cells in vivo. Combining the 2 vectors unexpectedly resulted in preferential transduction with the eGFP vector, such that only about 15% of the MSC were transduced with the pFVIII-encoding vector, as assessed by qPCR. Once the transduced MSC had been sufficiently expanded, the first animal to be transplanted was treated with a dose of hFVIII calculated to correct the levels to 200%, to ensure no procedure-related bleeding occurred. The animal was then sedated, and 30x10^6 transduced MSC were transplanted into the peritoneal cavity under ultrasound guidance in the absence of any preconditioning.

Following transplantation, FVIII activity (assessed by chromogenic assay) was undetectable in the circulation, but this animal's clinical picture improved dramatically. All spontaneous bleeding events ceased, and he enjoyed an event-free clinical course, devoid of spontaneous bleeds, enabling us to cease hFVIII infusions. Existing hemarthroses resolved, the animal's joints recovered fully and resumed normal appearance, and he regained normal posture and gait, resuming a normal activity level. To our knowledge, this represents the first report of phenotypic correction of severe hemophilia A in a large animal model following transplantation of cells engineered to produce FVIII, and the first time that reversal of chronic debilitating hemarthroses has been achieved.

Based on the remarkable clinical improvement we had achieved in this first animal, we transplanted a second animal with 120x10^6 paternal MSC, >95% of which were transduced and expressing pFVIII. We anticipated that by transplanting 4x's the number of cells with roughly 6x's the transduction efficiency, we would achieve pronounced improvement and therapeutic levels of FVIII in the circulation of this animal. In similarity to the first animal, hemarthroses present in this second animal at the time of transplant resolved, and he resumed normal activity shortly after transplantation. This second animal also became factor-independent following the transplant. These results thus confirm the ability of this MSC-based approach to provide phenotypic correction in this large animal model of hemophilia A. However, just as we had observed in the first animal, no FVIII was detectable in the circulation of this animal, making the mechanism by which this procedure mediated such pronounced clinical improvement uncertain.

Despite the pronounced clinical improvement we observed in the first animal, he mounted a rapid and fairly robust immune response to FVIII, in similarity to prior studies performed with hemophilia A mice [237]. Before transplant, this first animal had Bethesda titers against hFVIII of only ~3, yet this lifesaving procedure resulted in a rise in Bethesda titer to ~800 against the vector-encoded pFVIII and nearly 700 to hFVIII. The formation of such high titer inhibitors with cross-reactivity to the human protein was surprising, given the well established ability to successfully use porcine FVIII products in human patients to bypass existing anti-hFVIII inhibitors [238-241]. Similarly, despite having no detectable inhibitors prior to transplant, the second animal receiving the higher FVIII-expressing cell dose developed titers of ~150 Bethesda units against the vector-encoded pFVIII following transplantation which also exhibited cross-reactivity to the human protein.

Following euthanasia of these animals, we performed a detailed tissue analysis to begin deciphering the mechanism whereby this novel MSC-based gene delivery produced its pronounced therapeutic effect at a systemic level. PCR analysis demonstrated readily detectable levels of MSC engraftment in nearly all tissues analyzed, including liver, lymph nodes, intestine, lung, kidney, omentum, and thymus. These molecular analyses thereby proved that it is possible to achieve widespread durable engraftment of MSC following transplantation in a postnatal setting in a large animal model without the need for preconditioning/ablation, and in the absence of any selective advantage for the donor cells.

Confocal immunofluorescence analysis revealed large numbers of FVIII-expressing MSC within the synovium of the joints which exhibited hemarthrosis at the time of transplant, demonstrating (just as we had hoped/predicted) that the transplanted MSC possessed the intrinsic ability to home to and persist within sites of ongoing injury/inflammation, releasing FVIII locally within the joint, providing an explanation for the dramatic improvement we observed in the animal's joints. This finding is in agreement with prior studies [242], show-ing that local delivery of FIX-AAV to the joints of mice with injury-induced hemarthroses led to resolution of the hemarthroses in the absence of any detectable FIX in the circulation. While this finding provides an explanation for the reversal of the joint pathology present in these animals at transplant, it cannot explain the observed systemic benefits such as the ces-sation of spontaneous bleeding events.

Confocal analysis also revealed engrafted cells within the small intestine, demonstrating that MSC can still engraft within the intestine following postnatal transplantation, just as we had observed in prior studies in fetal recipients [232]. Given the ease with which proteins secreted from cells within the intestine can enter the circulation, future studies aimed at im-proving the levels of engraftment within the intestine have the potential to greatly improve the systemic release of FVIII. In addition to the intestine and hemarthrotic joints, significant levels of engraftment were also seen within the thymus of this animal. While the ability of the transplanted MSC to traffic to the thymus could clearly have important implications for the likelihood of long-term correction with this approach to hemophilia A treatment, addi-tional studies are required to determine with which cells within the thymus these MSC are interacting to ascertain the immunologic ramifications of thymic engraftment.

The marked phenotypic improvement and improvement in quality of life we have observed in our studies, to date, in the sheep model thus support the further development of thera-peutic strategies for hemophilia A and, perhaps, other coagulation disorders, employing MSC as cellular vehicles to deliver the required transgene.

8. MSC as anti-cancer gene delivery vehicles

As alluded to earlier, a large number of preclinical animal studies examining the differentia-tive potential of MSC isolated from a variety of adult tissues have also highlighted another interesting and clinically valuable characteristic of MSC; their ability to selectively navigate to sites of injury and/or inflammation within the body [192, 193, 243-247]. Once reaching these specific sites, the MSC then mediate repair both by engrafting and generating tissue-specific cells within the injured tissue (but contributing very little if at all to other tissues that are functionally normal [188-190]), and by releasing trophic factors that blunt the in-flammatory response and often promote healing by activating the tissue's own endogenous repair mechanisms. While the mechanisms responsible for this trafficking to sites of injury are currently not well understood, this observation has raised the exciting prospect of using MSC to treat a wide array of diseases in which inflammation plays a key role such as stroke [87, 88, 92, 248-255], rheumatoid arthritis [256], asthma [257-259] and allergic rhinitis [260], and both acute and chronic lung injury [261].

Cancer represents another condition in which there is a selective need for new cells created by the forming tumor, and a chronic state of insult/inflammation within the surrounding tumor microenvironment. Studies over the last several years have now revealed that MSC have the ability to "sense" this need for cells and the perceived injury to the tissue surrounding the tumor. As a result, both endogenous bone marrow- and adipose-resident MSC, as well as intravenously infused MSC, all appear to have the ability to efficiently migrate to the forming tumor, and contribute to the newly forming tumor "stroma" [191, 262-266]. Clearly, this may not seem ideal, since the MSC could, in fact, provide support to the growing tumor, potentially worsening the prognosis. Indeed, unraveling the role played by MSC within the tumor microenvironment is currently an area of active research [191, 192, 262-265, 267-269]. Irrespective of their role in the tumor's health/biology, however, the ability of MSC to selectively traffic to and integrate into the tumor microenvironment can be viewed as a double-edged sword, since this ability has now been recognized to present a very powerful and unique means of selectively delivering anti-cancer gene products to tumor cells in vivo [270-274]. Four of the gene products which have thus far received the most attention are IL-2 [275, 276], IL-12 [277-284], IFN-β [270, 271, 285, 286], and tumor necrosis factor-related apoptosis-inducing ligand (TRAIL) [287-298]. Unfortunately, the utility of these and many other biological agents that could be used for cancer therapy is often limited by both their short half-life in vivo and their pronounced toxicity due to effects on normal, non-malignant cells within the body. Using MSC to deliver these therapeutics promises to solve both of these problems, since the MSC can selectively migrate to the tumor site and release their therapeutic payload locally. This would be predicted to greatly increase the agent's concentration within the tumor and significantly lower its systemic toxicity. In addition, by genetically modifying the MSC with viral vectors, the engrafted MSC will steadily release the therapeutic agent, allowing a single administration to result in long-lasting effects. Other studies have now provided evidence that MSC have the ability to not only selectively home to solid tumors [270, 271, 287, 299], but also to actively seek out metastases at sites far removed from the primary site of the tumor [271, 288, 290, 299, 300]. This ability has recently been proven to be of great therapeutic value in the treatment of lung metastases arising from both breast cancer and melanoma in a murine xenograft model [271, 299]. Given the difficulty and frequent lack of success using traditional approaches such as surgery, radiotherapy, and chemotherapeutic agents to treat tumors which are either highly invasive or prone to metastasis, this property of MSC will likely prove to be of great clinical value in the near future.

One form of cancer for which the use of MSC is receiving a great deal of attention is glioblastoma multiforme (GBM). GBM represents the most common form of malignant glioma. Despite decades of research and many advances in the treatment of this disease with conventional surgery, radiotherapy, and chemotherapy, there is no cure, and the current prognosis is abysmal, with a median survival of only 6-18 months. The failure of current therapies to cure this disease arises predominantly from the highly invasive nature of this cancer and the inability of these agents to effectively target tumor cells which have disseminated into the normal parenchyma of the brain, at sites distant from the main tumor mass. Given the ability of MSC to home to tumors and their ability to track to metastases throughout the body, gene-modified MSC are receiving a great deal of attention as a possible therapy for GBM. Studies have now shown that MSC migrate through the normal brain parenchyma towards gliomas and appear to possess the uncanny ability to track microscopic tumor deposits and individual tumor cells which have infiltrated the normal brain parenchyma [276, 282, 289, 290, 301-310]. While these migratory properties are certainly interesting, even more exciting are the dramatic therapeutic benefits these same studies have shown, with reduction in tumor size, and pronounced improvements in survival. It is important to note that, in most of these studies, MSC were used as the sole therapy, and definite benefits were observed. In the clinical setting, the current plan is to use gene-modified MSC as an adjunct after surgical resection. In this scenario, the vast majority of the tumor mass would be surgically removed, and the MSC would then be transplanted, in the hopes that they would then remove the residual malignant cells at the site of the tumor, and then hunt down and eliminate any invasive tumor cells that have migrated away from the site of the primary tumor. In this context, one would imagine that the therapeutic benefit of the MSC will likely be even more pronounced, since their anti-tumor effects could be focused only on the small number of residual tumor cells that evaded removal during surgery. The remarkable success seen in studies aimed at treating GBM, one of the most devastating forms of cancer, thus serve to highlight the tremendous potential MSC harbor as gene delivery vehicles for the treatment of many forms of cancer for which current therapeutic strategies are ineffective.

9. Conclusions

Numerous investigators around the globe have now provided compelling evidence that MSC from a variety of tissues possess a far broader differentiative capacity than anyone would have foreseen at the time Friedenstein originally described his bone marrow-derived stromal cells. Extrapolating the work thus far on using MSC to deliver FVIII to treat hemophilia A, and the rapidly growing number of studies showing the tremendous potential of MSC as anti-cancer gene delivery vehicles, and combining this with the relative ease with which MSC can be isolated, propagated in culture, and modified with a variety of viral-based vectors, and their intrinsic ability to seek out sites of injury/inflammation within the body, one can readily see why MSC are widely viewed as being ideally suited not only as cellular therapeutics, but as vehicles to deliver gene therapy vectors to numerous tissues in the body, thus promising to provide a permanent cure for a diverse range of diseases.

Author details

Christopher D. Porada and Graça Almeida-Porada

Wake Forest Institute for Regenerative Medicine, Winston-Salem, NC, USA

References

[1] Friedenstein, A.J., *Osteogenic stem cells in the bone marrow.* Bone and Mineral, 1991. 7: p. 243-72.

[2] Friedenstein, A.J., et al., *Stromal cells responsible for transferring the microenvironment of the hemopoietic tissues. Cloning in vitro and retransplantation in vivo.* Transplantation, 1974. 17(4): p. 331-40.

[3] Caplan, A.I., *Mesenchymal stem cells.* J Orthop Res, 1991. 9(5): p. 641-50.

[4] Galotto, M., et al., *Stromal damage as consequence of high-dose chemo/radiotherapy in bone marrow transplant recipients.* Exp Hematol, 1999. 27(9): p. 1460-6.

[5] Kassem, M., *Mesenchymal stem cells: biological characteristics and potential clinical applications.* Cloning Stem Cells, 2004. 6(4): p. 369-74.

[6] Luria, E.A., A.F. Panasyuk, and A.Y. Friedenstein, *Fibroblast colony formation from monolayer cultures of blood cells.* Transfusion, 1971. 11(6): p. 345-9.

[7] Pittenger, M.F., et al., *Multilineage potential of adult human mesenchymal stem cells.* Science, 1999. 284(5411): p. 143-7.

[8] Simmons, P.J. and B. Torok-Storb, *Identification of stromal cell precursors in human bone marrow by a novel monoclonal antibody, STRO-1.* Blood, 1991. 78(1): p. 55-62.

[9] Airey, J.A., et al., *Human mesenchymal stem cells form Purkinje fibers in fetal sheep heart.* Circulation, 2004. 109(11): p. 1401-7.

[10] Almeida-Porada, M.G., Porada, C., ElShabrawy, D., Simmons, P.J., Zanjani, E.D., *Human marrow stromal cells (MSC) represent a latent pool of stem cells capable of generating long-term hematopoietic cells..* Blood, 2001. 98((Part 1)): p. 713a.

[11] Chamberlain, J., et al., *Efficient generation of human hepatocytes by the intrahepatic delivery of clonal human mesenchymal stem cells in fetal sheep.* Hepatology, 2007. 46(6): p. 1935-45.

[12] Colletti, E., Zanjani, E. D., Porada, C. D., Almeida-Porada, M. G., *Tales from the Crypt: Mesenchymal Stem Cells for Replenishing the Intestinal Stem Cell Pool..* Blood 2008. 112:. p. Abstract 390.

[13] Colletti E.J., A.J.A., Zanjani E.D., Porada C.D., Almeida-Porada G., *Human Mesenchy-mal Stem Cells differentiate promptly into tissue-specific cell types without cell fusion, mito-chondrial or membrane vesicular transfer in fetal sheep.*. Blood, 2007. 110(11): p. 135a.

[14] Colletti, E.J., et al., *Generation of tissue-specific cells from MSC does not require fusion or donor-to-host mitochondrial/membrane transfer.* Stem Cell Res, 2009. 2(2): p. 125-38.

[15] Colletti, E.J., et al., *The time course of engraftment of human mesenchymal stem cells in fetal heart demonstrates that Purkinje fiber aggregates derive from a single cell and not multi-cell homing.* Exp Hematol, 2006. 34(7): p. 926-33.

[16] Bruder, S.P., et al., *Mesenchymal stem cell surface antigen SB-10 corresponds to activated leukocyte cell adhesion molecule and is involved in osteogenic differentiation.* J Bone Miner Res, 1998. 13(4): p. 655-63.

[17] Haynesworth, S.E., M.A. Baber, and A.I. Caplan, *Cell surface antigens on human mar-row-derived mesenchymal cells are detected by monoclonal antibodies.* Bone, 1992. 13(1): p. 69-80.

[18] Mitchell, J.B., et al., *Immunophenotype of human adipose-derived cells: temporal changes in stromal-associated and stem cell-associated markers.* Stem Cells, 2006. 24(2): p. 376-85.

[19] Almeida-Porada, G., et al., *Differentiative potential of human metanephric mesenchymal cells.* Exp Hematol, 2002. 30(12): p. 1454-62.

[20] Fan, C.G., et al., *Characterization and neural differentiation of fetal lung mesenchymal stem cells.* Cell Transplant, 2005. 14(5): p. 311-21.

[21] Gotherstrom, C., et al., *Difference in gene expression between human fetal liver and adult bone marrow mesenchymal stem cells.* Haematologica, 2005. 90(8): p. 1017-26.

[22] in 't Anker, P.S., et al., *Mesenchymal stem cells in human second-trimester bone marrow, liver, lung, and spleen exhibit a similar immunophenotype but a heterogeneous multilineage differentiation potential.* Haematologica, 2003. 88(8): p. 845-52.

[23] Lee, O.K., et al., *Isolation of multipotent mesenchymal stem cells from umbilical cord blood.* Blood, 2004. 103(5): p. 1669-75.

[24] Morizono, K., et al., *Multilineage cells from adipose tissue as gene delivery vehicles.* Hum Gene Ther, 2003. 14(1): p. 59-66.

[25] Zuk, P.A., et al., *Human adipose tissue is a source of multipotent stem cells.* Mol Biol Cell, 2002. 13(12): p. 4279-95.

[26] Zuk, P.A., et al., *Multilineage cells from human adipose tissue: implications for cell-based therapies.* Tissue Eng, 2001. 7(2): p. 211-28.

[27] Garol, N.J., Yamagami, T., Osborne C., Porada, C.D., Zanjani, E.D., Almeida-Porada, G., *Tissue-specific molecular signature may explain differentiative bias of human MSC from different tissues.*. Blood, 2007. 110(11): p. 570a.

[28] Mazhari, S., Desai, J., Chamberlain, J., Porada, C., Zanjani, E.D., Almeida-Porada, G., *Proteomic Analysis Reveals Intrinsic Differences between Phenotypically Identical Mesenchymal Stem Cells.* Blood, 2005. 106(11).

[29] Mazhari, S.M., Porada, C.D., Chamberlain, J., Zanjani, E.D., Almeida-Porada, G., *Characterization of membrane proteins of mesenchymal stem cells from human liver* Experimental Hematology, 2006. 34(9, Suppl. 1): p. 80.

[30] Lee, R.H., et al., *Characterization and expression analysis of mesenchymal stem cells from human bone marrow and adipose tissue.* Cell Physiol Biochem, 2004. 14(4-6): p. 311-24.

[31] Kern, S., et al., *Comparative analysis of mesenchymal stem cells from bone marrow, umbilical cord blood, or adipose tissue.* Stem Cells, 2006. 24(5): p. 1294-301.

[32] Chamberlain, J., Frias, A., Porada, C., Zanjani, E. D., Almeida-Porada, G., *Neural Generation in vivo differs with route of administration and source of mesenchymal stem cells.* Experimental Hematology, 2005. 33(7): p. 47a.

[33] Almeida-Porada, M.G., Chamberlain, J., Frias, A., Porada, C.D., Zanjani, E.D., *Tissue of Origin Influences In Vivo Differentiative Potential of Mesenchymal Stem Cells..* Blood 2003. 102(11): p. abstract #1304.

[34] Bernardo, M.E., et al., *Human bone marrow derived mesenchymal stem cells do not undergo transformation after long-term in vitro culture and do not exhibit telomere maintenance mechanisms.* Cancer Res, 2007. 67(19): p. 9142-9.

[35] Bochkov, N.P., et al., *Chromosome variability of human multipotent mesenchymal stromal cells.* Bull Exp Biol Med, 2007. 143(1): p. 122-6.

[36] Buyanovskaya, O.A., et al., *Spontaneous aneuploidy and clone formation in adipose tissue stem cells during different periods of culturing.* Bull Exp Biol Med, 2009. 148(1): p. 109-12.

[37] Rubio, D., et al., *Human mesenchymal stem cell transformation is associated with a mesenchymal-epithelial transition.* Exp Cell Res, 2008. 314(4): p. 691-8.

[38] Rubio, D., et al., *Spontaneous human adult stem cell transformation.* Cancer Res, 2005. 65(8): p. 3035-9.

[39] Altanerova, V., et al., *Genotoxic damage of human adipose-tissue derived mesenchymal stem cells triggers their terminal differentiation.* Neoplasma, 2009. 56(6): p. 542-7.

[40] Crop, M., et al., *Potential of mesenchymal stem cells as immune therapy in solid-organ transplantation.* Transpl Int, 2009. 22(4): p. 365-76.

[41] Caplan, A.I. and J.E. Dennis, *Mesenchymal stem cells as trophic mediators.* J Cell Biochem, 2006. 98(5): p. 1076-84.

[42] Chen, T.S., et al., *Mesenchymal stem cell secretes microparticles enriched in pre-microRNAs.* Nucleic Acids Res, 2010. 38(1): p. 215-24.

[43] Dai, W., S.L. Hale, and R.A. Kloner, *Role of a paracrine action of mesenchymal stem cells in the improvement of left ventricular function after coronary artery occlusion in rats.* Regen Med, 2007. 2(1): p. 63-8.

[44] Gnecchi, M., et al., *Paracrine action accounts for marked protection of ischemic heart by Akt-modified mesenchymal stem cells.* Nat Med, 2005. 11(4): p. 367-8.

[45] Haynesworth, S.E., M.A. Baber, and A.I. Caplan, *Cytokine expression by human marrow-derived mesenchymal progenitor cells in vitro: effects of dexamethasone and IL-1 alpha.* J Cell Physiol, 1996. 166(3): p. 585-92.

[46] Huang, N.F., et al., *Bone marrow-derived mesenchymal stem cells in fibrin augment angiogenesis in the chronically infarcted myocardium.* Regen Med, 2009. 4(4): p. 527-38.

[47] Kuo, T.K., et al., *Stem cell therapy for liver disease: parameters governing the success of using bone marrow mesenchymal stem cells.* Gastroenterology, 2008. 134(7): p. 2111-21, 2121 e1-3.

[48] Ladage, D., et al., *Mesenchymal stem cells induce endothelial activation via paracine mechanisms.* Endothelium, 2007. 14(2): p. 53-63.

[49] Lai, R.C., et al., *Exosome secreted by MSC reduces myocardial ischemia/reperfusion injury.* Stem Cell Res, 2010. 4(3): p. 214-22.

[50] Li, Z., et al., *Paracrine role for mesenchymal stem cells in acute myocardial infarction.* Biol Pharm Bull, 2009. 32(8): p. 1343-6.

[51] Mias, C., et al., *Mesenchymal stem cells promote matrix metalloproteinase secretion by cardiac fibroblasts and reduce cardiac ventricular fibrosis after myocardial infarction.* Stem Cells, 2009. 27(11): p. 2734-43.

[52] Ohnishi, S., et al., *Mesenchymal stem cells attenuate cardiac fibroblast proliferation and collagen synthesis through paracrine actions.* FEBS Lett, 2007. 581(21): p. 3961-6.

[53] Parekkadan, B., et al., *Immunomodulation of activated hepatic stellate cells by mesenchymal stem cells.* Biochem Biophys Res Commun, 2007. 363(2): p. 247-52.

[54] Parekkadan, B., et al., *Mesenchymal stem cell-derived molecules reverse fulminant hepatic failure.* PLoS One, 2007. 2(9): p. e941.

[55] Shabbir, A., et al., *Heart failure therapy mediated by the trophic activities of bone marrow mesenchymal stem cells: a noninvasive therapeutic regimen.* Am J Physiol Heart Circ Physiol, 2009. 296(6): p. H1888-97.

[56] Timmers, L., et al., *Reduction of myocardial infarct size by human mesenchymal stem cell conditioned medium.* Stem Cell Res, 2007. 1(2): p. 129-37.

[57] van Poll, D., et al., *Mesenchymal stem cell-derived molecules directly modulate hepatocellular death and regeneration in vitro and in vivo.* Hepatology, 2008. 47(5): p. 1634-43.

[58] Xiang, M.X., et al., *Protective paracrine effect of mesenchymal stem cells on cardiomyocytes.* J Zhejiang Univ Sci B, 2009. 10(8): p. 619-24.

[59]   Yu, X.Y., et al., *The effects of mesenchymal stem cells on c-kit up-regulation and cell-cycle re-entry of neonatal cardiomyocytes are mediated by activation of insulin-like growth factor 1 receptor.* Mol Cell Biochem, 2009. 332(1-2): p. 25-32.

[60]   Ozawa, K., et al., *Cell and gene therapy using mesenchymal stem cells (MSCs).* J Autoimmun, 2008. 30(3): p. 121-7.

[61]   Reiser, J., et al., *Potential of mesenchymal stem cells in gene therapy approaches for inherited and acquired diseases.* Expert Opin Biol Ther, 2005. 5(12): p. 1571-84.

[62]   Bosch, P., et al., *Efficient adenoviral-mediated gene delivery into porcine mesenchymal stem cells.* Mol Reprod Dev, 2006. 73(11): p. 1393-403.

[63]   Bosch, P. and S.L. Stice, *Adenoviral transduction of mesenchymal stem cells.* Methods Mol Biol, 2007. 407: p. 265-74.

[64]   Roelants, V., et al., *Comparison between adenoviral and retroviral vectors for the transduction of the thymidine kinase PET reporter gene in rat mesenchymal stem cells.* J Nucl Med, 2008. 49(11): p. 1836-44.

[65]   Gnecchi, M. and L.G. Melo, *Bone marrow-derived mesenchymal stem cells: isolation, expansion, characterization, viral transduction, and production of conditioned medium.* Methods Mol Biol, 2009. 482: p. 281-94.

[66]   Meyerrose, T.E., et al., *In vivo distribution of human adipose-derived mesenchymal stem cells in novel xenotransplantation models.* Stem Cells, 2007. 25(1): p. 220-7.

[67]   Piccoli, C., et al., *Transformation by retroviral vectors of bone marrow-derived mesenchymal cells induces mitochondria-dependent cAMP-sensitive reactive oxygen species production.* Stem Cells, 2008. 26(11): p. 2843-54.

[68]   Sales, V.L., et al., *Endothelial progenitor and mesenchymal stem cell-derived cells persist in tissue-engineered patch in vivo: application of green and red fluorescent protein-expressing retroviral vector.* Tissue Eng, 2007. 13(3): p. 525-35.

[69]   Fan, L., et al., *Transplantation with survivin-engineered mesenchymal stem cells results in better prognosis in a rat model of myocardial infarction.* Eur J Heart Fail, 2009. 11(11): p. 1023-30.

[70]   Meyerrose, T.E., et al., *Lentiviral-transduced human mesenchymal stem cells persistently express therapeutic levels of enzyme in a xenotransplantation model of human disease.* Stem Cells, 2008. 26(7): p. 1713-22.

[71]   Wang, F., et al., *Transcriptional profiling of human mesenchymal stem cells transduced with reporter genes for imaging.* Physiol Genomics, 2009. 37(1): p. 23-34.

[72]   Xiang, J., et al., *Mesenchymal stem cells as a gene therapy carrier for treatment of fibrosarcoma.* Cytotherapy, 2009. 11(5): p. 516-26.

[73] Zhang, X.Y., V.F. La Russa, and J. Reiser, *Transduction of bone-marrow-derived mesen-chymal stem cells by using lentivirus vectors pseudotyped with modified RD114 envelope glycoproteins.* J Virol, 2004. 78(3): p. 1219-29.

[74] Zhang, X.Y., et al., *Lentiviral vectors for sustained transgene expression in human bone marrow-derived stromal cells.* Mol Ther, 2002. 5(5 Pt 1): p. 555-65.

[75] Kumar, S., et al., *Osteogenic differentiation of recombinant adeno-associated virus 2-trans-duced murine mesenchymal stem cells and development of an immunocompetent mouse mod-el for ex vivo osteoporosis gene therapy.* Hum Gene Ther, 2004. 15(12): p. 1197-206.

[76] Stender, S., et al., *Adeno-associated viral vector transduction of human mesenchymal stem cells.* Eur Cell Mater, 2007. 13: p. 93-9; discussion 99.

[77] Deuse, T., et al., *Hepatocyte growth factor or vascular endothelial growth factor gene trans-fer maximizes mesenchymal stem cell-based myocardial salvage after acute myocardial infarc-tion.* Circulation, 2009. 120(11 Suppl): p. S247-54.

[78] Guo, Y.H., et al., *Hepatocyte growth factor and granulocyte colony-stimulating factor form a combined neovasculogenic therapy for ischemic cardiomyopathy.* Cytotherapy, 2008. 10(8): p. 857-67.

[79] Liu, X.H., et al., *Therapeutic potential of angiogenin modified mesenchymal stem cells: an-giogenin improves mesenchymal stem cells survival under hypoxia and enhances vasculogen-esis in myocardial infarction.* Microvasc Res, 2008. 76(1): p. 23-30.

[80] Tang, J., et al., *Mesenchymal stem cells over-expressing SDF-1 promote angiogenesis and improve heart function in experimental myocardial infarction in rats.* Eur J Cardiothorac Surg, 2009. 36(4): p. 644-50.

[81] Wang, Y., et al., *Adenovirus-mediated hypoxia-inducible factor 1alpha double-mutant pro-motes differentiation of bone marrow stem cells to cardiomyocytes.* J Physiol Sci, 2009. 59(6): p. 413-20.

[82] Wang, Y., et al., *Bone marrow derived stromal cells modified by adenovirus-mediated HIF-1alpha double mutant protect cardiac myocytes against CoCl2-induced apoptosis.* Toxi-col In Vitro, 2009. 23(6): p. 1069-75.

[83] Huang, J., et al., *Genetic Modification of Mesenchymal Stem Cells Overexpressing CCR1 Increases Cell Viability, Migration, Engraftment, and Capillary Density in the Injured Myo-cardium.* Circ Res, 2010. Apr 8. [Epub ahead of print].

[84] Zhu, K., et al., *Novel vascular endothelial growth factor gene delivery system-manipulated mesenchymal stem cells repair infarcted myocardium.* Exp Biol Med (Maywood), 2012. 237(6): p. 678-87.

[85] Cho, Y.H., et al., *Enhancement of MSC adhesion and therapeutic efficiency in ischemic heart using lentivirus delivery with periostin.* Biomaterials, 2012. 33(5): p. 1376-85.

[86] Holladay, C.A., et al., *Recovery of cardiac function mediated by MSC and interleukin-10 plasmid functionalised scaffold.* Biomaterials, 2012. 33(5): p. 1303-14.

[87]   Kurozumi, K., et al., *Mesenchymal stem cells that produce neurotrophic factors reduce is-chemic damage in the rat middle cerebral artery occlusion model.* Mol Ther, 2005. 11(1): p. 96-104.

[88]   Kurozumi, K., et al., *BDNF gene-modified mesenchymal stem cells promote functional re-covery and reduce infarct size in the rat middle cerebral artery occlusion model.* Mol Ther, 2004. 9(2): p. 189-97.

[89]   Lu, Z., et al., *Overexpression of CNTF in Mesenchymal Stem Cells reduces demyelination and induces clinical recovery in experimental autoimmune encephalomyelitis mice.* J Neuro-immunol, 2009. 206(1-2): p. 58-69.

[90]   Lu, Z.Q., et al., *[Bone marrow stromal cells transfected with ciliary neurotrophic factor gene ameliorates the symptoms and inflammation in C57BL/6 mice with experimental allergic en-cephalomyelitis].* Nan Fang Yi Ke Da Xue Xue Bao, 2009. 29(12): p. 2355-61.

[91]   Zhao, M.Z., et al., *Novel therapeutic strategy for stroke in rats by bone marrow stromal cells and ex vivo HGF gene transfer with HSV-1 vector.* J Cereb Blood Flow Metab, 2006. 26(9): p. 1176-88.

[92]   Nomura, T., et al., *I.V. infusion of brain-derived neurotrophic factor gene-modified human mesenchymal stem cells protects against injury in a cerebral ischemia model in adult rat.* Neuroscience, 2005. 136(1): p. 161-9.

[93]   Glavaski-Joksimovic, A., et al., *Glial cell line-derived neurotrophic factor-secreting geneti-cally modified human bone marrow-derived mesenchymal stem cells promote recovery in a rat model of Parkinson's disease.* J Neurosci Res, 2010. 88(12): p. 2669-81.

[94]   Olson, S.D., et al., *Examination of mesenchymal stem cell-mediated RNAi transfer to Hun-tington's disease affected neuronal cells for reduction of huntingtin.* Mol Cell Neurosci, 2012. 49(3): p. 271-81.

[95]   Aquino, J.B., et al., *Mesenchymal stem cells as therapeutic tools and gene carriers in liver fibrosis and hepatocellular carcinoma.* Gene Ther, 2010. March 12. [epub ahead of print].

[96]   Ishikawa, T., et al., *Fibroblast growth factor 2 facilitates the differentiation of transplanted bone marrow cells into hepatocytes.* Cell Tissue Res, 2006. 323(2): p. 221-31.

[97]   McGinley, L., et al., *Lentiviral vector mediated modification of mesenchymal stem cells & enhanced survival in an in vitro model of ischaemia.* Stem Cell Res Ther, 2011. 2(2): p. 12.

[98]   Li, Y.L., et al., *[Effect of mesenchymal stem cells transfected with human vegf-165 gene car-ried by adenovirus on revascularization for hind limb ischemic necrosis in rat model].* Zhongguo Shi Yan Xue Ye Xue Za Zhi, 2011. 18(6): p. 1568-73.

[99]   Hagiwara, M., et al., *Kallikrein-modified mesenchymal stem cell implantation provides en-hanced protection against acute ischemic kidney injury by inhibiting apoptosis and inflamma-tion.* Hum Gene Ther, 2008. 19(8): p. 807-19.

[100] Jiang, Y.B., et al., *[Effects of autologous mesenchymal stem cells transfected with heme oxy-genase-1 gene transplantation on ischemic Swine hearts]*. Zhonghua Xin Xue Guan Bing Za Zhi, 2009. 37(8): p. 692-5.

[101] Manning, E., et al., *Interleukin-10 delivery via mesenchymal stem cells: a novel gene therapy approach to prevent lung ischemia-reperfusion injury*. Hum Gene Ther, 2010. 21(6): p. 713-27.

[102] Cao, H., et al., *Mesenchymal stem cells derived from human umbilical cord ameliorate ische-mia/reperfusion-induced acute renal failure in rats*. Biotechnol Lett, 2010. 32(5): p. 725-32.

[103] Huang, Z.Y., et al., *Infusion of mesenchymal stem cells overexpressing GDNF ameliorates renal function in nephrotoxic serum nephritis*. Cell Biochem Funct, 2012. 30(2): p. 139-44.

[104] Zhen-Qiang, F., et al., *Localized expression of human BMP-7 by BM-MSCs enhances renal repair in an in vivo model of ischemia-reperfusion injury*. Genes Cells, 2012. 17(1): p. 53-64.

[105] Yuan, L., et al., *VEGF-modified human embryonic mesenchymal stem cell implantation en-hances protection against cisplatin-induced acute kidney injury*. Am J Physiol Renal Physi-ol, 2011. 300(1): p. F207-18.

[106] Van Damme, A., et al., *Bone marrow mesenchymal cells for haemophilia A gene therapy us-ing retroviral vectors with modified long-terminal repeats*. Haemophilia, 2003. 9(1): p. 94-103.

[107] Chuah, M.K., et al., *Long-term persistence of human bone marrow stromal cells transduced with factor VIII-retroviral vectors and transient production of therapeutic levels of human factor VIII in nonmyeloablated immunodeficient mice*. Hum Gene Ther, 2000. 11(5): p. 729-38.

[108] Chuah, M.K., et al., *Bone marrow stromal cells as targets for gene therapy of hemophilia A*. Hum Gene Ther, 1998. 9(3): p. 353-65.

[109] Doering, C.B., *Retroviral modification of mesenchymal stem cells for gene therapy of hemo-philia*. Methods Mol Biol, 2008. 433: p. 203-12.

[110] Porada, C.D., Sanada, C., Kuo, E., Colletti, E.J., Moot, R., Doering, C., Spencer, H.T., Almeida-Porada, G., *Phenotypic Correction of Hemophilia A by Postnatal Intraperitoneal Transplantation of FVIII-Expressing MSC*. Blood, 2010. 116(21): p. 249a.

[111] Porada, C.D., Sanada, C., Kuo, E., Colletti, E.J., Moot, R., Doering, C., Spencer, H.T., Almeida-Porada, G., *Phenotypic Correction of Hemophilia A by Postnatal Intraperitoneal Transplantation of FVIII-Expressing MSC.*. Molecular Therapy, 2011. 19(Suppl 1): p. 873a.

[112] Porada, C.D., et al., *Phenotypic correction of hemophilia A in sheep by postnatal intraperito-neal transplantation of FVIII-expressing MSC*. Exp Hematol, 2011. 39(12): p. 1124-1135.

[113] Mannucci, P.M. and E.G. Tuddenham, *The hemophilias--from royal genes to gene thera-py*. N Engl J Med, 2001. 344(23): p. 1773-9.

[114] Agaliotis, D., *Hemophilia, Overview*. 2006.

[115] High, K.A., *Gene transfer as an approach to treating hemophilia*. Semin Thromb Hemost, 2003. 29(1): p. 107-20.

[116] Kay, M.A. and K. High, *Gene therapy for the hemophilias*. Proc Natl Acad Sci U S A, 1999. 96(18): p. 9973-5.

[117] Kaveri, S.V., et al., *Factor VIII inhibitors: role of von Willebrand factor on the uptake of factor VIII by dendritic cells*. Haemophilia, 2007. 13 Suppl 5: p. 61-4.

[118] High, K.A., *Gene therapy for haemophilia: a long and winding road*. J Thromb Haemost, 2011. 9 Suppl 1: p. 2-11.

[119] Arruda, V.R., *Toward gene therapy for hemophilia A with novel adenoviral vectors: successes and limitations in canine models*. J Thromb Haemost, 2006. 4(6): p. 1215-7.

[120] Doering, C.B., et al., *Directed Engineering of a High-expression Chimeric Transgene as a Strategy for Gene Therapy of Hemophilia A*. Mol Ther, 2009.

[121] Doering, C.B., et al., *Hematopoietic stem cells encoding porcine factor VIII induce pro-coagulant activity in hemophilia A mice with pre-existing factor VIII immunity*. Mol Ther, 2007. 15(6): p. 1093-9.

[122] Ide, L.M., et al., *Hematopoietic stem-cell gene therapy of hemophilia A incorporating a porcine factor VIII transgene and nonmyeloablative conditioning regimens*. Blood, 2007. 110(8): p. 2855-63.

[123] Lipshutz, G.S., et al., *Short-term correction of factor VIII deficiency in a murine model of hemophilia A after delivery of adenovirus murine factor VIII in utero*. Proc Natl Acad Sci U S A, 1999. 96(23): p. 13324-9.

[124] Nichols, T.C., et al., *Protein replacement therapy and gene transfer in canine models of hemophilia A, hemophilia B, von willebrand disease, and factor VII deficiency*. ILAR J, 2009. 50(2): p. 144-67.

[125] Ponder, K.P., *Gene therapy for hemophilia*. Curr Opin Hematol, 2006. 13(5): p. 301-7.

[126] Shi, Q., et al., *Syngeneic transplantation of hematopoietic stem cells that are genetically modified to express factor VIII in platelets restores hemostasis to hemophilia A mice with pre-existing FVIII immunity*. Blood, 2008. 112(7): p. 2713-21.

[127] Lee, K.D., et al., *In vitro hepatic differentiation of human mesenchymal stem cells*. Hepatology, 2004. 40(6): p. 1275-84.

[128] Sato, Y., et al., *Human mesenchymal stem cells xenografted directly to rat liver are differentiated into human hepatocytes without fusion*. Blood, 2005. 106(2): p. 756-63.

[129] Schwartz, R.E., et al., *Multipotent adult progenitor cells from bone marrow differentiate into functional hepatocyte-like cells*. J Clin Invest, 2002. 109(10): p. 1291-302.

[130] Almeida-Porada, G., C. Porada, and E.D. Zanjani, *Adult stem cell plasticity and methods of detection.* Rev Clin Exp Hematol, 2001. 5(1): p. 26-41.

[131] Almeida-Porada, G., C. Porada, and E.D. Zanjani, *Plasticity of human stem cells in the fetal sheep model of human stem cell transplantation.* Int J Hematol, 2004. 79(1): p. 1-6.

[132] Almeida-Porada, G. and E.D. Zanjani, *A large animal noninjury model for study of human stem cell plasticity.* Blood Cells Mol Dis, 2004. 32(1): p. 77-81.

[133] Aurich, H., et al., *Hepatocyte differentiation of mesenchymal stem cells from human adipose tissue in vitro promotes hepatic integration in vivo.* Gut, 2008.

[134] Aurich, I., et al., *Functional integration of hepatocytes derived from human mesenchymal stem cells into mouse livers.* Gut, 2007. 56(3): p. 405-15.

[135] Banas, A., et al., *Rapid hepatic fate specification of adipose-derived stem cells and their therapeutic potential for liver failure.* J Gastroenterol Hepatol, 2008.

[136] Banas, A., et al., *IFATS collection: in vivo therapeutic potential of human adipose tissue mesenchymal stem cells after transplantation into mice with liver injury.* Stem Cells, 2008. 26(10): p. 2705-12.

[137] Banas, A., et al., *Adipose tissue-derived mesenchymal stem cells as a source of human hepatocytes.* Hepatology, 2007. 46(1): p. 219-28.

[138] di Bonzo, L.V., et al., *Human mesenchymal stem cells as a two-edged sword in hepatic regenerative medicine: engraftment and hepatocyte differentiation versus profibrogenic potential.* Gut, 2008. 57(2): p. 223-31.

[139] Enns, G.M. and M.T. Millan, *Cell-based therapies for metabolic liver disease.* Mol Genet Metab, 2008. 95(1-2): p. 3-10.

[140] Fang, B., et al., *Systemic infusion of FLK1(+) mesenchymal stem cells ameliorate carbon tetrachloride-induced liver fibrosis in mice.* Transplantation, 2004. 78(1): p. 83-8.

[141] Higashiyama, R., et al., *Bone marrow-derived cells express matrix metalloproteinases and contribute to regression of liver fibrosis in mice.* Hepatology, 2007. 45(1): p. 213-22.

[142] Luk, J.M., et al., *Hepatic potential of bone marrow stromal cells: development of in vitro coculture and intra-portal transplantation models.* J Immunol Methods, 2005. 305(1): p. 39-47.

[143] Lysy, P.A., et al., *Persistence of a chimerical phenotype after hepatocyte differentiation of human bone marrow mesenchymal stem cells.* Cell Prolif, 2008. 41(1): p. 36-58.

[144] Muraca, M., et al., *Liver repopulation with bone marrow derived cells improves the metabolic disorder in the Gunn rat.* Gut, 2007. 56(12): p. 1725-35.

[145] Oyagi, S., et al., *Therapeutic effect of transplanting HGF-treated bone marrow mesenchymal cells into CCl4-injured rats.* J Hepatol, 2006. 44(4): p. 742-8.

[146] Popp, F.C., et al., *Therapeutic potential of bone marrow stem cells for liver diseases.* Curr Stem Cell Res Ther, 2006. 1(3): p. 411-8.

[147] Sakaida, I., et al., *Transplantation of bone marrow cells reduces CCl4-induced liver fibrosis in mice.* Hepatology, 2004. 40(6): p. 1304-11.

[148] Sgodda, M., et al., *Hepatocyte differentiation of mesenchymal stem cells from rat peritoneal adipose tissue in vitro and in vivo.* Exp Cell Res, 2007. 313(13): p. 2875-86.

[149] Talens-Visconti, R., et al., *Hepatogenic differentiation of human mesenchymal stem cells from adipose tissue in comparison with bone marrow mesenchymal stem cells.* World J Gastroenterol, 2006. 12(36): p. 5834-45.

[150] Theise, N.D. and D.S. Krause, *Bone marrow to liver: the blood of Prometheus.* Semin Cell Dev Biol, 2002. 13(6): p. 411-7.

[151] Zhao, D.C., et al., *Bone marrow-derived mesenchymal stem cells protect against experimental liver fibrosis in rats.* World J Gastroenterol, 2005. 11(22): p. 3431-40.

[152] Zheng, J.F. and L.J. Liang, *Intra-portal transplantation of bone marrow stromal cells ameliorates liver fibrosis in mice.* Hepatobiliary Pancreat Dis Int, 2008. 7(3): p. 264-70.

[153] Almeida-Porada G. ElShabrawy D, P.C., Ascensao JL,, Zanjani ED., *Clonally Derived MSCs Populations are able to Differentiate into Blood Liver and Skin Cells..* Blood, 2001. 98: p. abstract.

[154] Almeida-Porada G., P.C.D., Brouard N., Simmons P.J., Ascensao J.L., Zanjani E.D., *Generation of hematopoietic and hepatic cells by human bone marrow stromal cells in vivo..* Blood, 2000. 96(1): p. 570a.

[155] Almeida-Porada, M., et al., *Intra-Hepatic Injection of Clonally Derived Mesenchymal Stem Cell (MSC) Populations Results in the Successful and Efficient Generation of Liver Cells.* Blood, 2003. 102(11): p. abstract #1229.

[156] Chamberlain, J., Frias, A., Porada, C., Zanjani, E. D., Almeida-Porada, G., *Clonally derived mesenchymal stem cell (MSC) populations generate liver cells by intra-hepatic injection without the need for a hematopoietic intermediate..* Exp. Hematol., 2004. 32(7): p. 48.

[157] Porada, C.D. and G. Almeida-Porada, *Mesenchymal stem cells as therapeutics and vehicles for gene and drug delivery.* Adv Drug Deliv Rev, 2010.

[158] Porada CD, Z.E., Almeida-Porada G, *Adult mesenchymal stem cells: a pluripotent population with multiple applications..* Current Stem Cell Research and Therapy, 2006. 1(1): p. 231-238.

[159] Aiuti, A. and M.G. Roncarolo, *Ten years of gene therapy for primary immune deficiencies.* Hematology Am Soc Hematol Educ Program, 2009: p. 682-9.

[160] Nienhuis, A.W., C.E. Dunbar, and B.P. Sorrentino, *Genotoxicity of retroviral integration in hematopoietic cells.* Mol Ther, 2006. 13(6): p. 1031-49.

[161] Persons, D.A., *Lentiviral vector gene therapy: effective and safe?* Mol Ther, 2010. 18(5): p. 861-2.

[162] Pipe, S.W., et al., *Progress in the molecular biology of inherited bleeding disorders.* Haemophilia, 2008. 14 Suppl 3: p. 130-7.

[163] Bartholomew, A., et al., *Baboon mesenchymal stem cells can be genetically modified to secrete human erythropoietin in vivo.* Hum Gene Ther, 2001. 12(12): p. 1527-41.

[164] Devine, S.M., et al., *Mesenchymal stem cells are capable of homing to the bone marrow of non-human primates following systemic infusion.* Exp Hematol, 2001. 29(2): p. 244-55.

[165] Le Blanc, K. and O. Ringden, *Immunobiology of human mesenchymal stem cells and future use in hematopoietic stem cell transplantation.* Biol Blood Marrow Transplant, 2005. 11(5): p. 321-34.

[166] Le Blanc, K., et al., *Mesenchymal stem cells inhibit and stimulate mixed lymphocyte cultures and mitogenic responses independently of the major histocompatibility complex.* Scand J Immunol, 2003. 57(1): p. 11-20.

[167] Puissant, B., et al., *Immunomodulatory effect of human adipose tissue-derived adult stem cells: comparison with bone marrow mesenchymal stem cells.* Br J Haematol, 2005. 129(1): p. 118-29.

[168] Batten, P., et al., *Human mesenchymal stem cells induce T cell anergy and downregulate T cell allo-responses via the TH2 pathway: relevance to tissue engineering human heart valves.* Tissue Eng, 2006. 12(8): p. 2263-73.

[169] Di Nicola, M., et al., *Human bone marrow stromal cells suppress T-lymphocyte proliferation induced by cellular or nonspecific mitogenic stimuli.* Blood, 2002. 99(10): p. 3838-43.

[170] Groh, M.E., et al., *Human mesenchymal stem cells require monocyte-mediated activation to suppress alloreactive T cells.* Exp Hematol, 2005. 33(8): p. 928-34.

[171] Krampera, M., et al., *Bone marrow mesenchymal stem cells inhibit the response of naive and memory antigen-specific T cells to their cognate peptide.* Blood, 2003. 101(9): p. 3722-9.

[172] Jones, S., et al., *The antiproliferative effect of mesenchymal stem cells is a fundamental property shared by all stromal cells.* J Immunol, 2007. 179(5): p. 2824-31.

[173] Klyushnenkova, E., et al., *T cell responses to allogeneic human mesenchymal stem cells: immunogenicity, tolerance, and suppression.* J Biomed Sci, 2005. 12(1): p. 47-57.

[174] Tse, W.T., et al., *Suppression of allogeneic T-cell proliferation by human marrow stromal cells: implications in transplantation.* Transplantation, 2003. 75(3): p. 389-97.

[175] Djouad, F., et al., *Mesenchymal stem cells inhibit the differentiation of dendritic cells through an interleukin-6-dependent mechanism.* Stem Cells, 2007. 25(8): p. 2025-32.

[176] Jiang, X.X., et al., *Human mesenchymal stem cells inhibit differentiation and function of monocyte-derived dendritic cells.* Blood, 2005. 105(10): p. 4120-6.

[177]   Nauta, A.J., et al., *Mesenchymal stem cells inhibit generation and function of both CD34+-derived and monocyte-derived dendritic cells.* J Immunol, 2006. 177(4): p. 2080-7.

[178]   Zhang, W., et al., *Effects of mesenchymal stem cells on differentiation, maturation, and function of human monocyte-derived dendritic cells.* Stem Cells Dev, 2004. 13(3): p. 263-71.

[179]   Corcione, A., et al., *Human mesenchymal stem cells modulate B-cell functions.* Blood, 2006. 107(1): p. 367-72.

[180]   Aggarwal, S. and M.F. Pittenger, *Human mesenchymal stem cells modulate allogeneic immune cell responses.* Blood, 2005. 105(4): p. 1815-22.

[181]   Maccario, R., et al., *Interaction of human mesenchymal stem cells with cells involved in alloantigen-specific immune response favors the differentiation of CD4+ T-cell subsets expressing a regulatory/suppressive phenotype.* Haematologica, 2005. 90(4): p. 516-25.

[182]   Prevosto, C., et al., *Generation of CD4+ or CD8+ regulatory T cells upon mesenchymal stem cell-lymphocyte interaction.* Haematologica, 2007. 92(7): p. 881-8.

[183]   Sato, K., et al., *Nitric oxide plays a critical role in suppression of T-cell proliferation by mesenchymal stem cells.* Blood, 2007. 109(1): p. 228-34.

[184]   Nasef, A., et al., *Identification of IL-10 and TGF-beta transcripts involved in the inhibition of T-lymphocyte proliferation during cell contact with human mesenchymal stem cells.* Gene Expr, 2007. 13(4-5): p. 217-26.

[185]   Nasef, A., et al., *Immunosuppressive effects of mesenchymal stem cells: involvement of HLA-G.* Transplantation, 2007. 84(2): p. 231-7.

[186]   Hainz, U., B. Jurgens, and A. Heitger, *The role of indoleamine 2,3-dioxygenase in transplantation.* Transpl Int, 2007. 20(2): p. 118-27.

[187]   Meisel, R., et al., *Human bone marrow stromal cells inhibit allogeneic T-cell responses by indoleamine 2,3-dioxygenase-mediated tryptophan degradation.* Blood, 2004. 103(12): p. 4619-21.

[188]   Jiang, W., et al., *Homing and differentiation of mesenchymal stem cells delivered intravenously to ischemic myocardium in vivo: a time-series study.* Pflugers Arch, 2006. 453(1): p. 43-52.

[189]   Jiang, W., et al., *Intravenous transplantation of mesenchymal stem cells improves cardiac performance after acute myocardial ischemia in female rats.* Transpl Int, 2006. 19(7): p. 570-80.

[190]   Jiang, W.H., et al., *Migration of intravenously grafted mesenchymal stem cells to injured heart in rats.* Sheng Li Xue Bao, 2005. 57(5): p. 566-72.

[191]   Kidd, S., et al., *Direct evidence of mesenchymal stem cell tropism for tumor and wounding microenvironments using in vivo bioluminescent imaging.* Stem Cells, 2009. 27(10): p. 2614-23.

[192] Spaeth, E.L., S. Kidd, and F.C. Marini, *Tracking inflammation-induced mobilization of mesenchymal stem cells.* Methods Mol Biol, 2012. 904: p. 173-90.

[193] Spaeth, E.L. and F.C. Marini, *Dissecting mesenchymal stem cell movement: migration assays for tracing and deducing cell migration.* Methods Mol Biol, 2011. 750: p. 241-59.

[194] Turecek, P.L., et al., *Assessment of bleeding for the evaluation of therapeutic preparations in small animal models of antibody-induced hemophilia and von Willebrand disease.* Thromb Haemost, 1997. 77(3): p. 591-9.

[195] Hough, C., et al., *Aberrant splicing and premature termination of transcription of the FVIII gene as a cause of severe canine hemophilia A: similarities with the intron 22 inversion mutation in human hemophilia.* Thromb Haemost, 2002. 87(4): p. 659-65.

[196] Lozier, J.N., et al., *The Chapel Hill hemophilia A dog colony exhibits a factor VIII gene inversion.* Proc Natl Acad Sci U S A, 2002. 99(20): p. 12991-6.

[197] Bi, L., et al., *Targeted disruption of the mouse factor VIII gene produces a model of haemophilia A.* Nat Genet, 1995. 10(1): p. 119-21.

[198] Gallo-Penn, A.M., et al., *In vivo evaluation of an adenoviral vector encoding canine factor VIII: high-level, sustained expression in hemophiliac mice.* Hum Gene Ther, 1999. 10(11): p. 1791-802.

[199] Garcia-Martin, C., et al., *Therapeutic levels of human factor VIII in mice implanted with encapsulated cells: potential for gene therapy of haemophilia A.* J Gene Med, 2002. 4(2): p. 215-23.

[200] Moayeri, M., T.S. Hawley, and R.G. Hawley, *Correction of murine hemophilia A by hematopoietic stem cell gene therapy.* Mol Ther, 2005. 12(6): p. 1034-42.

[201] Moayeri, M., et al., *Sustained phenotypic correction of hemophilia a mice following oncoretroviral-mediated expression of a bioengineered human factor VIII gene in long-term hematopoietic repopulating cells.* Mol Ther, 2004. 10(5): p. 892-902.

[202] Reddy, P.S., et al., *Sustained human factor VIII expression in hemophilia A mice following systemic delivery of a gutless adenoviral vector.* Mol Ther, 2002. 5(1): p. 63-73.

[203] Sarkar, R., et al., *Total correction of hemophilia A mice with canine FVIII using an AAV 8 serotype.* Blood, 2004. 103(4): p. 1253-60.

[204] Ide, L.M., et al., *Functional aspects of factor VIII expression after transplantation of genetically-modified hematopoietic stem cells for hemophilia A.* J Gene Med, 2010. 12(4): p. 333-44.

[205] Gallo-Penn, A.M., et al., *Systemic delivery of an adenoviral vector encoding canine factor VIII results in short-term phenotypic correction, inhibitor development, and biphasic liver toxicity in hemophilia A dogs.* Blood, 2001. 97(1): p. 107-13.

[206] Scallan, C.D., et al., *Sustained phenotypic correction of canine hemophilia A using an adeno-associated viral vector.* Blood, 2003. 102(6): p. 2031-7.

[207] Nathwani, A.C., et al., *Adenovirus-associated virus vector-mediated gene transfer in hemophilia B*. N Engl J Med, 2011. 365(25): p. 2357-65.

[208] Neuenschwander, S., et al., *Inherited defect of blood clotting factor VIII (haemophilia A) in sheep*. Thromb Haemost, 1992. 68(5): p. 618-20.

[209] Backfisch, W., et al., *Carrier detection of ovine hemophilia A using an RFLP marker, and mapping of the factor VIII gene on the ovine X-chromosome*. J Hered, 1994. 85(6): p. 474-8.

[210] Neuenschwander, S. and V. Pliska, *Factor VIII in blood plasma of haemophilic sheep: analysis of clotting time-plasma dilution curves*. Haemostasis, 1994. 24(1): p. 27-35.

[211] Bormann C., L.C., Menges S., Hanna C., Foxworth G., Shin T., Westhusin M., Pliska V., Stranzinger G., Joerg H., Glimp H., Millsap L., Porada C., Almeida-Porada G., Kraemer D., *Reestablishment of an Extinct Strain of Sheep From a Limited Supply of Frozen Semen*. Reproduction, Fertility and Development 2005. 18(2): p. 201-202.

[212] Almeida-Porada, G., Desai, J., Long, C., Westhusin, M., Pliska, V., Stranzinger, G., Joerg, H., Thain, D., Glimp, H., Kraemer, D., Porada, C.D., *Re-establishment and characterization of an extinct line of sheep with a spontaneous bleeding disorder that closely recapitulates human hemophilia A*. Blood, 2007. 110(11): p. 347a.

[213] Sanada, C., Wood, J.A., Liu, W., Lozier, J.N., Almeida-Porada, G., Porada, C.D., *A Frame Shift-Induced Stop Codon Causes Hemophilia A in Sheep.*. Blood, 2008. 112: p. Abstract #3378.

[214] Porada, C.D., et al., *Clinical and molecular characterization of a re-established line of sheep exhibiting hemophilia A*. J Thromb Haemost, 2010. 8(2): p. 276-85.

[215] Bormann, C., Long, C., Menges, S., Hanna, C., Foxworth, G., Westhusin, M., Pliska, V., Stranzinger, G., Glimp, H., Millsap, L., Porada, C., Almeida-Porada, G., Kraemer, D., *Reestablishment of an extinct strain of sheep utilizing assisted reproductive technologies.*. Reproduction Fertility and Development 2007. 21(1): p. 153.

[216] Bormann C., L.C., Menges S., Hanna C., Foxworth G., Shin T., Westhusin M., Pliska V., Stranzinger G., Joerg H., Glimp H., Millsap L., Porada C., Almeida-Porada G., Kraemer D., *Reestablishment of an Extinct Strain of Sheep From a Limited Supply of Frozen Semen*. Reproduction, Fertility and Development 2006. 18(1): p. 201.

[217] Vidal, F., et al., *A novel mutation (2409delT) in exon 14 of the factor VIII gene causes severe haemophilia A*. Hum Hered, 2000. 50(4): p. 266-7.

[218] High, K., *Gene transfer for hemophilia: can therapeutic efficacy in large animals be safely translated to patients?* J Thromb Haemost, 2005. 3(8): p. 1682-91.

[219] Maddox, J.F., C.R. Mackay, and M.R. Brandon, *Ontogeny of ovine lymphocytes. I. An immunohistological study on the development of T lymphocytes in the sheep embryo and fetal thymus*. Immunology, 1987. 62(1): p. 97-105.

[220] Maddox, J.F., C.R. Mackay, and M.R. Brandon, *Ontogeny of ovine lymphocytes. III. An immunohistological study on the development of T lymphocytes in sheep fetal lymph nodes.* Immunology, 1987. 62(1): p. 113-8.

[221] Maddox, J.F., C.R. Mackay, and M.R. Brandon, *Ontogeny of ovine lymphocytes. II. An immunohistological study on the development of T lymphocytes in the sheep fetal spleen.* Immunology, 1987. 62(1): p. 107-12.

[222] Osburn, B.I., *The ontogeny of the ruminant immune system and its significance in the understanding of maternal-fetal-neonatal relationships.* Adv Exp Med Biol, 1981. 137: p. 91-103.

[223] Sawyer, M., J. Moe, and B.I. Osburn, *Ontogeny of immunity and leukocytes in the ovine fetus and elevation of immunoglobulins related to congenital infection.* Am J Vet Res, 1978. 39(4): p. 643-8.

[224] Silverstein, A.M., C.J. Parshall, Jr., and J.W. Uhr, *Immunologic maturation in utero: kinetics of the primary antibody response in the fetal lamb.* Science, 1966. 154(757): p. 1675-7.

[225] Tuboly, S., R. Glavits, and M. Bucsek, *Stages in the development of the ovine immune system.* Zentralbl Veterinarmed B, 1984. 31(2): p. 81-95.

[226] McCarroll, D.R., et al., *Canine platelet von Willebrand factor: quantification and multimeric analysis.* Exp Hematol, 1988. 16(11): p. 929-37.

[227] Parker, M.T., M.A. Turrentine, and G.S. Johnson, *von Willebrand factor in lysates of washed canine platelets.* Am J Vet Res, 1991. 52(1): p. 119-25.

[228] Montgomery, R.R. and Q. Shi, *Platelet and endothelial expression of clotting factors for the treatment of hemophilia.* Thromb Res, 2012.

[229] Shi, Q. and R.R. Montgomery, *Platelets as delivery systems for disease treatments.* Adv Drug Deliv Rev, 2010. 62(12): p. 1196-203.

[230] Shi, Q., et al., *Factor VIII ectopically targeted to platelets is therapeutic in hemophilia A with high-titer inhibitory antibodies.* J Clin Invest, 2006. 116(7): p. 1974-82.

[231] Almeida-Porada, G., E.D. Zanjani, and C.D. Porada, *Bone marrow stem cells and liver regeneration.* Exp Hematol, 2010. 38(7): p. 574-80.

[232] Colletti, E., Zanjani, E. D., Porada, C. D., Almeida-Porada, M. G., *Tales from the Crypt: Mesenchymal Stem Cells for Replenishing the Intestinal Stem Cell Pool.* Blood 2008. 112: p. abstract #390.

[233] Colletti, E., Airey, J.A., Liu, W., Simmons, P.J., Zanjani, E.D., Porada, C.D., Almeida-Porada, G., *Generation of tissue-specific cells by MSC does not require fusion or donor to host mitochondrial/membrane transfer.* Stem Cell Research, 2009. In Press.

[234] Yamagami, T., Colletti E, Wiendl, H, Zanjani, E, Porada, C, and Almeida-Porada, G, *Expression of Molecules Involved in Fetal-Maternal Tolerance Allows Human Mesenchymal*

Stem Cells to Engraft at High Levels across Immunologic Barriers Blood, 2008. 112(11): p. 3480.

[235] Fischer, U.M., et al., *Pulmonary passage is a major obstacle for intravenous stem cell delivery: the pulmonary first-pass effect.* Stem Cells Dev, 2009. 18(5): p. 683-92.

[236] Schrepfer, S., et al., *Stem cell transplantation: the lung barrier.* Transplant Proc, 2007. 39(2): p. 573-6.

[237] Gangadharan, B., et al., *High-level expression of porcine factor VIII from genetically modified bone marrow-derived stem cells.* Blood, 2006. 107(10): p. 3859-64.

[238] Barrow, R.T., et al., *Reduction of the antigenicity of factor VIII toward complex inhibitory antibody plasmas using multiply-substituted hybrid human/porcine factor VIII molecules.* Blood, 2000. 95(2): p. 564-8.

[239] Garvey, M.B., *Porcine factor VIII in the treatment of high-titre inhibitor patients.* Haemophilia, 2002. 8 Suppl 1: p. 5-8; discussion 28-32.

[240] Hermans, C., et al., *Single-dose pharmacokinetics of porcine factor VIII (Hyate C).* Haemophilia, 2002. 8 Suppl 1: p. 33-8.

[241] Kulkarni, R., et al., *Therapeutic choices for patients with hemophilia and high-titer inhibitors.* Am J Hematol, 2001. 67(4): p. 240-6.

[242] Sun, J., et al., *Intraarticular factor IX protein or gene replacement protects against development of hemophilic synovitis in the absence of circulating factor IX.* Blood, 2008. 112(12): p. 4532-41.

[243] Auletta, J.J., R.J. Deans, and A.M. Bartholomew, *Emerging roles for multipotent, bone marrow-derived stromal cells in host defense.* Blood, 2012. 119(8): p. 1801-9.

[244] Nurmenniemi, S., et al., *Toll-like receptor 9 ligands enhance mesenchymal stem cell invasion and expression of matrix metalloprotease-13.* Exp Cell Res, 2010. 316(16): p. 2676-82.

[245] Qiu, Y., L.A. Marquez-Curtis, and A. Janowska-Wieczorek, *Mesenchymal stromal cells derived from umbilical cord blood migrate in response to complement C1q.* Cytotherapy, 2012. 14(3): p. 285-95.

[246] Raheja, L.F., et al., *Hypoxic regulation of mesenchymal stem cell migration: the role of RhoA and HIF-1alpha.* Cell Biol Int, 2011. 35(10): p. 981-9.

[247] Teo, G.S., et al., *Mesenchymal Stem Cells Transmigrate Between and Directly Through TNF-alpha-activated Endothelial Cells.* Stem Cells, 2012.

[248] Honma, T., et al., *Intravenous infusion of immortalized human mesenchymal stem cells protects against injury in a cerebral ischemia model in adult rat.* Exp Neurol, 2006. 199(1): p. 56-66.

[249] Kang, S.K., et al., *Improvement of neurological deficits by intracerebral transplantation of human adipose tissue-derived stromal cells after cerebral ischemia in rats.* Exp Neurol, 2003. 183(2): p. 355-66.

[250] Chen, J., et al., *Intravenous bone marrow stromal cell therapy reduces apoptosis and promotes endogenous cell proliferation after stroke in female rat.* J Neurosci Res, 2003. 73(6): p. 778-86.

[251] Chen, J., et al., *Therapeutic benefit of intracerebral transplantation of bone marrow stromal cells after cerebral ischemia in rats.* J Neurol Sci, 2001. 189(1-2): p. 49-57.

[252] Chen, J., et al., *Intravenous administration of human bone marrow stromal cells induces angiogenesis in the ischemic boundary zone after stroke in rats.* Circ Res, 2003. 92(6): p. 692-9.

[253] Iihoshi, S., et al., *A therapeutic window for intravenous administration of autologous bone marrow after cerebral ischemia in adult rats.* Brain Res, 2004. 1007(1-2): p. 1-9.

[254] Li, Y., et al., *Human marrow stromal cell therapy for stroke in rat: neurotrophins and functional recovery.* Neurology, 2002. 59(4): p. 514-23.

[255] Zheng, W., et al., *Therapeutic benefits of human mesenchymal stem cells derived from bone marrow after global cerebral ischemia.* Brain Res, 2010. 1310: p. 8-16.

[256] Augello, A., et al., *Cell therapy using allogeneic bone marrow mesenchymal stem cells prevents tissue damage in collagen-induced arthritis.* Arthritis Rheum, 2007. 56(4): p. 1175-86.

[257] Park, H.K., et al., *Adipose-derived stromal cells inhibit allergic airway inflammation in mice.* Stem Cells Dev, 2010. March 17. [epub ahead of print].

[258] Weiss, D.J., et al., *Stem cells and cell therapies in lung biology and lung diseases.* Proc Am Thorac Soc, 2008. 5(5): p. 637-67.

[259] Nemeth, K., et al., *Bone marrow stromal cells use TGF-beta to suppress allergic responses in a mouse model of ragweed-induced asthma.* Proc Natl Acad Sci U S A, 2010. 107(12): p. 5652-7.

[260] Cho, K.S., et al., *IFATS collection: Immunomodulatory effects of adipose tissue-derived stem cells in an allergic rhinitis mouse model.* Stem Cells, 2009. 27(1): p. 259-65.

[261] Iyer, S.S., C. Co, and M. Rojas, *Mesenchymal stem cells and inflammatory lung diseases.* Panminerva Med, 2009. 51(1): p. 5-16.

[262] Kidd, S., et al., *Origins of the tumor microenvironment: quantitative assessment of adipose-derived and bone marrow-derived stroma.* PLoS One, 2012. 7(2): p. e30563.

[263] Klopp, A.H., et al., *Concise review: Dissecting a discrepancy in the literature: do mesenchymal stem cells support or suppress tumor growth?* Stem Cells, 2011. 29(1): p. 11-9.

[264] Marini, F.C., *The complex love-hate relationship between mesenchymal stromal cells and tumors.* Cytotherapy, 2009. 11(4): p. 375-6.

[265] Martin, F.T., et al., *Potential role of mesenchymal stem cells (MSCs) in the breast tumour microenvironment: stimulation of epithelial to mesenchymal transition (EMT).* Breast Cancer Res Treat, 2010. 124(2): p. 317-26.

[266] Spaeth, E., et al., *Inflammation and tumor microenvironments: defining the migratory itinerary of mesenchymal stem cells.* Gene Ther, 2008. 15(10): p. 730-8.

[267] Subramanian, A., et al., *Human umbilical cord Wharton's jelly mesenchymal stem cells do not transform to tumor-associated fibroblasts in the presence of breast and ovarian cancer cells unlike bone marrow mesenchymal stem cells.* J Cell Biochem, 2012. 113(6): p. 1886-95.

[268] Wong, R.S., *Mesenchymal stem cells: angels or demons?* J Biomed Biotechnol, 2011. 2011: p. 459510.

[269] Bergfeld, S.A. and Y.A. DeClerck, *Bone marrow-derived mesenchymal stem cells and the tumor microenvironment.* Cancer Metastasis Rev, 2010. 29(2): p. 249-61.

[270] Studeny, M., et al., *Bone marrow-derived mesenchymal stem cells as vehicles for interferon-beta delivery into tumors.* Cancer Res, 2002. 62(13): p. 3603-8.

[271] Studeny, M., et al., *Mesenchymal stem cells: potential precursors for tumor stroma and targeted-delivery vehicles for anticancer agents.* J Natl Cancer Inst, 2004. 96(21): p. 1593-603.

[272] Hall, B., et al., *Mesenchymal stem cells in cancer: tumor-associated fibroblasts and cell-based delivery vehicles.* Int J Hematol, 2007. 86(1): p. 8-16.

[273] Hall, B., M. Andreeff, and F. Marini, *The participation of mesenchymal stem cells in tumor stroma formation and their application as targeted-gene delivery vehicles.* Handb Exp Pharmacol, 2007(180): p. 263-83.

[274] Shah, K., *Mesenchymal stem cells engineered for cancer therapy.* Adv Drug Deliv Rev, 2012. 64(8): p. 739-48.

[275] Aboody, K.S., J. Najbauer, and M.K. Danks, *Stem and progenitor cell-mediated tumor selective gene therapy.* Gene Ther, 2008. 15(10): p. 739-52.

[276] Nakamura, K., et al., *Antitumor effect of genetically engineered mesenchymal stem cells in a rat glioma model.* Gene Ther, 2004. 11(14): p. 1155-64.

[277] Chen, X.C., et al., *Prophylaxis against carcinogenesis in three kinds of unestablished tumor models via IL12-gene-engineered MSCs.* Carcinogenesis, 2006. 27(12): p. 2434-41.

[278] Eliopoulos, N., et al., *Neo-organoid of marrow mesenchymal stromal cells secreting interleukin-12 for breast cancer therapy.* Cancer Res, 2008. 68(12): p. 4810-8.

[279] Elzaouk, L., K. Moelling, and J. Pavlovic, *Anti-tumor activity of mesenchymal stem cells producing IL-12 in a mouse melanoma model.* Exp Dermatol, 2006. 15(11): p. 865-74.

[280] Gao, P., et al., *Therapeutic potential of human mesenchymal stem cells producing IL-12 in a mouse xenograft model of renal cell carcinoma.* Cancer Lett, 2010. 290(2): p. 157-66.

[281] Hong, X., et al., *Antitumor treatment using interleukin- 12-secreting marrow stromal cells in an invasive glioma model.* Neurosurgery, 2009. 64(6): p. 1139-46; discussion 1146-7.

[282] Ryu, C.H., et al., *Gene therapy of intracranial glioma using interleukin 12-secreting human umbilical cord blood-derived mesenchymal stem cells.* Hum Gene Ther, 2011. 22(6): p. 733-43.

[283] Seo, S.H., et al., *The effects of mesenchymal stem cells injected via different routes on modified IL-12-mediated antitumor activity.* Gene Ther, 2011. 18(5): p. 488-95.

[284] Zhao, W.H., et al., *[Human umbilical cord mesenchymal stem cells with adenovirus-mediated interleukin 12 gene transduction inhibits the growth of ovarian carcinoma cells both in vitro and in vivo].* Nan Fang Yi Ke Da Xue Xue Bao, 2011. 31(5): p. 903-7.

[285] Kidd, S., et al., *Mesenchymal stromal cells alone or expressing interferon-beta suppress pancreatic tumors in vivo, an effect countered by anti-inflammatory treatment.* Cytotherapy, 2010. 12(5): p. 615-25.

[286] Ling, X., et al., *Mesenchymal Stem Cells Overexpressing IFN-beta Inhibit Breast Cancer Growth and Metastases through Stat3 Signaling in a Syngeneic Tumor Model.* Cancer Microenviron, 2010. 3(1): p. 83-95.

[287] Grisendi, G., et al., *Adipose-Derived Mesenchymal Stem Cells as Stable Source of Tumor Necrosis Factor-Related Apoptosis-Inducing Ligand Delivery for Cancer Therapy.* Cancer Res, 2010. Apr 13. [Epub ahead of print].

[288] Loebinger, M.R., et al., *Mesenchymal stem cell delivery of TRAIL can eliminate metastatic cancer.* Cancer Res, 2009. 69(10): p. 4134-42.

[289] Menon, L.G., et al., *Human bone marrow-derived mesenchymal stromal cells expressing S-TRAIL as a cellular delivery vehicle for human glioma therapy.* Stem Cells, 2009. 27(9): p. 2320-30.

[290] Sasportas, L.S., et al., *Assessment of therapeutic efficacy and fate of engineered human mesenchymal stem cells for cancer therapy.* Proc Natl Acad Sci U S A, 2009. 106(12): p. 4822-7.

[291] Ciavarella, S., et al., *In vitro anti-myeloma activity of TRAIL-expressing adipose-derived mesenchymal stem cells.* Br J Haematol, 2012. 157(5): p. 586-98.

[292] Grisendi, G., et al., *Adipose-derived mesenchymal stem cells as stable source of tumor necrosis factor-related apoptosis-inducing ligand delivery for cancer therapy.* Cancer Res, 2010. 70(9): p. 3718-29.

[293] Kim, S.M., et al., *Irradiation enhances the tumor tropism and therapeutic potential of tumor necrosis factor-related apoptosis-inducing ligand-secreting human umbilical cord blood-derived mesenchymal stem cells in glioma therapy.* Stem Cells, 2010. 28(12): p. 2217-28.

[294] Luetzkendorf, J., et al., *Growth inhibition of colorectal carcinoma by lentiviral TRAIL-transgenic human mesenchymal stem cells requires their substantial intratumoral presence.* J Cell Mol Med, 2010. 14(9): p. 2292-304.

[295] Moniri, M.R., et al., *TRAIL-engineered pancreas-derived mesenchymal stem cells: characterization and cytotoxic effects on pancreatic cancer cells.* Cancer Gene Ther, 2012. 19(9): p. 652-8.

[296] Mueller, L.P., et al., *TRAIL-transduced multipotent mesenchymal stromal cells (TRAIL-MSC) overcome TRAIL resistance in selected CRC cell lines in vitro and in vivo.* Cancer Gene Ther, 2011. 18(4): p. 229-39.

[297] Sun, X.Y., et al., *MSC(TRAIL)-mediated HepG2 cell death in direct and indirect co-cultures.* Anticancer Res, 2011. 31(11): p. 3705-12.

[298] Yang, B., et al., *Dual-targeted antitumor effects against brainstem glioma by intravenous delivery of tumor necrosis factor-related, apoptosis-inducing, ligand-engineered human mesenchymal stem cells.* Neurosurgery, 2009. 65(3): p. 610-24; discussion 624.

[299] Chen, X., et al., *A tumor-selective biotherapy with prolonged impact on established metastases based on cytokine gene-engineered MSCs.* Mol Ther, 2008. 16(4): p. 749-56.

[300] Hamada, H., et al., *Mesenchymal stem cells (MSC) as therapeutic cytoreagents for gene therapy.* Cancer Sci, 2005. 96(3): p. 149-56.

[301] Nakamizo, A., et al., *Human bone marrow-derived mesenchymal stem cells in the treatment of gliomas.* Cancer Res, 2005. 65(8): p. 3307-18.

[302] Ahmed, A.U., et al., *A comparative study of neural and mesenchymal stem cell-based carriers for oncolytic adenovirus in a model of malignant glioma.* Mol Pharm, 2011. 8(5): p. 1559-72.

[303] Doucette, T., et al., *Mesenchymal stem cells display tumor-specific tropism in an RCAS/Ntv-a glioma model.* Neoplasia, 2011. 13(8): p. 716-25.

[304] Fei, S., et al., *The antitumor effect of mesenchymal stem cells transduced with a lentiviral vector expressing cytosine deaminase in a rat glioma model.* J Cancer Res Clin Oncol, 2012. 138(2): p. 347-57.

[305] Choi, S.A., et al., *Human adipose tissue-derived mesenchymal stem cells: characteristics and therapeutic potential as cellular vehicles for prodrug gene therapy against brainstem gliomas.* Eur J Cancer, 2012. 48(1): p. 129-37.

[306] Kim, S.M., et al., *CXC chemokine receptor 1 enhances the ability of human umbilical cord blood-derived mesenchymal stem cells to migrate toward gliomas.* Biochem Biophys Res Commun, 2012. 407(4): p. 741-6.

[307] Kosaka, H., et al., *Therapeutic effect of suicide gene-transferred mesenchymal stem cells in a rat model of glioma.* Cancer Gene Ther, 2012. 19(8): p. 572-8.

[308] Park, S.A., et al., *CXCR4-transfected human umbilical cord blood-derived mesenchymal stem cells exhibit enhanced migratory capacity toward gliomas.* Int J Oncol, 2011. 38(1): p. 97-103.

[309] Wang, Q., et al., *Mesenchymal stem cells over-expressing PEDF decreased the angiogenesis of gliomas*. Biosci Rep, 2012.

[310] Yin, J., et al., *hMSC-mediated concurrent delivery of endostatin and carboxylesterase to mouse xenografts suppresses glioma initiation and recurrence*. Mol Ther, 2011. 19(6): p. 1161-9.

Chapter 4

Lentiviral Gene Therapy Vectors: Challenges and Future Directions

Hélio A. Tomás, Ana F. Rodrigues,
Paula M. Alves and Ana S. Coroadinha

Additional information is available at the end of the chapter

1. Introduction

Lentiviral vectors (LV) are efficient vehicles for gene transfer in mammalian cells due to their capacity to stably express a gene of interest in non-dividing and dividing cells. Their use has exponentially grown in the last years both in research and in gene therapy protocols, reaching 12% of the viral vector based clinical trials in 2011 [1]. This chapter reviews and discusses the state of the art on the production of HIV-1- based lentiviral vectors.

1.1. Lentiviruses

Lentiviruses are human and animal pathogens that are known to have long incubation periods and persistent infection. The time between the initial infection and the appearance of the first symptoms can reach several months or years [2]. Nowadays lentiviruses are classified as one of the seven genus of *Retroviridae* family. *Lentivirus* genus is composed by nine virus species that include primate and non-primate retroviruses (Figure 1) [3].

All Retroviruses share similarities in structure, genomic organization and replicative properties. Retroviruses are spherical viruses of around 80-120 nm in diameter [4] and are characterized by a genome comprising two positive-sense single stranded RNA. Also, they have a unique replicative strategy where the viral RNA is reverse transcribed into double stranded DNA that is integrated in the cellular genome [5]. Together with the RNA strands, the enzymes necessary for replication and the structural proteins form the nucleocapsid. The later is inside a proteic capsid that is surrounded by a double lipidic membrane [6]. Connecting the lipidic membrane and the capsid there are the matrix proteins. The lipidic membrane has its origin in the host cells and presents at surface the envelope viral glycoproteins (Env) (Figure 2).

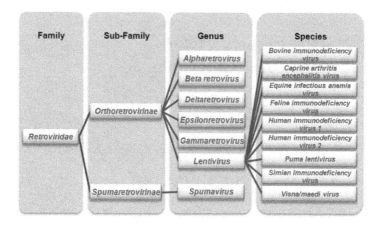

Figure 1. Lentiviruses taxonomy by the International Committee on Taxonomy of Viruses (ICTV).

Within the *Retroviridae* family, retroviruses can be classified as simple or complex. The complex retroviruses include the lentiviruses and spumaviruses presenting a more complex genome with additional regulation steps in their life cycle.

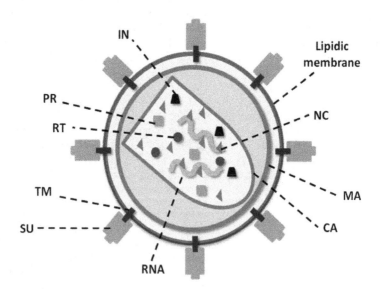

Figure 2. Schematic representation of a retrovirus particle. Abbreviations: NC – nucleopcapsid; MA – matrix; CA – capsid; SU – surface subunit of Env protein; TM – transmembrane subunit of Env protein; RT – reverse transcriptase; PR – protease; IN – integrase.

1.2. HIV-1 genome

HIV-1 genome has about 9-10 kb and is constituted by several non-coding sequences that control gene expression and protein synthesis, and genes that code for regulatory and accessory proteins in addition to the structural and enzymatic genes *gag*, *pol* and *env*, common to all retroviruses (Figure 3).

The *gag* gene codes for a polypeptide that is proteolytic cleaved by the viral protease (PR) originating three main structural proteins: matrix (MA), capsid (CA) and nucelocapsid (NC). The *pro* gene codes for a polypeptide that after cleavage by PR, during the virus maturation, originates PR, reverse transcriptase (RT) and integrase (IN). These enzymes play critical roles in the life cycle of retroviruses since their functions are the cleavage of viral polypeptides (also involved in virus maturation), the reverse transcription of viral RNA to double-stranded DNA (provirus) and the integration of the provirus into the cellular genome [7]. Finally the *env* gene encodes a polypeptide that is cleaved by cellular proteases in two proteins, the SU (surface) and TM (transmembrane) subunits. Together, these two proteins are the structural units of the Env protein that will interact with cellular receptors of the host cell allowing for virus entrance into the cell [10].

Flanking the retroviral provirus there are the 5' and 3' Long Terminal Repeats (LTRs) composed by the 3' untranslated region (U3), repeat elements (R) and 5' untranslated region (U5). The LTRs contain the enhancer/promoter sequence that allows for gene expression, the att repeats important for provirus integration and the polyadenylation signal (polyA).

The HIV-1 genome also has other six genes that code for two regulatory proteins (Tat and Rev), and four accessory proteins: Vif, Nef, Vpr, and Vpu. Tat protein interacts with cellular proteins and the mRNA TAR sequence acting by increasing the viral transcription hundreds of times. Rev interacts with Rev Responsive Element (RRE), a cis-acting sequence located in the middle of the *env* gene allowing the efficient nuclear export of unspliced or singly spliced messenger RNA. The functions of accessory proteins are related with pathogenesis of the virus and they are not crucial for the viral replication *in-vitro*.

The function of all HIV-1 proteins and their interactions with the host cells are not yet clearly understood but it is already reported that there are 2589 unique HIV-1–to–human protein interactions that are formed by 1448 human proteins [8,9].

Additionally to the coding sequences, the lentivirus genome also has several non-coding cis-acting sequences that play important roles in viral replication. The LTRs contains the Trans-activator Response element (TAR) for the interactions of the complex formed by the Tat protein and transcriptional factors. After the 5' LTR there are the primer binding site (PBS), where the reverse transcription starts, and the packaging signal (Ψ). Within the *pol* sequence there are also the central polypurine tract (cPPT) and the central termination sequence (CTS) contributing both for the efficient reverse transcription. Further there are the RRE in the middle of *env* gene and near the beginning of the 3'LTR the polypurine tract (PPT), a purine rich region where the synthesis of the plus strand DNA during the reverse transcription starts [10].

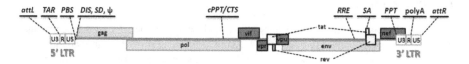

Figure 3. Schematic representation of HIV-1 provirus genome. Abbreviations: LTR - long terminal repeat; attL and attR - left and right attachment sites; U3 - 3' untranslated region; R - repeat element; U5 - 5' untranslated; TAR - transactivation response element; PBS - primer binding site; DIS - dimerization signal; SD - splice donor site; SA - splice acceptor site; ψ - packaging signal; cPPT - central polypurine tract; CTS - central termination sequence; RRE - Rev response element; PPT - 3' polypurine tract; polyA - polyadenylation signal.

1.3. HIV-1 life cycle

The HIV-1 Life cycle starts when the Env glycoproteins GP120 located at surface of the viral envelope bind the CD4 cellular receptor and co-receptor CCR5, CSCR4 or both. This binding induces conformational changes of Env glycoproteins that allows for the fusion of the viral envelope with the cell membrane and the consequent entry of the viral core into the cell. Once inside the cell the capsid starts to disintegrate and the RT enzyme begins the reverse transcription where a double-stranded proviral DNA is synthesized using one of the positive single-strand viral RNA molecules as template. When reverse transcription is completed the double-strand DNA now called provirus forms a complex with viral proteins (RT, IN, NC, Vpr and MA) and cellular proteins termed pre-integration complex (PIC) that is imported to the cell nucleus by an ATP-dependent manner. It is this energy-dependent mechanism that allows the transduction of non-dividing cells by lentiviruses, unlike γ-retrovirus.

In the nucleus the linear provirus is integrated into the cellular genome by the integrase. Now all the requisites to produce new viruses are filled and the proviral DNA is transcribed into mRNA by the cellular RNA polymerase II. Still inside the nucleus some transcripts suffer a splicing event. The mRNA transcripts are exported from the nucleus to cytoplasm to be transcribed and to start to form the viral particles; two full-length RNA transcripts will be packaged in the viral particles.

The assembly of the viral proteins and the viral RNA occurs near the cellular membrane, in specific regions called lipid-rafts that are rich in cholesterol and sphingolipds. The immature viral particles are released from cells by budding. After leaving the cells, the viral protease cleaves the Gag and Pol proteins precursors to finally generate a mature infectious virion (reviewed by [5,10]).

2. Lentiviral vector development

The development of lentiviral vectors (LVs) started in 1989 when an HIV-1 provirus with a*chloramphenicol acetyltransferase* (*cat*) reporter gene in place of the non-essential *nef* gene was constructed. The transfection of Jurkat cells with this modified provirus plasmid produced infectious replicative competent viruses, very similar with wild-type HIV-1, that could be used as a tool for study HIV infection [11]. Few months after, the same group presented the first replication-defective HIV-1 vector. In a trans-complementation assay for measuring the replicative potential of HIV-1 envelope glycoprotein mutants they used an identical HIV-1 provirus construction but with a deletion in the *env* gene. The Env glycoproteins were supplied by an independent expression plasmid. The co-transfection of these two plasmids allowed for the production of replication-defective viruses [12]. These vectors were structural identical to the wild-type virus, but lacked in their genome the *env* gene. They could only perform a single cycle of replication because their host cells, after infection, did not have the *env* gene to produce infectious virus. Although the principal aim of these studies was not the creation of viral vectors, they were the basis of lentiviral vector development, suggesting that lentiviruses could be adapted as a tool for genetic material transfer and permanent modification of animal cells.

Other preliminary studies were being conducted and several important discoveries or innovations had also contributed for the development of LVs. The introduction of the resistance marker gene *hypoxanthine–guanine phosphoribosyl-transferase* (*gpt*) under the expression control of SV40 promoter in the place of *env* gene deletion allowed the first quantification of infectious LVs produced [13]. Like it had been observed for other γ-retroviral vectors (γ-RVs) it was possible to produce infectious lentiviral particles with Env glycoproteins from other viruses (pseudotyping); for example the Moloney Murine Leukemia Virus amphotrophic envelope 4070A (A-MoMLV) [13], and Human T-cell Leukemia Virus Type I (HTLV-I) envelope [14] were successfully used suggesting that *env* gene was not necessary for virion particle formation. The localization and sequence of packaging signal was identified as the main responsible for the packaging of viral RNA [15] suggesting that modified RNAs with Ψ could also be packaged into virions. The discovery of the great stability conferred to LV pseudotyped with Vesicular Stomatitis Virus-G protein protein (VSV-G) allowed to concentrate the LV up to 10^9 by ultracentrifugation or ultrafiltration without significant loss of infectivity [16,17]. It was shown that LVs can transduce efficiently non-dividing cells, their principal advantage over the oncoretroviral vectors [16,18,19].

All these steps showed the potential of using modified lentiviruses as vectors, stimulating the iterative studies and the evolution of LVs in the next years. Their further development was based in safety principles (most of them already used in the development of oncoretroviral vectors) such as the splitting of the genome into several independent expression cassettes: the packaging cassette with the structural and enzymatic elements, the transfer cassettes with the gene of interest and the envelope expression cassette. In addition, the elimination of non-essential viral elements and the homology reduction among the expression cassettes also contributed to avoid the possibility of recombination, vector mobilization and the generation of replicative competent lentiviral vectors (RCLVs).

2.1. Four generations of packaging constructs

Four generations of LVs are currently considered; these differ from each other in terms of the number of genetic constructs used to drive the expression of the viral components, the number of wild-type genes retained as well as the number and type of heterologous *cis*-elements used to increase vector titers and promote vector safety.

The system of three expression cassettes developed in 1996 by Naldini *et al.* [16] is considered the first generation of LVs. In this system the packaging cassette has all structural proteins, with exception of Env glycoproteins, and all accessory and regulatory proteins. Later the 5′ LTR was substituted by a strong promoter (CMV or RSV) and the 3′ LTR by an SV40 or insulin poly(A) site to reduce the homology between the cassettes. To prevent the packaging of viral elements the Ψ and PBS were deleted. In the *env* expression cassette the gp120 from HIV-1 was replaced by other *env* genes as VSV-G or amphotrophic MLV envelope (Figure 4). Finally the transgene cassette was composed by the 5′ LTR, the ψ with a truncated *gag* gene, the RRE cis-acting region and the gene of interest under the control of a heterologous promoter (usually CMV) and the 3′LTR [16,20].This system allowed in an easy way to achieve good titers but its level of safety was not very high. RCL could be generated just with three recombination events by homologous recombination between the viral sequences in all cassettes or endogenous retroviral sequences in cells. In order to improve the safety and decrease the cytotoxicity of LVs, the three plasmid system was maintained, but all accessory genes not required for viral replication *in vitro* (vif, vpr, vpu, and nef) [21] were removed without negative effects on vector yield or infectivity. And in this way the second generation of LVs was developed (Figure 4) [22–25]. In the second generation, if by chance some RCL was generated, it would be unlikely to be pathogenic [26]. However the number of homologous events to generate RCL was the same as in the previous generation.

Reducing the lentiviral sequences by eliminating the *tat* and place the *rev* in an independent plasmid was the further step that originated the third generation of LV [27]. The *tar* sequence was replaced by a strong heterologous promoter. Therefore Tat protein was no longer necessary to increase the transgene transcription and *tat* gene was eliminated. This contributed for the reduction of lentiviral elements in the constructs. Rev was placed in an independent non-overlapping plasmid increasing the safety since now four events of homologous recombination were required for RCL formation [27]. With these new features, the vectors of third generation (Figure 4) presented a higher level of biosafety and, as the titers did not decreased, their use was widespread. Today they are the most commonly used LVs.

Although the formation of RCL was improbable, homologous recombination between the constructs was still possible since RRE sequence and part of packaging sequence in *gag* gene was in both transfer and structural packaging constructs. To solve these problems other solutions were developed originating the fourth generation of LV. The first approach used consisted in the replacement of the RRE sequences by heterologous sequences with similar functions that do not need the Rev protein. Some of these sequences were the Mason-Pfizer monkey virus constitutive transport element (CTE), the posttranscriptional control element (PCE) of the spleen necrosis virus and the human nuclear protein Sam68 [28–31]. The heterologous sequences increased the stability of the transcripts allowing their nuclear export. However the titers have decreased.

In 2000 a different approach based on codon optimization was implemented in lentiviral vector design [33]. This approach consists in perform silent mutations, changing the codon that codes for a certain aminoacid for other that codes for the same aminoacid, in principle, with a higher intracellular availability [32]. Applying this to the packaging and transfer constructs the homology between them was eliminated. These changes also allowed an independent expression of Rev since the sequences with suboptimal codon usage in HIV-1 genome, that conferred RNA instability and consequently lower expression, disappeared [32]. In the fourth generation (Figure 4) the homology between constructs were severely reduced but the titers had also been affected comparing with systems with the Rev/RRE [32]. Also, with the independence of Rev/RRE system, the level of biosafety decreased since the number of homologous recombination events for RCL formation was again three. Maybe due to these drawbacks the fourth generation has not been extensively used. However the codon optimization technology had been used to decrease the homology between sequences, improve the expression of viral components and viral titers [33].

Regarding the biosafety concerns about RNA mobilization and the possibility of generating RCLs, other improvements in packaging constructs were used and tested in transient LVs productions. These improvements relied on the concept of *split-genome* used for retroviral and lentiviral vector development but this time applied to the packaging construct. The *gag-pol* sequences were divided by two or three independent expression cassettes, disarming the functional *gag-pol* structure that is essential for vector mobilization [34]. In these systems additional recombination events between the several expression cassettes are necessary to generate RCLs which seems to contribute to a significant decrease of recombinant vectors formation with a functional *gag-pol* structure [35,36]. Although this increased LV safety the transduction efficiency and the LV production are challenged by the higher number of plasmids required [37].

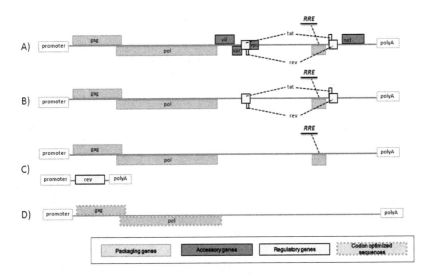

Figure 4. Schematic representation of the four generations of lentiviral packaging constructs: A) First generation packaging vector. B) Second generation packaging vector. C) Third generation packaging vector. D) Fourth generation packaging vector.

2.2. Transfer vector

The transfer vector is the expression cassette of the transgene that will be packaged into the viral vector and integrated in the cellular genome of the target cells. Besides the gene of interest and the commonly heterologous promoter for transgene expression, the transfer expression cassette must have: the sequences responsible for the expression of the full-length transcript and its packaging into the newly formed virions in the producer cells; the sequences that will interact with viral and cellular proteins to allow an efficient reverse transcription, transport into the cellular nucleus and proviral integration into target cells genome. Despite the simple design and the lack of sequences that code for viral proteins, the transfer vector also evolved over the time. This evolution was primarily focused on safety by reducing and replacing the viral sequences by heterologous elements and in optimizing both safety and efficiency by the addition of several cis-acting elements to the transfer cassette [10].

The transfer vectors usually used in the first and second generation of packaging constructs LVs were composed by the 5' LTR which include the TAR sequence, the PBS, the SD, the Ψ, the 5' part of gag gene, the RRE sequence, the SA, an heterologous promoter followed by the gene of interest, the PPT and polyA within the 3' LTR. The first hundreds of base pairs of gag are included after the packaging signal to increase the packaging efficiency (Figure 5). To avoid gag translation the initiation codon is usually mutated or cloned out of frame [16,20]. However, like it was previously found for γ-RVs, this transfer vector design with both wild-type LTRs can lead to integration genotoxicity and facilitates the mobilization of the transgene in the case of posterior infection of transduced cells [38]. To overcome these biosafety problems the LTRs of the transfer vector suffered additional changes. One of the first modifications was the replacement of the enhancer/promoter and Tar sequence of the 5' LTR by a strong heterologous promoter allowing the transcription of the full-length viral RNA in a Tat-independent manner [25]. In addition the wild-type enhancer/promoter sequences in the U3 region of the 3'LTR were deleted originating the self-inactivating (SIN) LVs [27,39,40], as it had already been done for γ-RVs [41].

The SIN design (Figure 5) generates in the target cells a proviral vector without enhancer/promoter sequences in both LTRs. In producer cells the packaged RNA transcript does have the heterologous promoter in the 5' end. Afterwards, in the target cells, during the reverse transcription, the U3 region of 3' LTR is copied and transferred to the 5'LTR. This transcriptional inactivation offered by the SIN design presents several safety advantages: prevents the formation of potentially packageable viral transcripts from the 5'LTR and consequently prevents vector mobilization by prior infection with a replicative retrovirus [39,42]; reduces the risk of insertional mutagenesis induced by the transcriptional interference of the LTRs in the neighboring sequences that can lead to the activation or up-regulation of oncogenes [43]; and lowers the risk of RCL formation by the reduction of the sequences with homology with wild-type virus.

The adoption of SIN design did not affected LV production as it happened with γ-RVs [27,39,40,44]. However both LVs and γ-RVs displayed high frequencies of read-through of the 3' polyadenylation signal which can lead to the transcription of cellular sequences as oncogenes. This inefficient termination of transcription could suggest that some of the enhancer/promoter sequences deleted can have a role in an efficient transcription termination [45]. In this context several improvements were done by the addition of heterologous elements to increase safety, expression and efficacy of LVs: heterologous polyadenylation signals in the 3′LTR could increase the efficiency of LVs and are particularly beneficial in the case of SIN LVs avoiding the read-through of cellular genes [40,46]; the chromatin insulators as the chicken hypersensitive site 4 (cHS4) sequence core from the β-globin locus control region (LCR) can reduce the interference from the neighboring regions in the vector and transgene expression [48]. Also these can improve the LV safety avoiding the full-length vector transcription or reducing long-distance effects of the integrated transgene promoter on neighboring cellular genes in the target cells. Additionally to the increased safety, insulators can help to maintain the gene expression over time preventing transcriptional silencing events in both producer and target cells [47–49]; incorporation of certain post-transcriptional regulatory elements (PRE) like the woodchuck hepatitis virus posttranscriptional regulatory element (WPRE) near the 3′ untranslated region can also decrease the read-through in SIN vectors increasing the transgene expression and viral titers, [50–53]. The firsts WPRE sequences used contained part of a sequence that codes for a protein (WHV X) that has been reported a few times as related with carcinoma formation, posing safety concerns. However a further improved WPRE was created without this potential harmful sequence [54]; The cPPT sequence contributes for efficient reverse transcription and the proviral nuclear import processes. Although this non-essential sequence was not used in the firsts transfer vectors, its re-insertion increased the gene transfer efficiency [55–57].

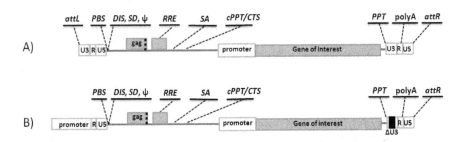

Figure 5. Schematic representation of a non-SIN transfer vector (A) and a SIN transfer vector (B).

3. Pseudotyping

LVs, as other retroviral vectors, can incorporate in their viral particles Env glycoproteins from other enveloped viruses, a feature denominated pseudotyping. This was firstly demonstrated for the HIV-1-based lentiviral vector using a Moloney Murine Leukemia Virus amphotropic envelope 4070A (A-MoMLV) [13] and an Human T-cell Leukemia Virus Type I (HTLV-I) envelope [14].

In general the pseudotyped LVs have the tropism of the virus where glycoproteins are derived from, but there are some exceptions such as the glycoprotein of the Mokola virus, where the pseudotyped vectors did not presented the specific neurotropism of the parental virus [58]. This ability of LVs to be pseudotyped showed to be advantageous since several glycoproteins could be tested to improve the transduction of cells with different receptors. As an example, HIV-based LVs pseudotyped with glycoprotein derived from the Rabies virus PV strain exhibited a great efficiency and neuronal tropism among the tested envelopes [59].

In addition to the tropism of LVs, the Env glycoproteins also affect vector structure and stability, the interactions with the target cells and the LV behavior during the infection. One example is LVs pseudotyped with rabies virus glycoprotein which allow for the retrograde axonal transport and access to the nervous system after peripheral infection [60]. Another example is the stability conferred to LVs by the VSV-G glycoproteins. The VSV-G glycoproteins are one of the most used Env proteins due to their wide tropism, with high titers achieved, great stability and resistance conferred to the LVs that allows for their concentration by ultracentrifugation. In addition they resist to freeze-thaw cycles, an important factor for storage of the vectors [16,18,19,61]. Despite these positive characteristics, the VSV-G protein is toxic for producer cells if expressed constitutively [17] and is inactivated by human serum complement [62], although this inactivation can be minimized using VSV-G conjugated with poly(ethylene glycol) [63].

Up to the present, several glycoproteins were used to pseudotype LVs (Table 1) each one presenting specific advantages and disadvantages that also depend on the LV application.

Although LVs pseudotyped with different Env glycoproteins present different tropisms, being some tropisms more selective than others, in general these are not specific for a particular cell type as happens with HIV-1 glycoproteins [80,81]. For instance, the Ebola Zaire (EboZ) glycoprotein seems to be superior to other glycoproteins in the transduction of apical airway epithelia [72]. However also has been shown to transduce liver, heart, and muscle tissues [82].

This lack of specificity is not ideal from a clinical point of view, especially for *in vivo* gene therapy applications since it can lead to the infection of cells that do not need to be transduced [83].

Several strategies have been used to increase the specificity of infection in order to retarget the LVs to a cell of interest. These strategies consisted in genetic engineering of virus envelops by deletion of some domains or fusing molecule-ligands (growth factors, hormones, peptides or single-chain antibodies) in several locations of the viral glycoproteins. The purpose is to choose cellular receptors specifically expressed on the target cells that will interact with the chimeric glycoproteins, restricting this way the vector tropism. A successful example was the removal of the heparan sulfate binding domain from the Sindbis virus envelope protein which effectively restricted the tropism of pseudotyped LVs to dendritic cells. This genetic modified Env protein interacts solely with the C-type lectin-like receptor almost exclusively on primary dendritic cells unlike its natural counterpart [84].

Species/Envelope	Vectors	Comments	References
Vesicular stomatitis virus (VSV-G)	HIV-1 HIV-2 FIV EIAV SIV BIV JDV CAEV	Very wide tropism. Presents resistance to high-speed centrifugation. Cytotoxic for producer cells if expressed constitutively. Susceptible to complement-mediated degradation which can be minimized by PEGylation	[16][64][65][66][66][66][67 - 67][67 – 69]
Feline endogenous retrovirus (RD114)	HIV-1 SIV	More efficient and less toxic than VSV-G in cells of the hematopoietic system	[70][71]
Ebola	HIV-1	Efficiently transduces airway epithelium	[72]
Lymphocytic choriomeningitis virus (LCMV)	SIV HIV-1 FIV	Low toxicity	[73]
Rabies	HIV-1	Rabies confers retrograde transport in neuronal axons	[24]
Mokola	EIAV	Mokola selectively transduces RPE upon subretinal injection	[24][74]
Ross River virus	HIV-1 FIV	Transduces hepatocytes, glia cells and neurons	[75][76]
Sindbis virus	HIV-1	pH-dependentendosomal entry. Useful for vector targeting	[77]
Influenza virus hemagglutinin	HIV-1	Transduces airway epithelium	[72]
Moloney murine leukemia virus 4070 envelope	HIV-1 SIV	Able to transduce most cells	[18][16]

Table 1. Lentiviral Vectors pseudotyped with various heterologous viral glycoproteins. Adapted from [78,79].

The envelope proteins engineered by fusion of natural ligands were in general able to bind to target cells. However the fusion domain of Env resulted generally in low vector titers since the ligand inhibits the fusogenic properties of the Env protein that allows for viral entry [85]. This approach seems to be more challenging but there are already improvements. One example is the LV pseudotyped with a chimeric glycoprotein of Sindbis virus covalently linked with mouse/human chimerical CD20-specific antibody which resulted in specific and stable transduction of CD20+ human lymphoid B cells. In this case the membrane fusion is triggered by the glycoprotein, in a pH-dependent manner, and it happens inside endocytic vesicles formed after antibody binding [86].

Other glycoproteins and ligands are being tested and used as well as alternative strategies to improve infection specificity of LVs [87–91].

4. Lentiviral vector production

The continuous research in LV development in the last twenty years and the acquired knowledge from the previous development of γ-RVs allowed the production of LVs with a significant biosafety level. However to apply LVs to clinical use they need to be easily and inexpensively produced and purified at a large-scale since, high concentrations of lentiviral particles are usually needed for efficient gene transfer in primary cells and the treatment of a single patient may require several liters of viral supernatant [92,93]

For large-scale and clinical-grade LV productions, a stable LV producer cell line seems to be the best approach for increased safety and well characterized production process. However, unlike γ-RVs, the development of LV packaging cell lines has been more challenging because of the cytotoxicity of some viral proteins like Tat, Nef, Vpr, Rev and PR [94]. Also VSV-G envelope, the typically envelope of choice for LV production because of its wide tropism and stability conferred to viral particles, is toxic for the producer cells. The VSV-G envelope can however be replaced by other non-toxic envelopes as the feline endogenous virus RD114 or the amphotropic MLV 4070A Env glycoproteins [33,95] and thus among the cytotoxic lentiviral proteins just the protease is still necessary for lentiviral vector production with the current packaging systems [93].

HIV protease mediates its toxicity *in vitro* and *in vivo* by cleaving procaspase 8, originating the casp8p41 fragment. This fragment induces mitochondrial depolarization leading to mitochondrial release of cytochrome C, activation of the downstream caspases 9 and 3 and nuclear fragmentation [96–98]. This cytotoxicity has hampered the development of stable cell lines.

The most used cells for LV production are the human embryonic kidney HEK-293 cell line and its genetic derivates the 293T (expressing the SV40 large-T antigen) and 293E (expressing the Epstein-Barr virus nuclear antigen-1, EBNA-1) cell lines. For clinical application human 293 and 293T cells have been the exclusive cell substrates [93]. Both cell lines can be used to produce LV in adherent systems and both can be easily adapted to serum-free suspension cultures. The 293T cells are most widely used because presents superior LV productivities compared with HEK-293 cells. However the HEK-293 cell line may have an advantage in terms of safety as it lacks the SV40 large T antigen encoding gene (expressed in 293T cells) which is oncogenic [93,99,100]. In some research works other human or monkey derived cells have been used (other 293 derived clones, HeLa, HT1080, TE671, COS-1, COS-7, CV-1), although most of them showed lower LV titers [101]. However, COS-1 cells have shown to be capable of producing 3-4 times improved vector quality (expressed in infectious vector titer per ng of CA protein, p24), comparing with 293T cells, under serum-containing conditions [102].

4.1. Transient lentiviral vector production

Commonly LVs are produced by co-transfecting cells with the several expression cassettes harboring the transgene and the viral elements using chemical agents (e.g. calcium phosphate or polyethylenimine) and after 24 to 72 hours the LV are harvested [93]. This production system is fast and can be easily adapted to produce LVs with new genes of interest or with other Env glycoproteins. It is a simple process to apply at small scales commonly used in research, unlike the laborious development of a packaging cell line. However transient production is not the ideal choice for large and clinical LV productions since it is difficult to scale-up and requires large amounts of Good Manufacturing Practices (GMP) grade plasmid expressions cassettes turning the production more expensive [93,103]. In addition, transient LV production brings some biosafety problems like recombination between expression cassettes that could originate or facilitate the RCL formation. The recombination can occur in the mixture of transfection, inside the producer cells or during reverse transcription in the target cells since, generally after transfection cells have several copies of the plasmids which can contribute for the co-packaging of RNA transcripts [33,104]. Also batch to batch variability is common in transient productions since a population of transfected cells that expresses viral elements from episomal cassettes is generated. This can further complicate biosafety validation steps.

Nevertheless transient LV production is commonly used and recently it was shown that high titers of HIV-based LVs for clinical applications can be obtained by transient calcium phosphate transfection at large-scale under GMP conditions (Table 2) [99].

Cell origin	Vector	Packaging generation	Envelope	Maximal titers (I.P./ml)	Observations	Reference
293 E	SIN HIV-1 based	3rd	VSV-G	1x10^6	PEI-mediated transfection	[107]
HEK293	HIV-1 based	3rd	VSV-G	1x10^8	PEI-mediated transfection	[101]
293T	HIV-1 based	3rd	VSV-G	2x10^9	Transfection with calcium phosphate	[99]
293T	HIV-1 based	3rd	VSV-G	1x10^8	Transfection by Flow Electroporation	[105]

Table 2. Transient LV productions. In this table they are presented several features of recent lentiviral productions in a transient manner.

There are several transfection agents that can be used to transfect mammalian cells as calcium phosphate, polyethylenimine (PEI) and cationic molecules (such as LipofectAMINE® and FuGENE®). For large scale only Ca-phosphate and PEI are used since the others are much more expensive. Both reagents are efficient but PEI is usually preferred since Ca-phosphate efficiency is highly sensitive to pH variations and can require serum or albumin to reduce Ca-phosphate cytotoxicity, unlike PEI [93]. However their use can raise some purity problems and can be cost-ineffective. Recently a method that does not use chemicals for transfection, flow electroporation, was used for transiently LV production at large-scale [105]. The electroporation systems are normally used to transfect small volumes but flow electroporation addresses this limitation by continuously passing the desired volume of a cell and DNA suspension between two electrodes [106]. The procedure can be effectively scaled up for large bioprocessing avoiding additional costs and purification problems (Table 2) [105].

4.2. Stable lentiviral vector production

To overcome the biosafey problems in LV transient productions, inducible packaging cells lines have been developed (Table 3). The development of these systems is more time-consuming since after insertion of each expression cassette the population of stably transfected cells is usually screened for the best producer clone, like for γ-RVs, to maximize the LV production. However, these packaging cell lines are derived from one clone, therefore all the cells have the same growth and LV production behavior being the LV productions reproducible. This allows the generation of GMP cell banks, increasing safety conditions.

Cell origin	Vector	Packaging generation	Envelope	Maximal titers (I.P./ml)	Observations	Reference
293T	HIV-1 based	2nd	VSV-G	1×10^7	Tet-off	[108]
293T	HIV-1 based	3rd	VSV-G	1.8×10^5	Ecdysone inducible system. Codon-optimized gag-pol	[109]
293T	SIV-based	3rd	VSV-G	1×10^5	Ponasterone inducible system. Codon-optimized gag-pol	[110]
293T	HIV-1 based	2nd	VSV-G	3×10^5	Tet-off. Codon-optimized gag-pol	[103]
293T	HIV-1 based	3rd	VSV-G	3.4×10^7	Tet-on	[111]
293T	EIAV based	3rd	VSV-G	7.4×10^5	Tet-on	[112]
293T	SIV-based	3rd	VSV-G	5×10^7	Introduction of vector by concatemeric array transfection. Tet-off	[113]
293T	HIV-1 based	2nd	Ampho GaLV RDpro	1.2×10^7 1.6×10^6 8.5×10^6	Continuous system. Codon-optimized gag-pol	[33]

Table 3. Lentiviral vector packaging cell lines. In this table they are presented several features of available packaging cell lines for LV production.

In conditional packaging cell lines the expression of cytotoxic proteins is under control of inducible promoters and the number ofcells and growth conditions can be controlled, starting the LV production at a defined moment by adding an inductor or removing the suppressor from the culture medium. Originally the titers were low but further improvements in the expression cassettes design and optimization of the induction parameters led to similar levels of transient productions. However, such systems can only produce LV for a few days because of the activity of the cytotoxic viral proteins. In addition these packaging cells have often shown to be instable due to leaky expression of the cytotoxic viral elements that are under control of the inducible promoters and the need to add an inductor to the medium in some systems can add further difficulties to the purification process [93].

In 2003 Ikeda and co-workers have reported the development of a non-inducible packaging cell line that continuously produces LV for three months in culture (Table 3). However, significant titers could only be obtained after MLV-based vector transduction. This procedure raises serious problems from the biosafety point of view, since it increases the chances of RCL by homologous recombination, posing further concerns of co-packaging [37]. Nevertheless it was shown that it is possible to establish a cell line that can continuously produce LV although, until now no additional reports for this system appeared.

5. Lentiviral vector applications

Lentiviral vectors have emerged as powerful and versatile vectors for *ex vivo* and *in vivo* gene transfer into dividing and non-dividing cells. The particular characteristics of LVs allied to their marked development during the last years have triggered the attention of different fields, consequently a vast range of applications for these vectors, from fundamental biological research to human gene therapy have appeared. One of the applications of LVs is in genome-wide functional studies. The combination of synthetic siRNAs (small interfering RNA) or shRNAs (short hairpin RNAs) that can suppress the expression of genes of interest in mammalian cells [114], with engineered LVs allowed the formation of libraries like the Netherlands Cancer Institute (NKI) libraries, the RNAi consortium (TRC) libraries, the Hannon–Elledge libraries, and the System Biosciences (SystemBio) libraries for high-throughput loss-of-function screens in a wide range of mammalian cells [115]. For example, the TRC shRNA library has nearly 300,000 shRNAs targeting for 60,000 human and mouse genes [116]. The ability of LVs to achieve stable high-efficiency gene silencing in a wide variety of cells including primary cells, that are difficult to transduce, or non-dividing cells such as neurons thus greatly expanded the possibility of the RNAi screens [117].

Other application for LVs is in animal transgenesis. Genetic-modified animals can be created by infection of fertilized or unfertilized oocytes, single-cell embryos, early blastocysts, embryonic stem cells or by transduction of cells that are used as donors of nucleus for somatic cell nuclear transfer (SCNT) [10]. These animals (transgenic mices, rats, pigs, cows, chicken, monkeys) are used to understand gene function or biological processes, for validation of drug targets, for production of human therapeutic proteins and as preclinical models for human diseases [118].

Lentiviral vectors are being increasingly used for the cell genetic modification leading to cell-engineering applications. Stable gene transduction can be used for *in vivo* imaging of vector infected cells. *In vivo* imaging studies of cells, including stem cells, have become increasingly important to understand cell distribution, differentiation, migration, function, and transgene expression in animal models. As an example, LVs expressing the firefly luciferase gene were used to monitor human embryonic stem cell (hESC) engraftment and proliferation in live mice after transplantation [119]. LVs can also be used to cellular reprogramming of somatic cells. More specifically, the promising induced pluripotent stem cells (iPS) can be generated from a somatic cell by transduction of four key transcription factors, Oct4, Sox2, Klf4, and c-Myc, using LVs[120,121]. iPS can be used to study stem cell biology, as a cellular platform for pharmacological and toxicological [122] and are considered a possible source of autologous stem cells for use in regenerative medicine. LVs also have been used in biotechnology to engineer cell lines for the production of proteins of interest [123].

The main goal of LV technology is their use in clinical gene therapy applications. Within this purpose considerable efforts have been made to increase the safety and efficacy of LVs. Proof-of-concept has been established in preclinical animal models since several research groups have reported that LVs could treat or cure a disease including β-thalassaemia[124], sickle cell anemia [125], hemophilia B [126] and ζ-chain-associated protein kinase of 70 kDa immunodeficiency [127]. Moreover, improvements in other genetic disorders like Parkinson's disease [128], cystic fibrosis [129] and spinal muscular atrophy [130] have been reported.

LVs have more recently moved beyond the preclinical stage into the clinical arena. The first human clinical trial using LVs was initiated in 2003. In this, a VSV-G-pseudotyped HIV-based vector was engineered to conditionally express an antisense RNA against envelope glycoprotein in the presence of regulatory proteins provided by wild-type virus. Five subjects with chronic HIV infection received a single dose of gene-modified autologous CD4+ T cells which resulted in an increase of CD4+ T cells (in four out of the five subjects) and decrease in the viral load (in all five participants) after 1 year. Further studies over 2 years have not detected any adverse clinical events [131].

Since this first gene therapy clinical trial until June 2012, about 54 gene therapy clinical trial using LVs are ongoing or have been approved. Among them there are 12 trials for the treatment of HIV infection, 22 for the treatment of monogenic diseases (X linked cerebral adrenoleukodystrophy, Sickle cell anemia, Wiskott-Aldrich Syndrome, Metachromatic Leukodystrophy, X-Linked Chronic Granulomatous Disease, Inherited Skin Disease Netherton Syndrome, mucopolysaccharidosis type VII, β-thalassemia, Fanconi Anemia Complementation Group A, X-Linked Severe Combined Deficiency, Adenosine Deaminase Deficient Severe Combined Immunodeficiency, Hemophilia A), 15 against various cancers, 2 for Parkinson's disease, 3 for ocular diseases and 1 for patients with Stargardt Macular Degeneration [1].

6. Conclusions and outlook

The major concerns associated with the use of all retroviral vectors are the formation of replication competent retroviral vectors (RCR), the mutational integration of the provirus into the host cellular genome and mobilization of structural viral genes to target cells. In addition, the majority of developed LVs are HIV-derived raising further safety concerns since this is a well known human pathogen. Significant efforts have been made to develop LVs with improved biosafety and increased transduction efficiency. Some of those biosafety features include the splitting of viral elements by several expression cassettes, the use of self-inactivating vectors (SIN), decreasing to a minimum the number of viral elements and reducing homology between them.

Lentiviral vectors have already won its place as valuable and flexible tool for gene delivery, being used in several applications but further research is still ongoing towards the development of a lentiviral vector providing higher titers, higher robustness, lower toxicity and higher biosafety.

Lentiviral vector gene therapy is becoming a real alternative vector for therapy with dozens of clinical trials either been already performed or ongoing. These, together with the future incoming clinical trials, will enable to assess overall the pros and cons of the newcomer lentiviral vectors and will provide insights to further vector innovations that will be important to increase their productivity, quality and safety.

Acknowledgments

The authors acknowledge the financial support received from the Fundaçãopara a Ciência e a Tecnologia-Portugal (FCT) (PTDC/EBB-BIO/100491/2008 and PTDC/EBB-BIO/118621/2010). Hélio Antunes Tomás and Ana F. Rodrigues acknowledge FCT for their PhD grants (SFRH/BD/79022/2011 and SFRH/BD/48393/2008).

Author details

Hélio A. Tomás[1,2], Ana F. Rodrigues[1,2], Paula M. Alves[1,2] and Ana S. Coroadinha[1,2]

1 Instituto de Tecnologia Química e Biológica, Universidade Nova de Lisboa, Oeiras, Portugal

2 Instituto de Biologia Experimental Tecnológica, Oeiras, Portugal

References

[1] The Journal of Gene Medicine: Gene Therapy Clinical Trials Worldwide www.wiley.com/legacy/wileychi/genmed/clinical/ (accessed 1 August 2012)

[2] Campbell RS, Robinson WF. The comparative pathology of the lentiviruses. Journalof comparative pathology. 1998; 119(4):333–95.

[3] International Committee on Taxonomy of Viruses(ICTV) http://ictvonline.org/virusTaxonomy.asp?version=2011(accessed 1 August 2012)

[4] Vogt VM, Simon MN. Mass determination of rous sarcoma virus virions by scanning transmission electron microscopy. Journal of virology. 1999;73(8):7050–5. jvi.asm.org/content/73/8/7050.full.pdf+html (accessed 1 August 2012)

[5] Coffin JM, Hughes SH, Varmus H. 1997. Retroviruses: Cold Spring Harbor. www.ncbi.nlm.nih.gov/books/NBK19376/(accessed 1 August 2012)

[6] Adamson CS, Jones IM. The molecular basis of HIV capsid assembly--five years of progress. Reviews in medical virology. ;14(2):107–21. onlinelibrary.wiley.com/doi/10.1002/rmv.418/citedby (accessed 1 August 2012)

[7] Katz RA, Skalka AM. The retroviral enzymes. Annual review of biochemistry. 1994;63:133–73.   www.annualreviews.org/doi/abs/10.1146/annurev.bi.63.070194.001025 (accessed 1 August 2012)

[8] Ptak RG, Fu W, Sanders-Beer BE, Dickerson JE, Pinney JW, Robertson DL, et al. Cataloguing the HIV type 1 human protein interaction network. AIDS research and human retroviruses. 2008;24(12):1497–502. online.liebertpub.com/doi/abs/10.1089/aid.2008.0113(accessed 1 August 2012)

[9] Fu W, Sanders-Beer BE, Katz KS, Maglott DR, Pruitt KD, Ptak RG. Human immunodeficiency virus type 1, human protein interaction database at NCBI. Nucleic acids research. 2009;37 (Database issue) :D417–22. nar.oxfordjournals.org/content/37/suppl_1/D417 (accessed 1 August 2012)

[10] Pluta K, Kacprzak MM. Use of HIV as a gene transfer vector. Acta biochimica Polonica. 2009;56(4):531–95. www.actabp.pl/pdf/4_2009/531.pdf (accessed 1August 2012)

[11] Terwilliger EF, Godin B, Sodroski JG, Haseltine W a. Construction and use of a replication-competent human immunodeficiency virus (HIV-1) that expresses the chloramphenicol acetyltransferase enzyme. Proceedings of the National Academy of Sciences of the United States of America. 1989 May;86(10):3857–61. http://www.pnas.org/content/86/10/3857.full.pdf+html (accessed 1 August 2012)

[12] Helseth E, Kowalski M, Gabuzda D, Olshevsky UDY, Haseltine W, Sodroskil J. Rapid complementation assays measuring replicative potential of human immunodeficiency virus type 1 envelope glycoprotein mutants. Rapid Complementation Assays Measuring Replicative Potential of Human Immunodeficiency Virus Type 1 Enve-

lope Glycoprotein M. Journal of Virology. 1990;64(5):2416–20. jvi.asm.org/content/64/5/2416.full.pdf+html (accessed 1 August 2012)

[13] Page K a, Landau NR, Littman DR. Construction and use of a human immunodeficiency virus vector for analysis of virus infectivity. Journal of virology. 1990;64(11): 5270–6. jvi.asm.org/content/64/11/5270.full.pdf+html (accessed 1 August 2012)

[14] Landau NR, Page K a, Littman DR. Pseudotyping with human T-cell leukemia virus type I broadens the human immunodeficiency virus host range. Journal of virology. 1991;65(1):162–9. jvi.asm.org/content/65/1/162 (accessed 1 August 2012)

[15] Clever J, Sassetti C, Parslow TG. RNA secondary structure and binding sites for gag gene products in the 5 ′ packaging signal of human immunodeficiency virus type 1. Journal of Virology. 1995;69(4):2101–9. jvi.asm.org/content/69/4/2101.full.pdf (accessed 1 August 2012)

[16] Naldini L, Blömer U, Gallay P, Ory D, Mulligan R, Gage FH, et al. In vivo gene delivery and stable transduction of nondividing cells by a lentiviral vector. Science (New York, N.Y.). 1996;272(5259):263–7. www.sciencemag.org/content/272/5259/263.long (accessed 1 August 2012)

[17] Burns JC, Friedmann T, Driever W, Burrascano M, Yee JK. Vesicular stomatitis virus G glycoprotein pseudotyped retroviral vectors: concentration to very high titer and efficient gene transfer into mammalian and nonmammalian cells. Proceedings of the National Academy of Sciences of the United States of America. 1993;90(17):8033–7. www.pnas.org/content/90/17/8033.full.pdf (accessed 1 August 2012)

[18] Reiser J, Harmison G, Kluepfel-Stahl S, Brady RO, Karlsson S, Schubert M. Transduction of nondividing cells using pseudotyped defective high-titer HIV type 1 particles. Proceedings of the National Academy of Sciences of the United States of America. 1996;93(26):15266–71. www.pnas.org/content/93/26/15266.long (accessed 1 August 2012)

[19] Akkina RK, Walton RM, Chen ML, Li QX, Planelles V, Chen IS. High-efficiency gene transfer into CD34+ cells with a human immunodeficiency virus type 1-based retroviral vector pseudotyped with vesicular stomatitis virus envelope glycoprotein G. Journal of virology. 1996;70(4):2581–5. jvi.asm.org/content/70/4/2581.long (accessed 1 August 2012)

[20] Naldini L, Blömer U, Gage FH, Trono D, Verma IM. Efficient transfer, integration, and sustained long-term expression of the transgene in adult rat brains injected with a lentiviral vector. Proceedings of the National Academy of Sciences of the United States of America. 1996;93(21):11382–8. www.pnas.org/content/93/21/11382.full.pdf (accessed 1 August 2012)

[21] Gibbs JS, Regier DA, Desrosiers RC. Construction and in vitro properties of HIV-1 mutants with deletions in "nonessential" genes. AIDS research and human retroviruses. 1994;10(4):343–50.http://www.ncbi.nlm.nih.gov/pubmed/8068414(accessed 1 August 2012)

[22] Zufferey R, Nagy D, Mandel RJ, Naldini L, Trono D. Multiply attenuated lentiviral vector achieves efficient gene delivery in vivo. Nature biotechnology. 1997;15(9):871–5. www.nature.com/nbt/journal/v15/n9/full/nbt0997-871.html (accessed 1 August 2012)

[23] Kafri T, Blömer U, Peterson DA, Gage FH, Verma IM. Sustained expression of genes delivered directly into liver and muscle by lentiviral vectors. Nature genetics. 1997;17(3):314–7. www.nature.com/ng/journal/v17/n3/abs/ng1197-314.html (accessed 1 August 2012)

[24] Mochizuki H, Schwartz JP, Tanaka K, Brady RO, Reiser J. High-titer human immune deficiency virus type 1-based vector systems for gene delivery into nondividing cells. Journal of virology. 1998;72(11):8873–83. jvi.asm.org/content/72/11/8873.long (accessed 1 August 2012)

[25] Kim VN, Mitrophanous K, Kingsman SM, Kingsman a J. Minimal requirement for a lentivirus vector based on human immunodeficiency virus type 1. Journal of virology. 1998 Jan;72(1):811–6. jvi.asm.org/content/72/1/811(accessed 1 August 2012)

[26] Naldini L, Verma IM. Lentiviral vectors. Advances in virus research. 2000;55:599–609. http://www.ncbi.nlm.nih.gov/pubmed/11050959(accessed 1 August 2012)

[27] Dull T, Zufferey R, Kelly M, Mandel RJ, Nguyen M, Trono D, et al. A third-generation lentivirus vector with a conditional packaging system. Journal of virology. 1998;72(11):8463–71. jvi.asm.org/content/72/11/8463.long (accessed 1 August 2012)

[28] Bray M, Prasad S, Dubay JW, Hunter E, Jeang KT, Rekosh D, et al. A small element from the Mason-Pfizer monkey virus genome makes human immunodeficiency virus type 1 expression and replication Rev-independent. Proceedings of the National Academy of Sciences of the United States of America. 1994;91(4):1256–60. www.pnas.org/content/91/4/1256.full.pdf+html?sid=f828b8ae-496c-476c-bace-e85aeee47e57(accessed 1 August 2012)

[29] Reddy TR, Xu W, Mau JK, Goodwin CD, Suhasini M, Tang H, et al. Inhibition of HIV replication by dominant negative mutants of Sam68, a functional homolog of HIV-1 Rev. Nature medicine. 1999;5(6):635–42. www.nature.com/nm/journal/v5/n7/full/nm0799_849c.html (accessed 1 August 2012)

[30] Roberts TM, Boris-Lawrie K. The 5′ RNA terminus of spleen necrosis virus stimulates translation of nonviral mRNA. Journal of virology. 2000;74(17):8111–8. jvi.asm.org/content/74/17/8111.long (accessed 1 August 2012)

[31] Pandya S, Boris-Lawrie K, Leung NJ, Akkina R, Planelles V. Development of an Rev-independent, minimal simian immunodeficiency virus-derived vector system. Human gene therapy. 2001 May 1;12(7):847–57. online.liebertpub.com/doi/pdfplus/10.1089/104303401750148847 (accessed 1 August 2012)

[32] Kotsopoulou E, Kim VN, Kingsman AJ, Kingsman SM, Mitrophanous KA. A Rev-independent human immunodeficiency virus type 1 (HIV-1)-based vector that exploits

a codon-optimized HIV-1 gag-pol gene. Journal of virology. 2000;74(10):4839–52. jvi.asm.org/content/74/10/4839.long (accessed 1 August 2012)

[33] Ikeda Y, Takeuchi Y, Martin F, Cosset F-L, Mitrophanous K, Collins M. Continuous high-titer HIV-1 vector production. 2003. www.nature.com/nbt/journal/v21/n5/full/nbt815.html (accessed 1 August 2012)

[34] Kappes JC, Wu X. Safety considerations in vector development. Somatic cell and molecular genetics. 2001;26(1-6):147–58. www.springerlink.com/content/w93t23118464r17k/?MUD=MP (accessed 1 August 2012)

[35] Wu X, Wakefield JK, Liu H, Xiao H, Kralovics R, Prchal JT, et al. Development of a novel trans-lentiviral vector that affords predictable safety. Molecular therapy: the journal of the American Society of Gene Therapy. 2000;2(1):47–55 www.nature.com/mt/journal/v2/n1/pdf/mt2000140a.pdf (accessed 1 August 2012)

[36] Westerman KA, Ao Z, Cohen EA, Leboulch P. Design of a trans protease lentiviral packaging system that produces high titer virus. Retrovirology. 2007;4(96):1–14. www.retrovirology.com/content/pdf/1742-4690-4-96.pdf (accessed 1 August 2012)

[37] Pauwels K, Gijsbers R, Toelen J, Schambach A, Willard-Gallo K, Verheust C, et al. State-of-the-art Lentiviral Vectors for Research Use: Risk Assessment and Biosafety Recommendations. Current gene therapy. 2009;9(6):459–74. www.benthamdirect.org/pages/content.php?CGT/2009/00000009/00000006/0002Q.SGM (accessed 1 August 2012)

[38] Montini E, Cesana D, Schmidt M, Sanvito F, Bartholomae CC, Ranzani M, et al. The genotoxic potential of retroviral vectors is strongly modulated by vector design and integration site selection in a mouse model of HSC gene therapy. The Journal of clinical investigation. 2009;119(4):964–75. www.jci.org/articles/view/37630 (accessed 1 August 2012)

[39] Zufferey R, Dull T, Mandel RJ, Bukovsky A, Quiroz D, Naldini L, et al. Self-Inactivating Lentivirus Vector for Safe and Efficient In Vivo Gene Delivery. J. Virol.. 1998;72(12):9873–80. jvi.asm.org/cgi/content/abstract/72/12/9873(accessed 1 August 2012)

[40] Iwakuma T, Cui Y, Chang LJ. Self-inactivating lentiviral vectors with U3 and U5 modifications. Virology. 1999;261(1):120–32. www.sciencedirect.com/science/article/pii/S0042682299998501(accessed 1 August 2012)

[41] Yu S-F. Self-Inactivating Retroviral Vectors Designed for Transfer of Whole Genes into Mammalian Cells. Proceedings of the National Academy of Sciences. 1986;83(10):3194–8. www.pnas.org/cgi/content/abstract/83/10/3194(accessed 1 August2012)

[42] Bukovsky AA, Song JP, Naldini L. Interaction of human immunodeficiency virus-derived vectors with wild-type virus in transduced cells. Journal of virology. 1999;73(8):7087–92. jvi.asm.org/content/73/8/7087.long (accessed 1 August 2012)

[43] Bokhoven M, Stephen SL, Knight S, Gevers EF, Robinson IC, Takeuchi Y, et al. Insertional gene activation by lentiviral and gammaretroviral vectors. Journal of virology. 2009;83(1):283–94. jvi.asm.org/content/83/1/283 (accessed 1 August 2012)

[44] Miyoshi H, Blomer U, Takahashi M, Gage FH, Verma IM. Development of a Self-Inactivating Lentivirus Vector. J. Virol.. 1998;72(10):8150–7. jvi.asm.org/cgi/content/abstract/72/10/8150(accessed 1 August 2012)

[45] Yang Q, Lucas A, Son S, Chang L-J. Overlapping enhancer/promoter and transcriptional termination signals in the lentiviral long terminal repeat. Retrovirology. 2007;4:4. www.retrovirology.com/content/4/1/4 (accessed 1 August 2012)

[46] Schambach A, Galla M, Maetzig T, Loew R, Baum C. Improving transcriptional termination of self-inactivating gamma-retroviral and lentiviral vectors. Molecular therapy: the journal of the American Society of Gene Therapy. 2007;15(6):1167–73. www.nature.com/mt/journal/v15/n6/full/6300152a.html (accessed 1 August 2012)

[47] Hanawa H, Persons DA, Nienhuis AW. Mobilization and mechanism of transcription of integrated self-inactivating lentiviral vectors. Journal of virology. 2005;79(13): 8410–21. jvi.asm.org/content/79/13/8410.long (accessed 1 August 2012)

[48] Hino S, Fan J, Taguwa S, Akasaka K, Matsuoka M. Sea urchin insulator protects lentiviral vector from silencing by maintaining active chromatin structure. Gene therapy. 2004;11(10):819–28. www.nature.com/gt/journal/v11/n10/full/3302227a.html (accessed 1 August 2012)

[49] Arumugam PI, Scholes J, Perelman N, Xia P, Yee J-K, Malik P. Improved human beta-globin expression from self-inactivating lentiviral vectors carrying the chicken hypersensitive site-4 (cHS4) insulator element. Molecular therapy: the journal of the American Society of Gene Therapy. 2007;15(10):1863–71. www.nature.com/mt/journal/v15/n10/full/6300259a.html (accessed 1 August 2012)

[50] Zufferey R, Donello JE, Trono D, Hope TJ. Woodchuck Hepatitis Virus Posttranscriptional Regulatory Element Enhances Expression of Transgenes Delivered by Retroviral Vectors. J. Virol. 1999;73(4):2886–92. jvi.asm.org/cgi/content/abstract/73/4/2886(accessed 1 August 2012)

[51] Oh T, Bajwa A, Jia G, Park F. Lentiviral vector design using alternative RNA export elements. Retrovirology. 2007;4(1):38. www.retrovirology.com/content/4/1/38 (accessed 1 August 2012)

[52] Pistello M, Vannucci L, Ravani A, Bonci F, Chiuppesi F, del Santo B, et al. Streamlined design of a self-inactivating feline immunodeficiency virus vector for transducing ex vivo dendritic cells and T lymphocytes. Genetic vaccines and therapy. 2007;5(1):8. www.gvt-journal.com/content/5/1/8(accessed 1 August 2012)

[53] Salmon P, Kindler V, Ducrey O, Chapuis B, Zubler RH, Trono D. High-level transgene expression in human hematopoietic progenitors and differentiated blood lineages after transduction with improved lentiviral vectors. Blood. 2000;96(10):3392–8.

bloodjournal.hematologylibrary.org/content/96/10/3392.long (accessed 1 August 2012)

[54] Schambach A, Bohne J, Baum C, Hermann FG, Egerer L, von Laer D, et al. Wood chuck hepatitis virus post-transcriptional regulatory element deleted from X protein and promoter sequences enhances retroviral vector titer and expression. Gene therapy. 2006;13(7):641–5. www.nature.com/gt/journal/v13/n7/full/3302698a.html (accessed 1 August 2012)

[55] Manganini M, Serafini M, Bambacioni F, Casati C, Erba E, Follenzi A, et al. A human immunodeficiency virus type 1 pol gene-derived sequence (cPPT/CTS) increases the efficiency of transduction of human nondividing monocytes and T lymphocytes by lentiviral vectors. Human gene therapy. 2002;13(15):1793–807. online.liebertpub.com/doi/abs/10.1089/104303402760372909 (accessed 1 August 2012)

[56] Sirven A, Pflumio F, Zennou V, Titeux M, Vainchenker W, Coulombel L, et al. The human immunodeficiency virus type-1 central DNA flap is a crucial determinant for lentiviral vector nuclear import and gene transduction of human hematopoietic stem cells. Blood. 2000;96(13):4103–10. bloodjournal.hematologylibrary.org/content/96/13/4103.long (accessed 1 August 2012)

[57] Logan AC, Nightingale SJ, Haas DL, Cho GJ, Pepper K a, Kohn DB. Factors influencing the titer and infectivity of lentiviral vectors. Human gene therapy. 2004;15(10):976–88. online.liebertpub.com/doi/abs/10.1089/hum.2004.15.976 (accessed 1 August 2012)

[58] Desmaris N, Bosch A, Salaün C, Petit C, Prévost MC, Tordo N, et al. Production and neurotropism of lentivirus vectors pseudotyped with lyssavirus envelope glycoproteins. Molecular therapy: the journal of the American Society of Gene Therapy.;4(2):149–56. www.nature.com/mt/journal/v4/n2/abs/mt2001210a.html (accessed 1 August 2012)

[59] Federici T, Kutner R, Zhang X-Y, Kuroda H, Tordo N, Boulis NM, et al. Comparative analysis of HIV-1-based lentiviral vectors bearing lyssavirus glycoproteins for neuronal gene transfer. Genetic vaccines and therapy. 2009;7(1):1. www.gvt-journal.com/content/7/1/1(accessed 1 August 2012)

[60] Mazarakis ND. Rabies virus glycoprotein pseudotyping of lentiviral vectors enables retrograde axonal transport and access to the nervous system after peripheral delivery. Human Molecular Genetics. 2001;10(19):2109–21. hmg.oxfordjournals.org/cgi/content/abstract/10/19/2109(accessed 1 August 2012)

[61] Bartz SR, Rogel ME, Emerman M. Human immunodeficiency virus type 1 cell cycle control: Vpr is cytostatic and mediates G2 accumulation by a mechanism which differs from DNA damage checkpoint control. Journal of virology. 1996;70(4):2324–31. jvi.asm.org/content/70/4/2324.full.pdf+html?sid=9792589f-078b-4868-a8a5-f0926b6b2dee (accessed 1 August 2012)

[62] DePolo NJ, Reed JD, Sheridan PL, Townsend K, Sauter SL, Jolly DJ, et al. VSV-G pseudotypedlentiviral vector particles produced in human cells are inactivated by human serum. Molecular therapy: the journal of the American Society of Gene Therapy. 2000;2(3):218–22. www.nature.com/mt/journal/v2/n3/abs/mt2000164a.html (accessed 1 August 2012)

[63] Croyle MA, Callahan SM, Auricchio A, Schumer G, Linse KD, Wilson JM, et al. PE-Gylation of a vesicular stomatitis virus G pseudotypedlentivirus vector prevents inactivation in serum. Journal of virology. 2004;78(2):912–21. jvi.asm.org/content/78/2/912 (accessed 1 August 2012)

[64] Berkowitz R, Ilves H, Lin WY, Eckert K, Coward A, Tamaki S, et al. Construction and molecular analysis of gene transfer systems derived from bovine immunodeficiency virus. Journal of virology. 2001;75(7):3371–82. jvi.asm.org/content/75/7/3371. long (accessed 1 August 2012)

[65] Metharom P, Takyar S, Xia HQ, Ellem KA, Wilcox GE, Wei MQ. Development of disabled, replication-defective gene transfer vectors from the Jembrana disease virus, a new infectious agent of cattle. Veterinary microbiology. 2001;80(1):9–22. www.sciencedirect.com/science/article/pii/S037811350000376X (accessed 1 August 2012)

[66] Mselli-Lakhal L, Guiguen F, Greenland T, Mornex J-F, Chebloune Y. Gene transfer system derived from the caprine arthritis-encephalitis lentivirus. Journal of virological methods. 2006;136(1-2):177–84. http://www.sciencedirect.com/science/article/pii/S0166093406001571(accessed 1 August 2012)

[67] Duisit G, Conrath H, Saleun S, Folliot S, Provost N, Cosset F-L, et al. Five recombinant simian immunodeficiency virus pseudotypes lead to exclusive transduction of retinal pigmented epithelium in rat. Molecular therapy: the journal of the American Society of Gene Therapy. 2002;6(4):446–54. www.nature.com/mt/journal/v6/n4/pdf/mt2002197a.pdf (accessed 1 August 2012)

[68] Kobinger GP, Deng S, Louboutin J-P, Vatamaniuk M, Matschinsky F, Markmann JF, et al. Transduction of human islets with pseudotypedlentiviral vectors. Human gene therapy. 2004;15(2):211–9. online.liebertpub.com/doi/abs/10.1089/104303404772680010 (accessed 1August 2012)

[69] Mochizuki H, Schwartz JP, Tanaka K, Brady RO, Reiser J. High-Titer Human Immunodeficiency Virus Type 1-Based Vector Systems for Gene Delivery into Nondividing Cells. J. Virol.. 1998;72(11):8873–83. jvi.asm.org/cgi/content/abstract/72/11/8873(accessed 1 August 2012)

[70] Hanawa H, Kelly PF, Nathwani AC, Persons DA, Vandergriff JA, Hargrove P, et al. Comparison of various envelope proteins for their ability to pseudotypelentiviral vectors and transduce primitive hematopoietic cells from human blood. Molecular therapy: the journal of the American Society of Gene Therapy. 2002;5(3):242–51. www.nature.com/mt/journal/v5/n3/full/mt200238a.html (accessed 1 August 2012)

[71] Zhang X-Y, La Russa VF, Reiser J. Transduction of bone-marrow-derived mesenchymal stem cells by using lentivirus vectors pseudotyped with modified RD114 envelope glycoproteins. Journal of virology. 2004;78(3):1219–29 jvi.asm.org/content/78/3/1219.long (accessed 1 August 2012)

[72] Kobinger GP, Weiner DJ, Yu QC, Wilson JM. Filovirus-pseudotypedlentiviral vector can efficiently and stably transduce airway epithelia in vivo. Nature biotechnology. 2001;19(3):225–30. www.nature.com/nbt/journal/v19/n3/full/nbt0301_225.html (accessed 1 August 2012)

[73] Beyer WR, Westphal M, Ostertag W, von Laer D. Oncoretrovirus and lentivirus vectors pseudotyped with lymphocytic choriomeningitis virus glycoprotein: generation, concentration, and broad host range. Journal of virology. 2002;76(3):1488–95. jvi.asm.org/content/76/3/1488.long (accessed 1 August 2012)

[74] Wong L-F, Azzouz M, Walmsley LE, Askham Z, Wilkes FJ, Mitrophanous KA, et al. Transduction patterns of pseudotyped lentiviral vectors in the nervous system. Molecular therapy: the journal of the American Society of Gene Therapy.;9(1):101–11. www.nature.com/mt/journal/v9/n1/full/mt200415a.html (accessed 1 August 2012)

[75] Kahl CA, Marsh J, Fyffe J, Sanders DA, Cornetta K. Human immunodeficiency virus type 1-derived lentivirus vectors pseudotyped with envelope glycoproteins derived from Ross River virus and Semliki Forest virus. Journal of virology. 2004;78(3):1421–30. jvi.asm.org/content/78/3/1421.long (accessed 1 August 2012)

[76] Kang Y, Stein CS, Heth JA, Sinn PL, Penisten AK, Staber PD, et al. In vivo gene transfer using a nonprimatelentiviral vector pseudotyped with Ross River Virus glycoproteins. Journal of virology. 2002;76(18):9378–88. jvi.asm.org/content/76/18/9378.long (accessed 1 August 2012)

[77] Morizono K, Bristol G, Xie YM, Kung SK, Chen IS. Antibody-directed targeting of retroviral vectors via cell surface antigens. Journal of virology. 2001;75(17):8016–20. jvi.asm.org/content/75/17/8016 (accessed 1 August 2012)

[78] Cronin J, Zhang X-Y, Reiser J. Altering the Tropism of Lentiviral Vectors through Pseudotyping. Current gene therapy. 2005;5(4):387–98. www.benthamdirect.org/pages/content.php?CGT/2005/00000005/00000004/0003Q.SGM (accessed 1 August 2012)

[79] Felder JM, Sutton RE. Lentiviral Vectors. In: Gene and Cell Therapy: Therapeutic Mechanisms and Strategies. 2009.

[80] Lodge R, Subbramanian R a, Forget J, Lemay G, Cohen E a. MuLV-based vectors pseudotyped with truncated HIV glycoproteins mediate specific gene transfer in CD4+ peripheral blood lymphocytes. Gene therapy. 1998;5(5):655–64. www.nature.com/gt/journal/v5/n5/abs/3300646a.html (accessed 1 August 2012)

[81] Thaler S, Schnierle BS. A packaging cell line generating CD4-specific retroviral vectors for efficient gene transfer into primary human T-helper lymphocytes. Molecular

therapy: the journal of the American Society of Gene Therapy. 2001;4(3):273–9. www.nature.com/mt/journal/v4/n3/abs/mt2001227a.html (accessed 1 August 2012)

[82] MacKenzie TC, Kobinger GP, Kootstra NA, Radu A, Sena-Esteves M, Bouchard S, et al. Efficient transduction of liver and muscle after in utero injection of lentiviral vectors with different pseudotypes. Molecular therapy: the journal of the American Society of Gene Therapy. 2002;6(3):349–58. www.nature.com/mt/journal/v6/n3/pdf/mt2002180a.pdf (accessed 1 August 2012)

[83] Peng KW, Pham L, Ye H, Zufferey R, Trono D, Cosset FL, et al. Organ distribution of gene expression after intravenous infusion of targeted and untargeted lentiviral vectors. Gene therapy. 2001;8(19):1456–63. www.nature.com/gt/journal/v8/n19/full/3301552a.html (accessed 1 August 2012)

[84] Yang L, Yang H, Rideout K, Cho T, Joo KI, Ziegler L, et al. Engineered lentivector targeting of dendritic cells for in vivo immunization. Nature biotechnology. 2008;26(3):326–34. www.nature.com/nbt/journal/v26/n3/full/nbt1390.html (accessed 1 August 2012)

[85] Escors D, Breckpot K. Lentiviral vectors in gene therapy: their current status and future potential. Archivum immunologiaeettherapiaeexperimentalis. 2010;58(2):107–19. www.springerlink.com/content/725574uvq7552u2g/ (accessed 1 August 2012)

[86] Ziegler L, Yang L, Joo K il, Yang H, Baltimore D, Wang P. Targeting lentiviral vectors to antigen-specific immunoglobulins. Human gene therapy. 2008;19(9):861–72. online.liebertpub.com/doi/abs/10.1089/hgt.2007.149 (accessed 1 August 2012)

[87] Frecha C, Szécsi J, Cosset F-L, Verhoeyen E. Strategies for targeting lentiviral vectors. Current gene therapy. 2008;8(6):449–60. www.benthamdirect.org/pages/content.php?CGT/2008/00000008/00000006/0005Q.SGM (accessed 1 August 2012)

[88] Trimby C. STRATEGIES FOR TARGETING LENTIVIRAL VECTORS. http://uknowledge.uky.edu/gradschool_diss/157(accessed 1 August 2012)

[89] Zhang X-Y, Kutner RH, Bialkowska A, Marino MP, Klimstra WB, Reiser J. Cell-specific targeting of lentiviral vectors mediated by fusion proteins derived from Sindbis virus, vesicular stomatitis virus, or avian sarcoma/leukosis virus. Retrovirology. 2010;7(1):3. http://www.retrovirology.com/content/7/1/3(accessed 1 August 2012)

[90] Yang L, Bailey L, Baltimore D, Wang P. Targeting lentiviral vectors to specific cell types in vivo. Proceedings of the National Academy of Sciences of the United States of America. 2006;103(31):11479–84. www.pnas.org/cgi/content/abstract/103/31/11479(accessed 1 August 2012)

[91] Lei Y, Joo K-I, Zarzar J, Wong C, Wang P. Targeting lentiviral vector to specific cell types through surface displayed single chain antibody and fusogenic molecule. Virology journal. 2010;7:35. www.virologyj.com/content/7/1/35 (accessed 1 August 2012)

[92] Haas DL, Case SS, Crooks GM, Kohn DB. Critical factors influencing stable transduction of human CD34(+) cells with HIV-1-derived lentiviral vectors. Molecular therapy⊚: the journal of the American Society of Gene Therapy. 2000;2(1):71–80. www.nature.com/mt/journal/v2/n1/abs/mt2000143a.html (accessed 1 August 2012)

[93] Schweizer M, Merten O-W. Large-scale production means for the manufacturing of lentiviral vectors. Current gene therapy. 2010;10(6):474–86. www.benthamdirect.org/pages/content.php?CGT/2010/00000010/00000006/0006Q.SGM (accessed 1 August 2012)

[94] Gougeon M-L. Apoptosis as an HIV strategy to escape immune attack. Nature reviews. Immunology. 2003;3(5):392–404. www.nature.com/nri/journal/v3/n5/full/nri1087.html (accessed 1 August 2012)

[95] Bell AJ, Fegen D, Ward M, Bank A. RD114 envelope proteins provide an effective and versatile approach to pseudotypelentiviral vectors. Experimental biology and medicine (Maywood, N.J.). 2010;235(10):1269–76. ebm.rsmjournals.com/content/235/10/1269.long (accessed 1 August 2012)

[96] Sainski AM, Natesampillai S, Cummins NW, Bren GD, Taylor J, Saenz DT, et al. The HIV-1-specific protein Casp8p41 induces death of infected cells through Bax/Bak. Journal of virology. 2011;85(16):7965–75. jvi.asm.org/content/85/16/7965.long (accessed 1 August 2012)

[97] Algeciras-Schimnich A, Belzacq-Casagrande A-S, Bren GD, Nie Z, Taylor J a, Rizza S a, et al. Analysis of HIV Protease Killing Through Caspase 8 Reveals a Novel Interaction Between Caspase 8 and Mitochondria. The open virology journal. 2007;1:39–46. benthamscience.com/open/openaccess.php?tovj/articles/V001/39TOVJ.htm (accessed 1 August 2012)

[98] Nie Z, Phenix BN, Lum JJ, Alam a, Lynch DH, Beckett B, et al. HIV-1 protease processes procaspase 8 to cause mitochondrial release of cytochrome c, caspase cleavage and nuclear fragmentation. Cell death and differentiation. 2002;9(11):1172–84. www.nature.com/cdd/journal/v9/n11/full/4401094a.html (accessed 1 August 2012)

[99] Merten O-W, Charrier S, Laroudie N, Fauchille S, Dugué C, Jenny C, et al. Large-scale manufacture and characterization of a lentiviral vector produced for clinical ex vivo gene therapy application. Human gene therapy. 2011;22(3):343–56 online.liebertpub.com/doi/abs/10.1089/hum.2010.060 (accessed 1 August 2012)

[100] Gama-Norton L, Botezatu L, Herrmann S, Schweizer M, Alves PM, Hauser H, et al. Lentivirus production is influenced by SV40 large T-antigen and chromosomal integration of the vector in HEK293 cells. Human gene therapy. 2011;22(10):1269–79. online.liebertpub.com/doi/abs/10.1089/hum.2010.143 (accessed 1 August 2012)

[101] Ansorge S, Lanthier S, Transfiguracion J, Durocher Y, Henry O, Kamen A. Development of a scalable process for high-yield lentiviral vector production by transient transfection of HEK293 suspension cultures. The journal of gene medicine.

2009;11(10):868–76. onlinelibrary.wiley.com/doi/10.1002/jgm.1370/abstract (accessed 1 August 2012)

[102] Smith SL, Shioda T. Advantages of COS-1 monkey kidney epithelial cells as packaging host for small-volume production of high-quality recombinant lentiviruses. Journal of virological methods. 2009;157(1):47–54. www.sciencedirect.com/science/article/pii/S0166093408004412 (accessed 1 August 2012)

[103] Ni Y, Sun S, Oparaocha I, Humeau L, Davis B, Cohen R, et al. Generation of a packaging cell line for prolonged large-scale production of high-titer HIV-1-based lentiviral vector. The journal of gene medicine. 2005;7(6):818–34. onlinelibrary.wiley.com/doi/10.1002/jgm.726/abstract (accessed 1 August 2012)

[104] Mann R, Mulligan RC, Baltimore D. Construction of a retrovirus packaging mutant and its use to produce helper-free defective retrovirus. Cell. 1983;33(1):153–9. onlinelibrary.wiley.com/doi/10.1002/jgm.726/abstract (accessed 1 August 2012)

[105] Witting SR, Li L-H, Jasti A, Allen C, Cornetta K, Brady J, et al. Efficient large volume lentiviral vector production using flow electroporation. Human gene therapy. 2012;23(2):243–9. online.liebertpub.com/doi/abs/10.1089/hum.2011.088 (accessed 1 August 2012)

[106] Rols MP, Coulet D, Teissié J. Highly efficient transfection of mammalian cells by electric field pulses. Application to large volumes of cell culture by using a flow system. European journal of biochemistry / FEBS. 1992;206(1):115–21. onlinelibrary.wiley.com/doi/10.1111/j.1432-1033.1992.tb16908.x/abstract (accessed 1 August 2012)

[107] Segura M, Garnier A, Durocher Y, Coelho H. Production of Lentiviral Vectors by Large-Scale Transient Transfection of Suspension Cultures and Affinity Chromatography Purification. 2007;98(4):789–99. onlinelibrary.wiley.com/doi/10.1002/bit.21467/pdf (accessed 1 August 2012)

[108] Kafri T, van Praag H, Ouyang L, Gage FH, Verma IM. A Packaging Cell Line for Lentivirus Vectors. Journal of Virology. 1999;73(1):576–84. jvi.asm.org/cgi/content/abstract/73/1/576 (accessed 1 August 2012)

[109] Pacchiaa L, Adelson ME, Kaul M, Ron Y, Dougherty JP. An inducible packaging cell system for safe, efficient lentiviral vector production in the absence of HIV-1 accessory proteins. Virology. 2001 Mar 30;282(1):77–86. www.sciencedirect.com/science/article/pii/S0042682200907876 (accessed 1 August 2012)

[110] Kuate S, Wagner R, Uberla K. Development and characterization of a minimal inducible packaging cell line for simian immunodeficiency virus-based lentiviral vectors. The journal of gene medicine;4(4):347–55. onlinelibrary.wiley.com/doi/10.1002/jgm.290/abstract (accessed 1 August 2012)

[111] Broussau S, Jabbour N, Lachapelle G, Durocher Y, Tom R, Transfiguracion J, et al. Inducible packaging cells for large-scale production of lentiviral vectors in serum-free suspension culture. Molecular therapy©: the journal of the American Society of Gene

Therapy. 2008;16(3):500–7. www.nature.com/mt/journal/v16/n3/full/6300383a.html (accessed 1 August 2012)

[112] Stewart HJ, Leroux-Carlucci MA, Sion CJM, Mitrophanous KA, Radcliffe PA. Development of inducible EIAV-based lentiviral vector packaging and producer cell lines. Gene therapy. 2009;16(6):805–14. www.nature.com/gt/journal/v16/n6/full/gt200920a.html (accessed 1 August 2012)

[113] Throm RE, Ouma A a, Zhou S, Chandrasekaran A, Lockey T, Greene M, et al. Efficient construction of producer cell lines for a SIN lentiviral vector for SCID-X1 gene therapy by concatemeric array transfection. Blood. 2009;113(21):5104–10 bloodjournal.hematologylibrary.org/content/113/21/5104.long (accessed 1 August 2012)

[114] Paddison PJ, Caudy AA, Bernstein E, Hannon GJ, Conklin DS. Short hairpin RNAs (shRNAs) induce sequence-specific silencing in mammalian cells. Genes & development. 2002;16(8):948–58. genesdev.cshlp.org/content/16/8/948.long (accessed 1 August 2012)

[115] Hu G, Luo J. A primer on using pooled shRNA libraries for functional genomic screens. Acta biochimic et biophysica Sinica. 2012 ;44(2):103–12. abbs.oxford-journals.org/cgi/content/abstract/44/2/103(accessed 1 August 2012)

[116] Moffat J, Grueneberg DA, Yang X, Kim SY, Kloepfer AM, Hinkle G, et al. A lentiviralRNAi library for human and mouse genes applied to an arrayed viral high-content screen. Cell. 2006;124(6):1283–98. www.cell.com/retrieve/pii/S0092867406002388 (accessed 1 August 2012)

[117] Singer O, Verma IM. Applications of lentiviral vectors for shRNA delivery and transgenesis. Current gene therapy. 2008;8(6):483–8. www.benthamdirect.org/pages/content.php?CGT/2008/00000008/00000006/0008Q.SGM (accessed 1 August 2012)

[118] Pfeifer A. Lentiviral transgenesis--a versatile tool for basic research and gene therapy. Current gene therapy. 2006;6(4):535–42. www.benthamdirect.org/pages/content.php?CGT/2006/00000006/00000004/0006Q.SGM (accessed 1 August 2012)

[119] Pomper MG, Hammond H, Yu X, Ye Z, Foss CA, Lin DD, et al. Serial imaging of human embryonic stem-cell engraftment and teratoma formation in live mouse models. Cell research. 2009;19(3):370–9. www.nature.com/cr/journal/v19/n3/full/cr2008329a.html (accessed 1 August 2012)

[120] Welstead GG, Brambrink T, Jaenisch R. Generating iPS cells from MEFS through forced expression of Sox-2, Oct-4, c-Myc, and Klf4. Journal of visualized experiments©: JoVE.2008;(14). www.jove.com/video/734/generating-ips-cells-from-mefs-through-forced-expression-sox-2-oct-4 (accessed 1 August 2012)

[121] Brambrink T, Foreman R, Welstead GG, Lengner CJ, Wernig M, Suh H, et al. Sequential expression of pluripotency markers during direct reprogramming of mouse somatic cells. Cell stem cell. 2008;2(2):151–9. www.cell.com/cell-stem-cell/abstract/S1934-5909(08)00005-2 (accessed 1 August 2012)

[122] Lian Q, Chow Y, Esteban MA, Pei D, Tse H-F. Future perspective of induced pluripotent stem cells for diagnosis, drug screening and treatment of human diseases. Thrombosis and haemostasis. 2010;104(1):39–44. www.schattauer.de/en/magazine/subject-areas/journals-a-z/thrombosis-and-haemostasis/contents/archive/issue/1093/manuscript/13188.html (accessed 1 August 2012)

[123] Spencer HT, Denning G, Gautney RE, Dropulic B, Roy AJ, Baranyi L, et al. Lentiviral vector platform for production of bioengineered recombinant coagulation factor VIII. Molecular therapy: the journal of the American Society of Gene Therapy. 2011;19(2): 302–9. www.nature.com/mt/journal/v19/n2/full/mt2010239a.html (accessed 1 August 2012)

[124] Malik P, Arumugam PI, Yee J-K, Puthenveetil G. Successful correction of the human Cooley's anemia beta-thalassemia major phenotype using a lentiviral vector flanked by the chicken hypersensitive site 4 chromatin insulator. Annals of the New York Academy of Sciences. 2005;1054:238–49. onlinelibrary.wiley.com/doi/10.1196/annals. 1345.030/abstract (accessed 1 August 2012)

[125] Pawliuk R, Westerman KA, Fabry ME, Payen E, Tighe R, Bouhassira EE, et al. Correction of sickle cell disease in transgenic mouse models by gene therapy. Science (New York, N.Y.). 2001;294(5550):2368–71. www.sciencemag.org/content/294/5550/2368.abstract (accessed 1 August 2012)

[126] Brown BD, Cantore A, Annoni A, Sergi LS, Lombardo A, Della Valle P, et al. A microRNA-regulated lentiviral vector mediates stable correction of hemophilia B mice. Blood. 2007;110(13):4144–52. bloodjournal.hematologylibrary.org/content/110/13/4144.long (accessed 1 August 2012)

[127] Adjali O, Marodon G, Steinberg M, Mongellaz C, Thomas-Vaslin V, Jacquet C, et al. In vivo correction of ZAP-70 immunodeficiency by intrathymic gene transfer. The Journal of clinical investigation. 2005;115(8):2287–95. www.jci.org/articles/view/23966 (accessed 1 August 2012)

[128] Lo Bianco C, Schneider BL, Bauer M, Sajadi A, Brice A, Iwatsubo T, et al. Lentiviral vector delivery of parkin prevents dopaminergic degeneration in an alpha-synuclein rat model of Parkinson's disease. Proceedings of the National Academy of Sciences of the United States of America. 2004;101(50):17510–5. www.pnas.org/cgi/content/abstract/101/50/17510(accessed 1 August 2012)

[129] Wang G, Slepushkin V, Zabner J, Keshavjee S, Johnston JC, Sauter SL, et al. Feline immunodeficiency virus vectors persistently transduce nondividing airway epithelia and correct the cystic fibrosis defect. The Journal of clinical investigation. 1999;104(11):R55–62. www.jci.org/articles/view/8390 (accessed 1 August 2012)

[130] Azzouz M, Le T, Ralph GS, Walmsley L, Monani UR, Lee DCP, et al. Lentivector-mediated SMN replacement in a mouse model of spinal muscular atrophy. The Journal of clinical investigation. 2004;114(12):1726–31. www.jci.org/articles/view/22922(accessed 1 August 2012)

[131] Levine BL, Humeau LM, Boyer J, MacGregor R-R, Rebello T, Lu X, et al. Gene transfer in humans using a conditionally replicating lentiviral vector. Proceedings of the
National Academy of Sciences of the United States of America. 2006;103(46):17372–7.
www.pnas.org/cgi/content/abstract/103/46/17372 (accessed 1 August 2012)

Chapter 5

Transposons for Non-Viral Gene Transfer

Sunandan Saha and Matthew H. Wilson

Additional information is available at the end of the chapter

1. Introduction

DNA based transposon vectors offer a mechanism for non-viral gene delivery into mammalian and human cells. These vectors work via a cut-and-paste mechanim whereby transposon DNA containing a transgene(s) of interest is integrated into chromosomal DNA by a transposase enzyme. The first DNA based transposon system which worked efficienty in human cells was *sleeping beauty*. This was followed a few years later by the use of the *piggy-Bac* transposon system in mammalian and human cells. The advantages of transposon vectors include lower cost, less innate immunogenicity, and the ability to easily co-deliver multiple genes when compared to viral vectors. However, when compared to viral vectors, non-viral transposon systems are limited by delivery to cells, they are possibly still immunogenic, and they can be less efficient depending on the cell type of interest. Nonetheless, transposons have shown promise in genetic modification of clinical grade cell types such as human T lymphocytes, induced pluripotent stem cells, and stem cells. Recently generated hyperactive transposon elements have improved gene delivery to levels similar to that obtained with viral vectors. In addition, current research is focused on manipulating transposon systems to achieve user-selected and site-directed genomic integration of transposon DNA cargo to improve safety and efficacy of transgene delivery. DNA based transposon systems represent a powerful tool for gene therapy and genome engineering applications.

2. Transposons as gene delivery systems

Transposons or mobile genetic elements were first described by Barbara McClintock as "jumping genes" responsible for mosaicism in maize [1]. Transposons are found in the genome of all eukaryotes and in humans at least 45% of the genome is derived from such elements [2]. Transposons active in eukaryotes can work either by a "copy and paste" (Class I) or "cut and paste" (Class II) mechanism (Figure 1).

In the "copy and paste" mechanism, the transposon first makes a copy of itself via an RNA intermediate (hence also known as retrotransposons).Class II DNA-transposons work by a "cut and paste" mechanism in which the transposon is excised by the transposase upon expression and then relocates to a new locus by creating double strand breaks *in situ*. Most transposon systems used for gene delivery use a modified "cut and paste" system consisting of a transposon carrying the transgene of interest and a helper plasmid expressing the transposase (Figure 2). The "cut and paste" transposition mechanism involves recognition of the inverted terminal repeat sequences (IRs) by the transposase and excision of the transposon from the donor loci, usually a supplied plasmid. The two most commonly used transposon system for genetic modification of mammalian and human cells are *sleeping beauty* and *piggyBac*.

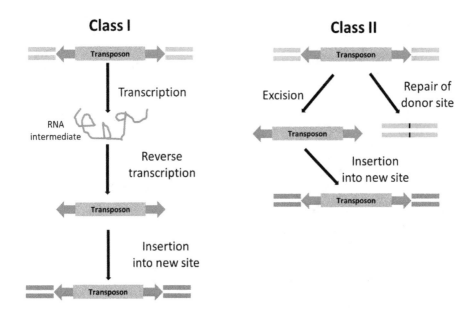

Figure 1. Class I and II transposons and mechanisms of integration.

The *sleeping beauty* (SB) transposon was reconstructed from the genome of salmonid fish using molecular phylogenetic data [3] and belongs to the Tc1/mariner superfamily of transposons. The sleeping beauty transposon is flanked by 230bp IRs which conatin within them non identical direct repeats (DRs).

The *piggyBac* transposon was isolated from cabbage looper moth *Trichoplusia ni*[4].One desirable feature of the *piggyBac* system is the precise excision of the transposon from the donor site without leaving behind any footprints [5], making it an attractive feature for cellular reprogramming. Excision of the transposon from the donor site, creates complimentary TTAA overhangs which undergo simple ligation to regenerate the donor site bypassing DNA synthesis during transposition [6].

In "cis" delivery the transposase is carried by the same plasmid backbone as the transposn. In "trans" delivery it is delivered by a separate circular plasmid. For gene therapy purposes transposase and transposon are delivered either in "cis" or in "trans" (Figure 2). In "cis" delivery the transposase is carried on the same vector backbone as the transposon carrying the gene of interest (GOI). In the "trans" configuration, the transposase is delivered by a separate non integrating plasmid. The "cis" configuration has been shown to improve transposition efficiency [7], but there is a question of whether the linearized backbone carrying the transposase may also get integrated and lead to residual transposase expression. A comparison of the properties of *sleeping beauty* and *piggyBac* is described in Table 1.

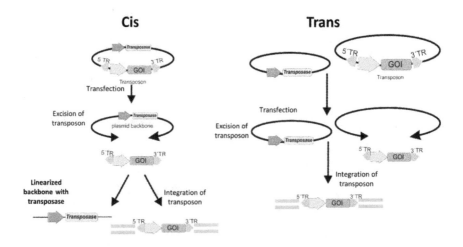

Figure 2. "Cis" and "Trans" transposon mediated gene delivery. GOI, gene of interest; 5′TR, 5′ terminal repeat; 3′TR, 3′ terminal repeat; the yellow and beige arrows indicate promoters to drive gene expression.

3. Advantages of transposon as gene delivery system

3.1. Lower cost compared to viral vectors

In spite of viral vectors having been successfully used in gene therapy clinical trials (e.g. generation of clinical grade T cells for immunotherapy [8], their use in extensive gene therapy regimens is constrained. Clinical grade viral vectors are very expensive to manufacture given the stringent regulatory oversight and limited number of GMP certified production facilities. A batch of clinical grade retroviral supernatant for treating patients costs between $400,000 to $500,000 (personal communciation, GMP facility director, Baylor College of Medicine). The production of clinical GMP (cGMP) grade viral supernatant is extremely time intensive as, in addition to optimization of culture conditions, the supernatant needs extensive testing for microbial contamination, presence of replication competent viral particles as well as validation of sequence and functionality. The entire production run and associated testing may require up to six months. These viral stocks also have limited shelf life. Upon release the desired cell type is transduced, selected and expanded which is then followed by quality assurance checks. This also requires extensive training of the personnel involved in production and testing and scaling up production as would be required for future gene therapy regimens will not be economical. In contrast, cGMP grade transposon plasmids can be manufactured more quickly. The production can be scaled up quickly and existing facilities can be upgraded and certified in a shorter time frame. The cost of manufacturing and release of cGMP grade plasmid DNA is between $20,000 and $ 40,000 [9]. The use of transposons drastically reduces both the time and cost of production of the gene delivery system. In the first clinical trial approved by the FDA for infusion of autologous *ex vivo sleeping beauty* modified T cells [10], the most time intensive step was the test for fungal and bacterial contamination (14 days).

	sleeping beauty	*piggyBac*
Cargo Capacity	~10 kb	>100 kb
Foot Print	Insertion site mutated upon excision	No "foot print" mutation
Needs titration for optimal activity	Yes	Yes
Hyper Active Versions	SB100X (most active SB version)	hyPBase
Effect of 'N' and 'C' terminal modifications	50% or more reduction in efficacy	No apparent reduction in efficiency
Integration site preference	More random	Slight increased preference for genes and TSS
Can be engineerd to bias integration sites	Yes	Yes

Table 1. Comparison of *sleeping beauty* and *piggyBac* properties. TSS, transcriptional start sites.

3.2. Delivery of large and multiple transgenes

Although retroviral and lentiviral vectors have been successfully used for delivering multiple transgenes, they are limited by their cargo capacity[11,12]. Both these vector systems can carry a limited cargo of up to 8kb which is limited by the packaging capacity of their capsid envelop [13]. Early reports demontrated the *sleeping beauty* system to have reduced efficiency beyond transposon size of 10kb [14]. In contrast the *piggyBac* system has been successfully utilized to modify primary human lymphocytes with 15 kb transposon with an initial transfection efficiency of 20% which increased up to 90% upon selection and expansion [15]. The *piggyBac* system has been successfully used for mobilizing transposons as large as 100 kb in mouse embryonic stem (ES) cells [16]. An increased cargo capacity also imparts the ability to deliver multiple transgenes to the same cell. For example, using the *piggyBac* system, human cells were efficiently modified to express a three subunit functional sodium channel which retained its electro-physiological properties even after 35 passages [17].

3.3. Less immunogenicity

One of the major concerns for viral gene delivery system is the associated immunogenicity as evidenced by the death of a patient receiving liver targeted adenoviral gene therapy for partial ornithine transcarbamylase deficiency in 1999 [13].The systemic delivery of the viral particles initiated a cytokine storm leading to multiple organ failure within four days of administration of the vector [18]. Attempts have been made to reduce the immunogenicity of viral vectors by stripping them of all endogenous viral genes ('gutted' or 'helper-dependent' vectors) [19], but even the use of modified viral delivery systems are potentially immunogenic as evidenced by long term inflammation of rat brains injected with replication deficient adenoviral vectors [20].

Transposons are circular plasmid DNA molecules and do not contain a viral shell or viral antigens. The host response to non-viral vectors has not been well characterized. Toll-like receptor (TLR)-9 is known to recognize DNA with unmethylated CpG dinucleotides in the endosome- which can lead to signalling via MyD88 and production of inflammatory mediators such as TNF and IFN-α [21]. Other mechanisms of innate immune sensing of naked DNA include DNA-dependent activator of interferon (IFN)-regulatory factors (DAI) (also called Z-DNA-binding protein 1, ZBP1), RNA polymerase III (Pol III), absent in melanoma 2 (AIM2), leucine-rich repeat (in Flightless I) interacting protein-1 (Lrrfip1), DExD/H box helicases (DHX9 and DHX36), and most recently, the IFN-inducible protein IFI16 [22]. These molecules use independent and sometimes overlapping signalling pathways to elicit immune response to delivered DNA. Nonetheless, much remains to be discovered about host immune response to delivered DNA and how to overcome such an obstacle for effective gene therapy.

3.4. Less propensity for oncogenic mutations

Human immunodeficiency virus (HIV) has been shown to prefer genes for integration in SupT1 and Jurkat cells [23]. Murine leukemia virus (MLV) derived vectors have been used for stable gene transfer for therapy but they have been shown to prefer transcriptional start sites (TSS) for integration [24]. Integrations near the promoter of the LMO2 proto-oncogene has been associated with leukemia in the French X-SCID gene therapy trial [25]. The genome wide mapping of *sleeping beauty* transposons in mammals have revealed a modest bias towards transcriptional units and upstream regulatory sequences which varies between cell types [26]. The integration site profiling of both *piggyBac* in primary human cells and cell lines have revealed no preferred chromosomal hotspots [7,27]. It also has no preference for genomic repeat elements and known proto-oncogenes. *PiggyBac* has a preference for integrating into RefSeq genes and near TSS and CpG enriched motifs although this may be influenced by the state of the cell or type of the cell. Both *sleeping beauty* and *piggyBac* are being engineered for site-directed gene delivery to improve the safety of gene transfer. True genotoxic risk for viral vectors was not discovered until they were used in humans. Transposons have not yet been used in humans, though one clinical trial has be approved.

4. Challenges of transposon as gene delivery system

Given the promise of transposons as gene delivery vehicle, it suffers from certain challenges e.g. reduced delivery, random integration profile and silencing of the integrated transgene.

4.1. Low delivery efficiency

Transposon systems are carried by naked DNA plasmids and there efficiency is limited to the efficiency of getting the plasmid into to the cell by chemical or physical means. Certain primary cells and cell lines are easy to transfect (e.g. HEK293, HeLa, Hepatocytes) and transposons have high transposition efficiency in these cells. But other clinically relevant cells (e.g. primary lymphocytes) are difficult to transfect. Often the method used for transfection (e.g. nucleofection and electroporation) is toxic to the cells and leads to excessive cell death thus reducing the efficiency of stable transfection. Efforts are on to circumvent these difficulties by developing novel delivery methods e.g. cell-penetrating peptides (CPP) –*piggyBac* fusions [28] or using polyethylenimine [29]. Some investigators have encapsulated transposon systems within viruses to use the virus to deliver the DNA from which transposition occurs [30-34] This may improve efficiency, however, the issues with immunogenicity of viruses remain.

4.2. Random integration profile

Transposons as described above have uncontrolled or relatively random integration preference with regards to genomic elements. This leaves the transposed transgene open to influence of the neighboring genomic region. Additional, uncontrolled or not site-directed integration increases the risk for possible genotoxicity.

4.3. Silencing of the integrated transgene

Gene silencing has been observed when using *sleeping beauty* in cultured cells [35]. Transgene silencing and epigenetic transgene modification has not been well studied with *piggyBac*.

5. Applications

Both *sleeping beauty* and *piggyBac* have demonstrated correct of disease phenotypes in animal models or in human cells (Table 2).

Disease	Transposon system	Reference
Hemophilia B	SB	[34,36]
Hemophilia A	SB	[37,38]
Tyrosinemia Type I	SB	[39]
JunctionalEpidermolysisBullosa	SB	[40]
Diabetes	SB	[41]
Huntington's disease	SB	[42]
Mucopolysaccharidosis I & VII	SB	[43,44]
α1-antitrypsin deficiency	PB	[45]

Table 2. List of diseases corrected with *Sleeping Beauty* (SB) and *piggyBac* (PB)

5.1. Genetic modification of human T lymphocytes

Peripheral blood and umbilical cord T cells have been extensively modified with both viral and non-viral gene delivery systems for immunotherapeutic purposes [10]. This therapeutic avenue has been successfully used for the treatment of viral infections and Epstein Barr virus (EBV) associated lymphoma post autologous bone marrow transplantation [46,47]. They also hold promise for treatment of other cancers [48-50]. But the use of of viral vectors for the generation of clinical grade T cells is expensive, time intensive and not free of risks. Non-viral gene delivery systems, including DNA transposons, are being increasingly explored as an alternative strategy.

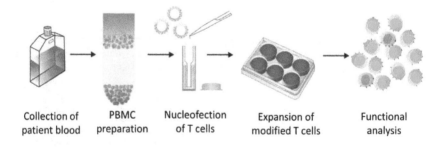

| Collection of patient blood | PBMC preparation | Nucleofection of T cells | Expansion of modified T cells | Functional analysis |

Figure 3. Schematic of transposon modificaiton of primary human T cells.

A schematic of how primary human T lymphocytes can be gene modified with transposons is shown in Figure 3. The *sleeping beauty* system was used to successfully modify peripheral blood mononuclear cells with a CD19-specific chimeric antigen receptor (CAR)[9]. These modified PBMCs were then used to generate CAR+ T cells which preserved their CD4+, CD8+, central memory and effector-effector cell phenotypes. The *piggyBac* system has also been optimized to achieve stable transgene expression in human T lymphocytes [51]. Further, primary lymphocytes have been modified with multiple transgenes to redirect their specificity for CD19 and make them resistant to off target effects of chemotherapeutic drugs like rapamycin [15]. Cytotoxic T lymphocytes specific for Epstein Barr Virus (EBV) have also been successfully modified with human epidermal growth factor receptor-2 specific CAR (HER2-CAR)[52]. The first clinical trial involving transposon modified autologous T cells with a second generation CD19-specific CAR has been approved by the Food and Drug Administration[10]. This trial will involve the infusion of *ex vivo* expanded autologous T cells in patients undergoing autologous hematopoietic stem cell (HSC) transplantation with high risk of relapsed B-cell malignancies.

5.2. Generation of induced pluripotent stem cells

Induced pluripotent stem cells (iPSCs) generated from a patient's own differentiated somatic cells holds promise for regenerative medicine. Early successful attempts involved delivery of defined reprogramming factors using retroviral vectors [11,53]. Unfortunately 20% of the chimeric offspring obtained from germline transmission of retrovirally reprogrammed clones developed tumors due to reactivation of the c-myc oncogene [54]. In addition, ectopic expression of the reprogramming factor(s) has been linked to tumors and skin dysplasia [55-56]. One way to circumvent the use of viral delivery systems is to deliver the programming factors as recombinant proteins [57] or by repeated plasmid transfections [58], both of which have proven to be extremely slow and inefficient. The higher gene delivery efficiency of transposons together with their ability of being excised from the cells post reprogramming and differentiation make them an attractive choice for generating iPSCs.

Somatic cells have been transfected with *piggyBac* transposons carrying reprogramming factors and transposase. Reprogrammed iPSCs are selected and propagated to obtain individual iPSC clones. To generate transgene-free iPSCs, the transposase is re-expressed to remove the reprogramming factors followed by negative selection to identify transgene-free iPSCs (Figure 4).

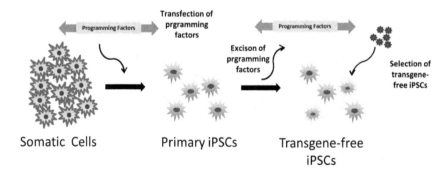

Figure 4. Generation of transgene-free iPSCs using the *piggyBac* system.

The *piggyBac* system seems to be ideally suited for this as it can undergo precise excision and does not leave behind "foot print" mutations [5]. In contrast, the *sleeping beauty* system has been shown to excise imprecisely leaving behind altered insertion sites [3]. The *piggyBac* system has been successfully used to generate transgene free iPSCs from both mouse and human embryonic fibroblasts with efficiency comparable to retroviral vectors [59-60]. *Piggy-Bac* has also been used to successfully reprogram murine tail tip fibroblasts into fully differentiated melanocytes which are more compatible with cell therapy regimens [61]. The use of a *piggyBac* based inducible reprogramming system also proved to be more stable and quicker than an inducible lentiviral system [62].

5.3. Genetic modification of stem cells

Transposons have been used for genetic modification of human embryonic stem cells [63]. More recently, transposons have been used to insert bacterial artificial chromosomes (BACs) in human ES cells [64]. Both *sleeping beauty* and *piggyBac* have been used to genetically modify hematopoietic stem cells [65]. Transposons provide an effective mechanism for permanent (or reversible in the case of *piggyBac*) genetic modification of a variety of stem cell types for eventual use in therapy.

6. Current hot topics and future directions

6.1. Generation of hyperactive transposon elements

SB100X and native *piggyBac* both have similar activity levels in human cells which is 100 fold more than the native *sleeping beauty*. The hyperactive *piggyBac* transposase (hyPBase) has been shown to have 2 to 3 fold more activity than SB100X or native PB [66] (Figure 5).

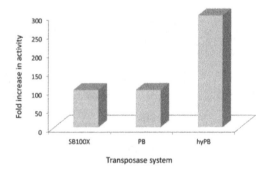

Figure 5. Comparison of transposase activity in human cells

Efficiency of transposition is perceived as a bottleneck to efficient gene delivery. Attempts to engineer hyperactive versions of transposase have resulted in versions with increasing transposition activity. Strategies employed include import of amino acids from related transposases [67], alanine scanning [68] and site directed mutagenesis [69]. The construction of the SB100X transposase with ~100 folds higher activity than the original *sleeping beauty* transposase employed a high throughput screen of mutant transposases obtained from DNA shuffling [70]. A hyperactive version of the *piggyBac* transposase (hyPBase) has also been engineered with 17-fold increase in excision and 9-fold increase in integration [71]. The hyPBase has 7 amino acid substitution identified from a screen of PBase mutants but none of the 7 substitutions are in the catalytic domain of the transposase. The hyPBase also has foot-print mutation frequency (<5%) comparable to the wild type transposase and no apparent effect on genomic integrity. Unlike SB100X which showed a 50% reduction, the addition of a 24 kDa ZFN tag did not significantly alter transposition efficiency [66]. In vivo, a mouse codon optimized version of hyPBase showed 10-fold greater long term gene expression than both native *piggyBac* and SB100X.

6.2. Engineering transposon systems for site-directed integration

Random integration of transgene during delivery have resulted in adverse events including leukemia [25,72]. Integration of transgenes at other genetic loci may also affect expression of critical genes. Engineering transposon systems for site-directed integration would allow transgene delivery to sites in the genome resulting in improved gene expression, reduced positional effects at the site of integration, and improved safety. Most studies have utilized fusion of DNA-binding domains to the transposase to achieve site directed integration, beginning with the engineering of the *sleeping beauty* system. *Sleeping beauty* has been engineered to bias integration into plasmids containing target sites [73-74] and near selected elements and repeat elements in the genome [75-76]. The *piggyBac* system seems to be more suited for transposase modifications as the addition of additional domains to the transposase does not alter the systems efficiency [7,77-79]. A Gal4-*piggyBac* fusion transposase has been shown to bias integration near Gal4 sites in episomal plasmids [80] and the genome [81]. A chimeric transposase containing an engineered zinc finger protein (ZFP) fused to the native *piggyBac* transposase has also been successfully used to bias integration at the genomic level [79]. Researchers have also used transcription factor DNA binding domains fused to the *piggyBac* transposase to label nearby transcription factor binding sites in the genomes of cells [82]. Current approaches are hampered by the ability of the transposase to integrate on its own without the targeting machinery which can lead to off-target integration. Futher engineering modifications to both the transposase and transposon may overcome this limitation.

7. Conclusion

Transposon systems are well suited for *ex vivo* gene therapy and *in vivo* delivery to target organs may also become a reality in the future. The advantages of lower cost and more widespread applicability than viral vectors, in combination with the potential for site-directed gene delivery, make transposons a promising non-viral gene delivery system as an alternative to viral vectors.

Acknowlegements

SS is supported in part by the Howard Hughes Medical Institute Med-Into-Grad Scholar grant to TBMM Program. MHW is supported in part by NIH R01 DK093660.

Author details

Sunandan Saha[2,3] and Matthew H. Wilson[1,2,3,4]

*Address all correspondence to: mhwilson@bcm.edu

1 Michael E. DeBakey VA Medical Center, Baylor College of Medicine, Houston TX, USA

2 Interdepartmental Program in Translational Biology & Molecular Medicine, Baylor College of Medicine, Houston TX, USA

3 Department of Medicine-Nephrology Division, Baylor College of Medicine, Houston TX, USA

4 Center for Cell and Gene Therapy, Baylor College of Medicine, Houston TX, USA

References

[1] McClintock B. The Origin and Behavior of Mutable Loci in Maize. *ProcNatlAcadSci* U S A. 1950 Jun;36(6):344–55.

[2] Lander ES, Linton LM, Birren B, Nusbaum C, Zody MC, Baldwin J, et al. Initial sequencing and analysis of the human genome. *Nature*. 2001 Feb 15;409(6822):860–921.

[3] Ivics Z, Hackett PB, Plasterk RH, Izsvák Z. Molecular Reconstruction of Sleeping Beauty, a Tc1-like Transposon from Fish, and Its Transposition in Human Cells. *Cell*. 1997 Nov 14;91(4):501–10.

[4] Cary LC, Goebel M, Corsaro BG, Wang H-G, Rosen E, Fraser MJ. Transposon mutagenesis of baculoviruses: Analysis of Trichoplusiani transposon IFP2 insertions within the FP-locus of nuclear polyhedrosis viruses. *Virology*. 1989 Sep;172(1):156–69.

[5] Fraser MJ, Clszczon T, Elick T, Bauser C. Precise excision of TTAA-specific lepidopteran transposons piggyBac (IFP2) and tagalong (TFP3) from the baculovirus genome

in cell lines from two species of Lepidoptera. *Insect Molecular Biology*. 1996;5(2):141–51.

[6] Mitra R, Fain-Thornton J, Craig NL. piggyBac can bypass DNA synthesis during cut and paste transposition. *The EMBO Journal*. 2008 Apr 9;27(7):1097–109.

[7] Wilson MH, Coates CJ, George AL. PiggyBac Transposon-mediated Gene Transfer in Human Cells. *Molecular Therapy*. 2007;15(1):139–45.

[8] Savoldo B, Ramos CA, Liu E, Mims MP, Keating MJ, Carrum G, et al. CD28 costimulation improves expansion and persistence of chimeric antigen receptor–modified T cells in lymphoma patients. *Journal of Clinical Investigation*. 2011 May 2;121(5):1822–6.

[9] Singh H, Manuri PR, Olivares S, Dara N, Dawson MJ, Huls H, et al. Redirecting Specificity of T-Cell Populations For CD19 Using the Sleeping Beauty System. *Cancer Res*. 2008 Apr 15;68(8):2961–71.

[10] Hackett PB, Largaespada DA, Cooper LJ. A Transposon and Transposase System for Human Application. *Molecular Therapy*. 2010;18(4):674–83.

[11] Takahashi K, Tanabe K, Ohnuki M, Narita M, Ichisaka T, Tomoda K, et al. Induction of Pluripotent Stem Cells from Adult Human Fibroblasts by Defined Factors. *Cell*. 2007 Nov 30;131(5):861–72.

[12] Yu J, Vodyanik MA, Smuga-Otto K, Antosiewicz-Bourget J, Frane JL, Tian S, et al. Induced Pluripotent Stem Cell Lines Derived from Human Somatic Cells. *Science*. 2007 Dec 21;318(5858):1917–20.

[13] Thomas CE, Ehrhardt A, Kay MA. Progress and problems with the use of viral vectors for gene therapy. *Nature Reviews Genetics*. 2003 May 1;4(5):346–58.

[14] Balciunas D, Wangensteen KJ, Wilber A, Bell J, Geurts A, Sivasubbu S, et al. Harnessing a High Cargo-Capacity Transposon for Genetic Applications in Vertebrates. *PLoS Genet*. 2006 Nov 10;2(11):e169.

[15] Huye LE, Nakazawa Y, Patel MP, Yvon E, Sun J, Savoldo B, et al. CombiningmTor Inhibitors With Rapamycin-resistant T Cells: A Two-pronged Approach to Tumor Elimination. *Molecular Therapy* [Internet]. 2011 [cited 2012 Jul 12]; Available from: http://www.nature.com.ezproxyhost.library.tmc.edu/mt/journal/vaop/ncurrent/full/mt2011179a.html

[16] Li MA, Turner DJ, Ning Z, Yusa K, Liang Q, Eckert S, et al. Mobilization of giant piggyBac transposons in the mouse genome. *Nucl. Acids Res*. 2011 Dec 1;39(22):e148–e148.

[17] Kahlig KM, Saridey SK, Kaja A, Daniels MA, George AL, Wilson MH. Multiplexed transposon-mediated stable gene transfer in human cells. *ProcNatlAcadSci* U S A. 2010 Jan 26;107(4):1343–8.

[18] Assessment of adenoviral vector safety and toxicity: report of the National Institutes of Health Recombinant DNA Advisory Committee. *Hum. Gene Ther.* 2002 Jan 1;13(1): 3–13.

[19] Morsy MA, Caskey CT. Expanded-capacity adenoviral vectors--the helper-dependent vectors. *Mol Med Today.* 1999 Jan;5(1):18–24.

[20] Thomas CE, Schiedner G, Kochanek S, Castro MG, Löwenstein PR. Peripheral infection with adenovirus causes unexpected long-term brain inflammation in animals injected intracranially with first-generation, but not with high-capacity, adenovirus vectors: Toward realistic long-term neurological gene therapy for chronic diseases. *PNAS.* 2000 Jun 20;97(13):7482–7.

[21] Baccala R, Gonzalez-Quintial R, Lawson BR, Stern ME, Kono DH, Beutler B, et al. Sensors of the innate immune system: their mode of action. *Nature Reviews Rheumatology.* 2009 Jul 14;5(8):448–56.

[22] Sharma S, Fitzgerald KA. Innate immune sensing of DNA. *PLoSPathog.* 2011 Apr; 7(4):e1001310.

[23] Bushman F, Lewinski M, Ciuffi A, Barr S, Leipzig J, Hannenhalli S, et al. Genome-wide analysis of retroviral DNA integration. *Nature Reviews Microbiology.* 2005 Nov 1;3(11):848–58.

[24] Wu X, Li Y, Crise B, Burgess SM. Transcription Start Regions in the Human Genome Are Favored Targets for MLV Integration. *Science.* 2003 Jun 13;300(5626):1749–51.

[25] Hacein-Bey-Abina S, Kalle CV, Schmidt M, McCormack MP, Wulffraat N, Leboulch P, et al. LMO2-Associated Clonal T Cell Proliferation in Two Patients after Gene Therapy for SCID-X1. *Science.* 2003 Oct 17;302(5644):415–9.

[26] Yant SR, Wu X, Huang Y, Garrison B, Burgess SM, Kay MA. High-Resolution Genome-Wide Mapping of Transposon Integration in Mammals. *Mol. Cell. Biol.* 2005 Mar 15;25(6):2085–94.

[27] Galvan DL, Nakazawa Y, Kaja A, Kettlun C, Cooper LJN, Rooney CM, et al. Genome-wide Mapping of PiggyBac Transposon Integrations in Primary Human T Cells. *Journal of Immunotherapy.* 2009 Oct;32(8):837–44.

[28] Lee C-Y, Li J-F, Liou J-S, Charng Y-C, Huang Y-W, Lee H-J. A gene delivery system for human cells mediated by both a cell-penetrating peptide and a piggyBactransposase. *Biomaterials.* 2011 Sep;32(26):6264–76.

[29] Kang Y, Zhang X, Jiang W, Wu C, Chen C, Zheng Y, et al. Tumor-directed gene therapy in mice using a composite nonviral gene delivery system consisting of the piggyBac transposon and polyethylenimine. *BMC Cancer.* 2009 Apr 27;9(1):126.

[30] Bak RO, Mikkelsen JG. Mobilization of DNA transposable elements from lentiviral vectors. *Mob Genet Elements.* 2011;1(2):139–44.

[31] Mikkelsen JG, Yant SR, Meuse L, Huang Z, Xu H, Kay MA. Helper-Independent Sleeping Beauty transposon-transposase vectors for efficient nonviral gene delivery and persistent gene expression in vivo. *Mol. Ther.* 2003 Oct;8(4):654–65.

[32] Staunstrup NH, Moldt B, Mátés L, Villesen P, Jakobsen M, Ivics Z, et al. Hybrid lentivirus-transposon vectors with a random integration profile in human cells. *Mol. Ther.* 2009 Jul;17(7):1205–14.

[33] Hausl M, Zhang W, Voigtländer R, Müther N, Rauschhuber C, Ehrhardt A. Development of adenovirus hybrid vectors for Sleeping Beauty transposition in large mammals. *Curr Gene Ther.* 2011 Oct;11(5):363–74.

[34] Yant SR, Ehrhardt A, Mikkelsen JG, Meuse L, Pham T, Kay MA. Transposition from a gutless adeno-transposon vector stabilizes transgene expression in vivo. *Nature Biotechnology.* 2002;20(10):999–1005.

[35] Garrison BS, Yant SR, Mikkelsen JG, Kay MA. Postintegrative gene silencing within the Sleeping Beauty transposition system. *Mol. Cell. Biol.* 2007 Dec;27(24):8824–33.

[36] Yant SR, Meuse L, Chiu W, Ivics Z, Izsvak Z, Kay MA. Somatic integration and long-term transgene expression in normal and haemophilic mice using a DNA transposon system. *Nature Genetics.* 2000 May 1;25(1):35–41.

[37] Ohlfest JR, Frandsen JL, Fritz S, Lobitz PD, Perkinson SG, Clark KJ, et al. Phenotypic correction and long-term expression of factor VIII in hemophilic mice by immunotolerization and nonviral gene transfer using the Sleeping Beauty transposon system. *Blood.* 2005 Apr 1;105(7):2691–8.

[38] Liu L, Mah C, Fletcher BS. Sustained FVIII Expression and Phenotypic Correction of Hemophilia A in Neonatal Mice Using an Endothelial-Targeted Sleeping Beauty Transposon. *Molecular Therapy.* 2006;13(5):1006–15.

[39] Montini E, Held PK, Noll M, Morcinek N, Al-Dhalimy M, Finegold M, et al. In Vivo Correction of Murine Tyrosinemia Type I by DNA-Mediated Transposition. *Molecular Therapy.* 2002;6(6):759–69.

[40] Ortiz-Urda S, Lin Q, Yant SR, Keene D, Kay MA, Khavari PA. Sustainable correction of junctionalepidermolysisbullosa via transposon-mediated nonviral gene transfer. *Gene Therapy.* 2003;10(13):1099–104.

[41] He C-X, Shi D, Wu W-J, Ding Y-F. Insulin expression in livers of diabetic mice mediated by hydrodynamics-based administration. *World J Gastroenterol.* 2004 Feb 15;10(4):567–72.

[42] Chen ZJ, Kren BT, Wong PY-P, Low WC, Steer CJ. Sleeping Beauty-mediated down-regulation of huntingtin expression by RNA interference. *Biochemical and Biophysical Research Communications.* 2005 Apr 8;329(2):646–52.

[43] Aronovich EL, Bell JB, Belur LR, Gunther R, Koniar B, Erickson DCC, et al. Prolonged expression of a lysosomal enzyme in mouse liver after Sleeping Beauty trans-

poson-mediated gene delivery: implications for non-viral gene therapy of mucopolysaccharidoses. *The Journal of Gene Medicine*. 2007;9(5):403–15.

[44] Aronovich EL, Bell JB, Khan SA, Belur LR, Gunther R, Koniar B, et al. Systemic Correction of Storage Disease in MPS I NOD/SCID Mice Using the Sleeping Beauty Transposon System. *Molecular Therapy*. 2009;17(7):1136–44.

[45] Yusa K, Rashid ST, Strick-Marchand H, Varela I, Liu P-Q, Paschon DE, et al. Targeted gene correction of α1-antitrypsin deficiency in induced pluripotent stem cells. *Nature*. 2011 Oct 12;478(7369):391–4.

[46] Leen AM, Myers GD, Sili U, Huls MH, Weiss H, Leung KS, et al. Monoculture-derived T lymphocytes specific for multiple viruses expand and produce clinically relevant effects in immunocompromised individuals. *Nature Medicine*. 2006 Oct 1;12(10): 1160–6.

[47] Rooney C., Ng CY., Loftin S, Smith C., Li C, Krance R., et al. Use of gene-modified virus-specific T lymphocytes to control Epstein-Barr-virus-related lymphoproliferation. *The Lancet*. 1995 Jan 7;345(8941):9–13.

[48] Straathof KCM, Bollard CM, Popat U, Huls MH, Lopez T, Morriss MC, et al. Treatment of nasopharyngeal carcinoma with Epstein-Barr virus–specific T lymphocytes. *Blood*. 2005 Mar 1;105(5):1898–904.

[49] Bollard CM, Gottschalk S, Leen AM, Weiss H, Straathof KC, Carrum G, et al. Complete responses of relapsed lymphoma following genetic modification of tumor-antigen presenting cells and T-lymphocyte transfer. *Blood*. 2007 Oct 15;110(8):2838–45.

[50] Dudley ME, Wunderlich JR, Yang JC, Sherry RM, Topalian SL, Restifo NP, et al. Adoptive Cell Transfer Therapy Following Non-Myeloablative but Lymphodepleting Chemotherapy for the Treatment of Patients With Refractory Metastatic Melanoma. *JCO*. 2005 Apr 1;23(10):2346–57.

[51] Nakazawa Y, Huye LE, Dotti G, Foster AE, Vera JF, Manuri PR, et al. Optimization of the PiggyBac Transposon System for the Sustained Genetic Modification of Human T Lymphocytes. *Journal of Immunotherapy*. 2009 Oct;32(8):826–36.

[52] Nakazawa Y, Huye LE, Salsman VS, Leen AM, Ahmed N, Rollins L, et al. PiggyBac-mediated Cancer Immunotherapy Using EBV-specific Cytotoxic T-cells Expressing HER2-specific Chimeric Antigen Receptor. *Molecular Therapy* [Internet]. 2011 [cited 2012   Jul   12];   Available   from: http:// www.nature.com.ezproxyhost.library   .tmc.edu/mt/journal/vaop/ncurrent/full/ mt2011131a.html

[53] Takahashi K, Yamanaka S. Induction of Pluripotent Stem Cells from Mouse Embryonic and Adult Fibroblast Cultures by Defined Factors. *Cell*. 2006 Aug 25;126(4):663–76.

[54] Okita K, Ichisaka T, Yamanaka S. Generation of germline-competent induced pluripotent stem cells. *Nature*. 2007 Jun 6;448(7151):313–7.

[55] Hochedlinger K, Yamada Y, Beard C, Jaenisch R. Ectopic Expression of Oct-4 Blocks Progenitor-Cell Differentiation and Causes Dysplasia in Epithelial Tissues. *Cell*. 2005 May 6;121(3):465–77.

[56] Foster KW, Liu Z, Nail CD, Li X, Fitzgerald TJ, Bailey SK, et al. Induction of KLF4 in basal keratinocytes blocks the proliferation–differentiation switch and initiates squamous epithelial dysplasia. *Oncogene*. 2005;24(9):1491–500.

[57] Zhou H, Wu S, Joo JY, Zhu S, Han DW, Lin T, et al. Generation of Induced Pluripotent Stem Cells Using Recombinant Proteins. *Cell Stem Cell*. 2009 May 8;4(5):381–4.

[58] Stadtfeld M, Nagaya M, Utikal J, Weir G, Hochedlinger K. Induced Pluripotent Stem Cells Generated Without Viral Integration. *Science*. 2008 Nov 7;322(5903):945–9.

[59] Yusa K, Rad R, Takeda J, Bradley A. Generation of transgene-free induced pluripotent mouse stem cells by the piggyBac transposon. *Nature Methods*. 2009;6(5):363–9.

[60] Woltjen K, Michael IP, Mohseni P, Desai R, Mileikovsky M, Hämäläinen R, et al. piggyBac transposition reprograms fibroblasts to induced pluripotent stem cells. *Nature*. 2009 Mar 1;458(7239):766–70.

[61] Yang R, Jiang M, Kumar SM, Xu T, Wang F, Xiang L, et al. Generation of Melanocytes from Induced Pluripotent Stem Cells. *Journal of Investigative Dermatology*. 2011;131(12):2458–66.

[62] Wernig M, Lengner CJ, Hanna J, Lodato MA, Steine E, Foreman R, et al. A drug-inducible transgenic system for direct reprogramming of multiple somatic cell types. *Nat. Biotechnol*. 2008 Aug;26(8):916–24.

[63] Wilber A, Linehan JL, Tian X, Woll PS, Morris JK, Belur LR, et al. Efficient and stable transgene expression in human embryonic stem cells using transposon-mediated gene transfer. *Stem Cells*. 2007 Nov;25(11):2919–27.

[64] Rostovskaya M, Fu J, Obst M, Baer I, Weidlich S, Wang H, et al. Transposon-mediated BAC transgenesis in human ES cells. *Nucleic acids research* [Internet]. 2012 Jun 30 [cited 2012 Aug 9]; Available from: http://www.ncbi.nlm.nih.gov/pubmed/22753106

[65] Grabundzija I, Irgang M, Mátés L, Belay E, Matrai J, Gogol-Döring A, et al. Comparative Analysis of Transposable Element Vector Systems in Human Cells. *Molecular Therapy*. 2010;18(6):1200–9.

[66] Doherty JE, Huye LE, Yusa K, Zhou L, Craig NL, Wilson MH. Hyperactive piggyBac gene transfer in human cells and in vivo. *Hum. Gene Ther*. 2012 Mar;23(3):311–20.

[67] Baus J, Liu L, Heggestad AD, Sanz S, Fletcher BS. Hyperactive Transposase Mutants of the Sleeping Beauty Transposon. *Molecular Therapy*. 2005;12(6):1148–56.

[68] Yant SR, Park J, Huang Y, Mikkelsen JG, Kay MA. Mutational Analysis of the N-Terminal DNA-Binding Domain of Sleeping Beauty Transposase: Critical Residues for DNA Binding and Hyperactivity in Mammalian Cells. *Mol. Cell. Biol*. 2004 Oct 15;24(20):9239–47.

[69] Zayed H, Izsvák Z, Walisko O, Ivics Z. Development of Hyperactive Sleeping Beauty Transposon Vectors by Mutational Analysis. *Molecular Therapy*. 2004;9(2):292–304.

[70] Mátés L, Chuah MKL, Belay E, Jerchow B, Manoj N, Acosta-Sanchez A, et al. Molecular evolution of a novel hyperactive Sleeping Beauty transposase enables robust stable gene transfer in vertebrates. *Nature Genetics*. 2009;41(6):753–61.

[71] Yusa K, Zhou L, Li MA, Bradley A, Craig NL. A hyperactive piggyBactransposase for mammalian applications. *PNAS*. 2011 Jan 25;108(4):1531–6.

[72] Check E. Gene therapy: A tragic setback. *Nature*. 2002 Nov 14;420(6912):116–8.

[73] Ivics Z, Katzer A, Stüwe EE, Fiedler D, Knespel S, Izsvák Z. Targeted Sleeping Beauty Transposition in Human Cells. *Molecular Therapy*. 2007;15(6):1137–44.

[74] Yant SR, Huang Y, Akache B, Kay MA. Site-directed transposon integration in human cells. *Nucleic Acids Res*. 2007;35(7):e50.

[75] Voigt K, Gogol-Döring A, Miskey C, Chen W, Cathomen T, Izsvák Z, et al. Retargeting Sleeping Beauty Transposon Insertions by Engineered Zinc Finger DNA-binding Domains. *Molecular therapy*: the journal of the American Society of Gene Therapy [Internet]. 2012 Jul 10 [cited 2012 Aug 10]; Available from: http://www.ncbi.nlm.nih.gov/pubmed/22776959

[76] Ammar I, Gogol-Döring A, Miskey C, Chen W, Cathomen T, Izsvák Z, et al. Retargeting transposon insertions by the adeno-associated virus Rep protein. *Nucleic Acids Res*. 2012 Aug 1;40(14):6693–712.

[77] Wu SC-Y, Meir Y-JJ, Coates CJ, Handler AM, Pelczar P, Moisyadi S, et al. piggyBac is a flexible and highly active transposon as compared to Sleeping Beauty, Tol2, and Mos1 in mammalian cells. *PNAS*. 2006 Oct 10;103(41):15008–13.

[78] Cadiñanos J, Bradley A. Generation of an inducible and optimized piggyBac transposon system. *Nucleic Acids Res*. 2007;35(12):e87.

[79] Kettlun C, Galvan DL, Jr ALG, Kaja A, Wilson MH. Manipulating piggyBac Transposon Chromosomal Integration Site Selection in Human Cells. *Molecular Therapy*. 2011;19(9):1636–44.

[80] Maragathavally KJ, Kaminski JM, Coates CJ. Chimeric Mos1 and piggyBactransposases result in site-directed integration. *FASEB J*. 2006 Sep;20(11):1880–2.

[81] Owens JB, Urschitz J, Stoytchev I, Dang NC, Stoytcheva Z, Belcaid M, et al. Chimeric piggyBactransposases for genomic targeting in human cells. *Nucl. Acids Res*. [Internet]. 2012 Apr 9 [cited 2012 Jul 5]; Available from: http://nar.oxfordjournals.org/content/early/2012/04/08/nar.gks309

[82] Wang H, Mayhew D, Chen X, Johnston M, Mitra RD. "Calling cards" for DNA-binding proteins in mammalian cells. *Genetics*. 2012 Mar;190(3):941–9.

Chapter 6

Lentiviral Vectors in Immunotherapy

Ines Dufait, Therese Liechtenstein, Alessio Lanna,
Roberta Laranga, Antonella Padella,
Christopher Bricogne, Frederick Arce,
Grazyna Kochan, Karine Breckpot and David Escors

Additional information is available at the end of the chapter

1. Introduction

Genetic immunotherapy can be defined as a therapeutic approach in which therapeutic genes are introduced into defined target cell types to modulate immune responses. A major challenge for this therapeutic strategy is the delivery of these genes into target cells in an efficient, stable manner. Possibly one of the best systems to achieve this is the use of lentiviral vectors (lentivectors) as gene carriers, as they are capable of transducing both dividing and resting cells [1].

Lentivectors are mainly derived from the human immunodeficiency virus (HIV-1) genome, a member of the *Retroviridae* family. The defining characteristic of retroviruses is their capacity to stably integrate their RNA genome into the host cell chromosomes, in the form of a cDNA copy (Figure 1). Therefore, retrovirus and lentivirus vectors have been used extensively in research since they are ideal gene carriers into target cells. Moreover, both retrovirus and lentivirus vectors have been successfully applied in human gene therapy for the treatment of several genetic/metabolic inherited diseases (Cartier et al, 2009; Cavazzana-Calvo et al, 2010; Gaspar et al, 2004; Grez et al, 2010; Ott et al, 2006; Thrasher et al, 2006).

Lentiviruses are spherical enveloped viruses with a diameter around 80 to 120 nm and contain two copies of a single-stranded RNA genome (Figure 2) [2]. The genome is enclosed within a core composed of the structural and enzymatic proteins nucleocapsid (NC), capsid (CA), reverse transcriptase (RT), integrase (IN) and protease (PR). The core is surrounded by a protein layer of matrix (MA) protein. The envelope protein (ENV) is embedded in the virion lipid envelope, and it binds to the target cellular receptor and mediates virion entry.

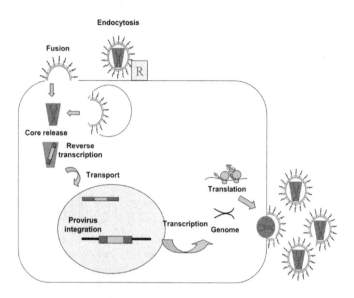

Figure 1. The retrovirus life cycle.The life cycle of retroviruses, including lentiviruses is shown in this figure as a multi-step mechanism, starting with virion binding to the cellular receptor (R), leading to direct fusion or endocytosis. Then, the internal core is released and the two RNA molecules undergo reverse transcription as indicated, ending up with a single cDNA molecule. The core is then transported to the nucleus (in the case of lentiviruses) and the cDNA is integrated into the cell chromosome. The integrated genome (provirus) undergoes transcription, producing more RNA genome copies (and also spliced mRNAs, not shown here), which are also translated into structural and enzymatic proteins. These are then assembled into virions that bud out of the infected cells.

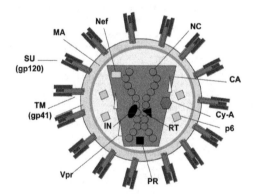

Figure 2. In this scheme, the lentivirus virion is represented as a sphere containing a genome made of two RNA molecules associated to the nucleocapsid (NC) protein. The nucleocapsid is enclosed by a core made of capsid (CA) protein, which is surrounded by a shell of matrix (MA) protein that associates to the virion envelope. The two subunits of the HIV-1 envelope are also indicated (SU and TM). In addition, other enzymatic (IN, RT, PR), accessory (Vpr, p6) and cellular (Cyclophilin A, Cy-A) proteins are shown, which are incorporated into lentivirus particles.

Lentivectors are classified as complex retroviruses according to their genome organisation, as it contains accessory and regulatory genes absent in other retroviruses. Nevertheless, the retrovirus genome shares a common 5' to the 3' gene organisation, with Gag, Pol and Env genes [1, 3]. Gag encodes MA, CA and NC as a polyprotein. Pol encodes enzymatic proteins associated to reverse transcription, that is, the reverse transcriptase (RT), integrase (IN) and protease (PR). RT synthesizes a single cDNA copy from the retrovirus genomic RNA [4]. IN mediates cDNA integration in the host cell chromosome, while PR cleaves Gag and Gag-Pol polyproteins during virion maturation.

The integrated cDNA genome is flanked by two long terminal repeats (LTRs) subdivided in U3, R and U5 regions. U3 is the HIV-1 promoter. The R region marks the starting point of transcription, and U5 region is critical for reverse transcription. The other key elements are the packaging signal (Ψ) and the polypurine tract (PPT). The packaging signal, as in many other virus species, allows RNA genome encapsidation during virion assembly in the cytoplasm. The PPT element is a key element for reverse transcription [5].

Lentivectors are usually obtained following a three-plasmid co-transfection in 293T cells (Figure 3) [6, 7]. The first one, the packaging plasmid, provides the structural and RT proteins (Gag-Pol). The second one, the envelope plasmid, encodes a glycoprotein to pseudotype the lentivector particles. This process consists on the incorporation of an heterologous Env in the viral lipid envelope. This will allow the lentivector to exhibit the specific cell tropism given by the Env used in pseudotyping. One of the most used Env is the Vesicular Stomatitis Virus (VSV) Glycoprotein (G). The VSV-G confers stability to the lentivector particles and a very broad tropism for human and non-human cells [8]. Lastly, the third one, the transfer plasmid, contains the cis-acting sequences for replication/transcription and packaging (Figure 3) [9]. By including promoters within the transfer plasmid, any gene of interest can be expressed either constitutively or inducibly, in a cell type-specific of unspecific manner (Figure 3) [1]. Therefore, lentiviral vectors can also incorporate genes with immunoregulatory properties in cells from the immune system.

Two main cell types of the immune system have been preferential targets for genetic immunotherapy: antigen presenting cells (APCs) and effector T lymphocytes. These two cell types are key controllers of immune responses. By expressing transgenes of interest in APCs, such as DCs, they can be processed and presented to antigen-specific T cells in the immunological synapse. This antigen presentation is the first step in either starting of suppressing immune responses. Therefore, if genes with modulating properties of APC functions can be co-expressed with antigens, the strength and type of immune response can be controlled. In fact, genetic modification of cells from the immune system can circumvent the limitations of current immunotherapeutic protocols. Using targeted lentiviral vectors, specificity and effectiveness can be achieved by targeting key cells that modulate and polarize immune responses.

Although more challenging than DCs, T lymphocytes can also be genetically modified using lentiviral vectors. Vectors expressing T cell receptors (TCRs) specific for antigens of interest can modify the specificity of T cell populations, or expand their antigen profile. Therefore, these genetically modified T cells can be adoptively transferred in the human patients. This strategy is particularly important to generate T cells with high affinity TCRs towards tumour-associated antigens.

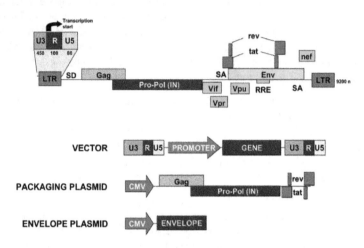

Figure 3. The HIV-1 genome is shown at the top of the figure. All structural, accessory and enzymatic genes are indicated throughout the genome. The two LTRs are shown as present in an integrated provirus. The three functional regions of the HIV LTR are shown on top of the 5- LTR. Numbers indicate nucleotide positions. The HIV genome is splitted in three different plasmids to engineer a gene vector. The transfer (vector) plasmid is indicated, with only the HIV-1 LTRs containing an internal promoter driving the expression of a gene of interest. In the packaging plasmid, only the Gag-Pro-Pol and Rev, Tat genes have been retained. This increases biosafety. Transcription of these genes takes place under the control of the cytomegalovirus promoter (CMV), as indicated in the figure. Lastly, a third plasmid encoding an envelope glycoprotein is shown on the bottom of the figure. This envelope pseudotypes the lentivector particle.

2. Genetic modification of DCs with lentivectors

For the elimination of cancer cells and chronic infections such as HIV, hepatitits B and malaria, a strong, effective T cell response is required. To initiate these strong T cell responses, the interaction between antigen-specific T cells and antigen-presenting APCs has to be strengthened[10]. Amongst APCs, DCs are most frequently the targets of immunotherapy protocols since they are probably the most immunogenic [10, 11].

To activate T cells during antigen presentation, these T cells have to receive at least three different signals from APCs (Figure 4) [10, 12-16]. The first signal, or signal 1, is the direct recognition of the peptide-major histocompatibility molecule complex (p-MHC) by the TCR. However, this interaction is not sufficient to confer T cells with effector activities. For this, a second co-stimulatory signal (signal 2) has to be co-delivered together with p-MHC recognition. This signal 2 is the consequence of the integration of activatory and inhibitory interactions between ligands/receptors on the surface of DCs and T cells (Figure 4)[16, 17]. For example, CD80 binding to CD28 is strongly activatory, while CD80 binding with CTLA-4, or

PD-L1 with PD-1, are strongly inhibitory[16, 17]. Apart from these two signals, T cells require a third signal which drives their differentiation into distinct subtypes that will regulate different types of immune responses [13, 18]. This third signal is usually provided by different combination of cytokines present within the immunological synapse (Figure 4). For example, the presence of high levels of IL12 will polarise T cell differentiation towards a Th1 type (cellular cytotoxic immunity). On the other hand, high levels of IL10 will drive polarisation towards Th2 (antibody responses).

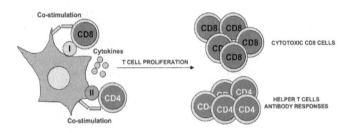

Figure 4. In this scheme, DCs (left) present antigens to specific CD8 and CD4 T cells (as indicated) in the context of MHC class I (I) or class II (II) molecules. These T cells receive further stimuli by co-stimulation through ligand-receptor interactions between the DC and T cells (as indicated in the figure). Simultaneously, activated DCs secrete cytokines and chemokines (indicated in the figure as spheres) that will drive T cell activation, proliferation and differentiation into either cytotoxic CD8 T cells or T helper cells, as shown on the right.

An ideal immunotherapeutic approach would be to use lentiviral vectors to deliver the antigen of interest together with the three signals required for the desired T cell polarisation. Lentivectors have been extensively used for this purpose, because they are particularly effective in transducing DCs without affecting their functionality, unlike other vectors such as those based on adenoviruses [8, 19-26]. In fact, the stable integration of the lentivector genome allows long-term, sustained transgene expression[1, 9]. In addition, the expressed transgene is processed and its antigen peptides loaded in MHC I and MHC II molecules [27]. This is of the outmost importance for immunotherapy, since expressed proteins can be processed and loaded onto MHC-II molecules through several pathways. While secreted proteins can enter the endocytic pathway and membrane proteins can be recycled towards the endosomal pathway, cytoplasmic proteins can still enter the MHC II pathway by autophagy[28]. Nevertheless, to improve MHC II loading of peptides from cytoplasmic proteins, endocytic localisation sequences can be fused to the transgene, with the lysosomal-associated membrane protein 1 or with the amino-terminal portion of the MHC II invariant chain [29-32].

The use of lentivectors to express whole trangenes rather than antigen petides circumvents the necessity of designing specific peptide/protein vaccines for loading into specific MHC genotypes [27]. Thus, lentivectors expressing model antigens have been extensively used as a proof of principle. Amongst others, the antigens chicken ovalbumin (OVA), tumour-tumour associated antigens such as MELAN-A, tyrosinase related protein (Trp), NY-ESO or antigens from infectious agents have been expressed in DCs. These modified DCs induced strong activation and proliferation of antigen-specific T cells. [17, 33-38].

3. Lentivector immunogenicity

Lentivectors have been extensively used in vaccination protocols, due to their capacity of raising strong transgene-specific immune responses [9, 17, 30, 38-40]. Interestingly, some reports suggest that lentivectors are incapable of inducing DC maturation *in vitro*, suggesting that some components of the lentivector preparations provide signals 2 and 3 through a mechanisms not well understood [40, 41].

DC maturation is a complex, step-wise process in which they up-regulate the surface expression of co-stimulatory molecules such as CD80, CD83, CD86, CD40, adhesion molecules such as ICAM-1 and also the expression of MHC molecules. In general terms, DC maturation can be triggered by recognition of pathogen-derived molecules by specific receptors on the DC surface, such as the family of toll-like receptors (TLRs) [42, 43]. DCs can also mature through the exposure of pro-inflammatory cytokines by a process called cytokine priming [13-15]. Matured DCs can effectively provide strong signals 1 and 2, leading to efficient T cell activation and proliferation. Thus, their administration *in vivo* induces DC maturation and production of type I interferon that can provide signal 3 [9, 39, 44, 45].

The capacity of lentivectors to induce DC maturation after vaccination is probably caused by either specific components of the lentivector particle or by contaminants present in the lentivector preparation. As a matter of fact, lentivector particles resemble viruses and therefore, some components have the potential to stimulate immune responses such as the RNA genome or the cDNA [46]. These are ligands for TLR7 and TLR9, respectively [41, 45]. In addition to specific components of the lentivector particle, contaminants can also alter their immunostimulatory properties. In fact, most lentivector preparations pseudotyped with VSV G contain VSV-G tubulo-vesicular structures enclosing plasmid DNA that stimulate TLR9 *in vitro*, leading to type I IFN production by pDCs [47]. In addition, foetal calf serum (FCS) contributes to immunogenicity by providing T cell epitopes with adjuvant capacities [48].

4. Control of DC maturation by expression of molecular activators with lentivectors

Lentivector preparations can induce DC maturation in vivo. However, in some circumstances this is not enough for effective therapeutic activities. This is the case for cancer immunotherapy, in which breaking tolerance towards TAAs is still a medical challenge. One possible solution is to co-express TAAs with molecular activators of DCs using lentivectors, particularly using activators of signalling cascades belonging to the TLR pathways.

This has been firstly achieved by over-expressing adaptor molecules, which associate with TLR cytoplasmic tails. These adaptor molecules recruit activatory protein kinases leading to DC maturation. Thus, lentivectors have been used to express MYD88 or TRIF1 in mouse myeloid DCs, which also increases secretion of pro-inflammatory cytokines IL-6, IL-12 and IFN-α, which enhanced T cell cytotoxicity [49]. The NF-κB pathway has also been an attractive target because it controls transcription of the majority of pro-inflammatory genes (Figure 5). Lentivectors have thus been used to express the Kaposi's sarcoma-associated herpes virus FLICE-like inhibitory protein (vFLIP), a constitutive activator of NF-κB by direct association and activation of NF-κB essential modulator (NEMO) [50-53]. In fact, vFLIP expression has resulted to be a strong adjuvant when expressed in DCs, leading to strong DC maturation and effective CD4 and CD8 T cell responses. Lentivector expression of vFLIP significantly improves anti-tumour activities in a lymphoma mouse model and anti-parasitic efficacy in an OVA-expressing leishmania model [38, 54]. Lentivectors have also been used to inhibit negative regulators of NF-κB activation, such as the ubiquitin ligase A20. Lentivectors have successfully delivered to DCs short hairpin RNAs (shRNAs) targeting A20. The abrogation of A20 expression caused DC maturation, effective CD8 cell responses and inihibition of regulatory T cells (Tregs) [55, 56].

Other molecular activators of mitogen activated protein kinases (MAPKs), activated after TLR engagement, have also been co-expressed in DCs with antigens of interest (Figure 5). MAPKs are mainly divided in three groups, ERK, p38 and JNK. While ERK is associated to survival and immune suppression, p38 and JNK are thought to stimulate DC maturation and inflammation (Figure 5). Constitutive p38 activation was achieved by expressing the MKK6 EE mutant using lentivectors, and it resulted in CD80, CD40 and ICAM-I up-regulation without significant secretion of pro-inflammatory cytokines [17, 40, 41]. A similar result was achieved by JNK1 activation, following expression of the MKK7-JNK1 fusion gene in DCs. Interestingly, although a full DC maturation phenotype was not achieved *ex vivo*, co-expression of these MAPK activators with an OVA-containing transgene or MELAN-A induced significant antigen-specific CD4 and CD8 T cell responses. Moreover, these lentivectors improved survival in a murine tumour model for lymphoma, both with integrating and non-integrating lentivectors [38].

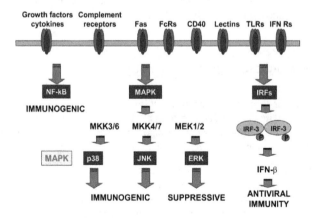

Figure 5. Intracellular signalling pathways regulating DC functions.

Other molecules have been applied for DC maturation. For example, CD40 ligand expression achieved human DC activation and up-regulated the expression of CD83, CD80, MHC-I and induced IL-12 secretion [57]. This strategy increased CD4 and CD8 responses towards influenza epitopes and the TAA gp100. Co-expression of DC-promoting cytokines such as GM-CSF- and IL-4 using lentivectors resulted in long-lasting immunity against melanoma when co-expressed with TAAs Trp-2 and Mart-1 [58].

In this scheme, the main signalling pathways triggered after the engagement of a wide range of receptors on the DC surface (see the indicated receptors embedded in the membrane) with their ligands. Engagement of these receptors starts a complicated cascade of signalling pathways that will converge in a few, well-characterised ones, the NK-κB, MAPKs and interferon regulatory factors (IRFs) (as indicated below the membrane). Some of these pathways, such as NK-κB, MAPKs p38 and JNK1 are pro-inflammatory and lead to DC maturation. Others, such as ERK, are clearly immunosuppressive.

5. Control of DC maturation by inhibiting negative co-stimulation using lentivectors

DC maturation can also up-regulate molecules that provide negative stimulation to T cells, such as programmed cell death receptor ligand 1 (PD-L1) and PD-L2, the ligands for the PD-1 receptor on T cells. Negative co-stimulation is part of a regulatory mechanism that controls the activation state of T cells following antigen presentation [17, 59, 60]. Thus, interference with negative co-stimulation could in principle reinforce T cell activation and enhance cytotoxic activities. Therefore, lentivectors have been used to deliver shRNAs in DC against PD-L1. PD-L1 silencing in antigen-presenting DCs hyperactivated T cells by preventing the up-regulation of Casitas B-lymphoma (Cbl)-b E3 ubiquitin ligase. This strategy co- accelerated anti-tumour immune responses, particularly if combined with a p38 activator or dominant negative mutant of MEK1, the upstream kinase of ERK [17, 59].

6. Lentivectors and cancer immunotherapy

Lentivectors are particularly promising in cancer immunotherapy, for which conventional immunization is largely ineffective due to two major barriers. Firstly, TAAs are generally self-proteins to which there is strong immunological tolerance. Secondly, that tumours are strongly immune-suppressive and they use several mechanisms to avoid immune responses [41].

Lentivectors can be used in cancer immunotherapy in two different ways. In the first one, DCs can be generated *ex vivo* from the patient, followed by lentivector transduction and *in vivo* administration. Thus, cellular vaccination with transduced DCs expressing HLA-Cw3 induced activation and proliferation of CD8 T cells in a mouse model [37]. Similarly, lentivector transduction was shown to be superior to peptide pulsing in inducing OVA-specific T cell responses [61], protected mice from OVA-expressing tumour cells and significantly inhibited tumour growth. The second strategy is direct lentivector vaccination, taking advantage of their intrinsic immuno-stimulatory capacities and their reduced cost [24, 26, 35].

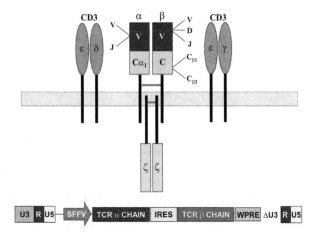

Figure 6. A scheme of the TCR is shown embedded in the cellular membrane. Both α and β chains are shown as indicated, subdivided in variable and constant regions (V, C). The other CD3 chains that associate with the TCR are also included in the figure. On the bottom, a lentivector co-expressing α and β TCR chains is shown, under the control of the spleen focus forming virus promoter (SFFV) and an internal ribosome entry site (IRES) [67]. This particular lentivector is self-inactivating (SIN) and presents a deletion of viral enhancers in the 3' LTR. When this construct is integrated, the 5' LTR disappears and it is replaced with the deleted version.

As mentioned above, a major issue with cancer immunotherapy is that most TAA-specific T cells may have been eliminated during thymic clonal deletion. Thus, even if effective and strong DC maturation is achieved, no effective responses will be achieved due to lack of TAA-specific T cells. To circumvent this, TAA-specific T cells can be generated by lentivector transduction *in vitro*, and adoptively transfered in patients (Figure 6) [62]. Clinical efficacy has been reported for melanoma, synovial cell sarcoma, colorectal, neuroblastoma and lymphoma, but using γ-retrovirus vectors instead of lentivectors [63-66].

T cells are largely refractory to transduction by VSV G-pseudotyped lentivectors, and they require some level of T cell stimulation [67]. Treatment with IL-2 and IL-7 allows lentivector transduction and preserves a functional T cell repertoire [68, 69]. As an example, Wilms tumour antigen (WT1)-specific T cells were generated by lentivector expression of a WT1-specific TCR in the presence of IL-15 and IL-21. These modified T cells were multifunctional and exhibited the expected antigen specificity [67]. This approach of T cell modification is rather promising. In a clinical trial with 15 terminally sick melanoma patients, 2 showed complete regression and long-term survival after transfer of T cells expressing a MART-1-specific TCR using γ-retrovirus vectors [70]. Interestingly, it has been recently demonstrated that entivectors pseudotyped with measles virus H/F glycoproteins effectively transduce quiescent adult T cells in the absence of any exogenous stimulus, whether cytokines or anti-CD3/anti-CD28 stimulation. In fact, transduction with these lentivectors did not affect T cells in any way [17, 71-73].

7. Lentivector gene immunotherapy for the treatment of autoimmune disorders

It is relatively "straightforward" to achieve immune stimulation using lentivectors. However, the induction of immune suppression or tolerance with lentivectors is rather challenging. Nevertheless, the induction and maintenance of immunological tolerance is critical for homeostasis. The organism is permanently and closely in contact with a very wide range of antigens of many origins. A large majority of them are innocuous and do not pose a direct threat. Thus, the immune system must not respond to these antigens, as an immune response is associated with significant collateral tissue damage. The immune system should be activated only if a real threat appears. Therefore, the immune system possesses several tolerogenic mechanisms in place to keep immunological homeostasis. As mentioned before, a key one is clonal deletion of auto-reactive T cells in the thymus [74]. However, there is a significant number of auto-reactive T cells that escape from clonal deletion. Many of them will differentiate towards natural Foxp3 CD4 regulatory T cells [74-77].

In addition to clonal deletion and differentiation of natural Tregs, there are a number of tolerogenic mechanisms in place that regulate immune responses towards peripheral antigens. The organism is in permanent direct contact with many substances and commensal organisms in mucosal areas and in peripheral tissues. In these situations, inducible Tregs differentiate from naïve CD4 T cells after antigen presentation by tolerogenic DCs. These regulatory T cell types are usually classified in Tr1 (CD4 CD25 IL10 or TGF-β) and Th3 (CD4 CD25 Foxp3) cells [78-82]. Therefore, DCs can also be converted in tolerogenic by expression of immunomodulatory genes with lentivectors. This strategy opens up the application of lentivectors for the treatment of autoimmune disorders.

8. Induction of tolerogenic DCs using lentivectors

It is relatively "straightforward" to achieve immune stimulation using lentivectors. However, the induction of immune suppression or tolerance with lentivectors is rather challenging. However, the induction and maintenance of immunological tolerance is critical for homeostasis. The organism is permanently and closely in contact with a very wide range of antigens of many origins. A large majority of them are innocuous and do not pose a direct threat. Thus, the immune system must not respond to these antigens, as an immune response is associated with significant collateral tissue damage. The immune system should be activated only if a real threat appears. Therefore, the immune system possesses several tolerogenic mechanisms in place to keep immunological homeostasis. As mentioned before, a key one is clonal deletion of auto-reactive T cells in the thymus [74]. However, there is a significant number of auto-reactive T cells that escape from clonal deletion. Many of them will differentiate towards natural Foxp3 CD4 regulatory T cells [74-77].

In addition to clonal deletion and differentiation of natural Tregs, there are a number of tolerogenic mechanisms in place that regulate immune responses towards peripheral antigens.

The organism is in permanent direct contact with many substances and commensal organisms in mucosal areas and in peripheral tissues. In these situations, inducible Tregs differentiate from naïve CD4 T cells after antigen presentation by tolerogenic DCs. These regulatory T cell types are usually classified in Tr1 (CD4 CD25 IL10 or TGF-β) and Th3 (CD4 CD25 Foxp3) cells [78-82]. Therefore, DCs can also be converted in tolerogenic by expression of immunomodulatory genes with lentivectors. This strategy opens up the application of lentivectors for the treatment of autoimmune disorders

9. Induction of tolerogenic DCs using lentivectors

DCs can induce immunological tolerance through a number of mechanisms. It is generally accepted that antigen presentation by immature DCs is poorly immunogenic, and results in Treg differentiation, T cell apoptosis and T cell anergy [83-86]. These immature tolerogenic DCs express low levels of co-stimulatory molecules CD80, CD86, CD83, CD40 and MHC molecules [10, 40, 41, 78, 87]. Resident mucosal DCs are intrinsically tolerogenic independently on their maturation phenotype as a consequence of the presence of retinoic-acid [88]. In addition, these DCs become strongly immunosuppressive due to contact with TLR agonists from commensal microbiota [88-90]. DCs can also become strongly immunosuppressive after treatment with lectin ligands or exposure to immunosuppressive cytokines such as IL-10, IL-4 or TGF-β[78, 87, 89-92]. Tolerogenic DCs usually express high levels of these immunosuppressive cytokines, even if they are phenotypically mature [10, 40, 78, 87, 89-93]. In this situation, they provide strong signals 1 and 2 to T cells, together with a simultaneous strong tolerogenic signal 3. For example, in the presence of bioactive TGF-β, strong antigen presentation leads to differentiation to antigen-specific Foxp3 Tregs, while secretion of IL-10 usually results in Tr1 differentiation [91, 93-95].

Tolerogenic DCs can also up-regulate molecules that provide an inhibitory signal to T cells, such as PD-L1 (or B7-H1), a member of the B7 co-stimulatory molecules [17, 96]. PD-L1 expression in DCs regulates T cell activities during antigen presentation and prevents T cell hyperactivation [17]. In addition, PD-L1-CD80 binding on T cells induces antigen-specific Treg differentiation [97]. Other members of the B7 family are immunosuppressive [98]. Immunosuppressive DCs also up-regulate aminoacid-metabolising enzymes, such as arginase or indoleamine 2,3-dioxygenase (IDO) [99-104]. It is thought that these enzymes deplete T cells of essential aminoacids.

Lentivectors can be used to confer tolerogenic activities to DCs by expression of immunoregulatory genes together with antigens of interest. The first strategy that was tested experimental was the expression of potent immunosuppressive cytokines. This approach was used with γ-retroviral vectors for inflammatory diseases [95, 105, 106], 105, 106]. Lentivectors have been applied in an experimental model of asthma by expressing IL-10, leading to expansion of IL-10-expressing Foxp3 Tregs with potent anti-inflammatory properties [107]. Alternatively, small immunosuppressive peptides can also be delivered with lentivectors, such as the vasointestinal peptide (VIP). Intraperitoneal administration of VIP-encoding lentivectors in mice effectively inhibited the development of experimental collagen-induced arthritis. This was achieved by a markedly reduction of pro-inflammatory cytokine secretion and the expansion of Foxp3 Tregs [108]. The administration of genetically modified VIP-expressing DCs also showed significant therapeutic effects in EAE and in the coecal ligation and puncture (CLP) model [109].

DCs can also be reprogrammed by direct modulation tolerogenic signalling pathways within DCs (Figure 5). Therefore, lentivector expression of a constitutively active MEK1 mutant resulted in sustained MAPK ERK phosphorylation, resulting in immunological tolerance [40, 90, 110-114]. These genetically modified DCs exhibit an immature phenotype with low levels of CD40 and secretion of bioactive TGF-β[40, 78]. Antigen presentation by these ERK-activated DCs differentiated antigen-specific Foxp3 Tregs both *ex vivo* and *in vivo* in a mouse model [78]. Direct lentivector vaccination encoding the ERK activator effectively controlled antigen-induced inflammatory arthritis in a mouse model [78].

Similarly, lentivector expression of a constitutively active IRF3 mutant induced high expression levels of IL-10, and expanded antigen-specific Foxp3 Tregs which inhibited immune responses (Figure 5) [40]. Activation of endogenous negative feedback mechanisms of DC maturation pathways has also been applied to induce immune suppression. In this way, by over-expressing the suppressor of cytokine signalling 3 (SOCS-3) in DCs, pro-inflammatory signalling pathways were severly impaired [115]. These genetically modified DCs significantly decreased secretion of pro-inflammatory cytokines IFN-γ, IL-12 and IL-23, and showed an enhanced IL-10 production, which effectively inhibited effectively inhibit experimental autoimmune encephalomyelitis (EAE) in mice [115].

An alternative strategy to generate tolerogenic DCs is the inhibition of pro-inflammatory signalling pathways instead of activating immunosuppressive pathways. As NF-κB is a critical inflammatory signalling pathway, its inhibition in promising for the induction of immunological tolerance [41]. To achieve this, Rel-B was silenced by the delivery of a shRNA targeted to Rel-B [116]. In this way, its inhibition could effectively prevent DC maturation after engagement with TLR ligands, and it was sufficient to treat autoimmune myasthenia gravis in a mouse model [116]. In an analogous manner, lentivectors have also been applied to silence B cell activating factor (BAFF) in the inflamed joint [117, 118], which was very effective for the treatment of experimental collagen-induced arthritis [119] without the need of targeting the arthritogenic antigen. These lentivectors were directly injected in the inflamed joint, where they preferentially transduced resident DCs. BAFF silencing in these DCs inhibited their maturation, and most importantly, inhibited differentiation of pathogenic Th17 [119].

10. Conclussions

Classical immunotherapeutic strategies for the treatment of cancer and infectious diseases rely on either administration of the antigen peptides together with adjuvants, or the inoculation with attenuated strains of pathogenic agents. This approach has been largely successful for the treatment of a wide range of infectious agents. However, for cancer immunotherapy, most potent and targeted immunotherapeutic approaches are required to break the natural tolerance towards TAAs. The targeted co-delivery of immunomodulatory genes with antigens of interests to DCs has opened the application of gene therapy for immunotherapy. Lentivectors exhibit a remarkable transduction capacity of DCs and also T cells, and thus, they are ideal tools to achieve immunodulation. In this way, the immune system can be strongly and specifically activated for the treatment of cancer and infectious diseases, but it can on the other hand be strongly immunosuppressed. This makes it possible the induction of immunological tolerance and treatment of autoimmune disorders.

Acknowledgements

Ines Dufait is funded by an ERASMUS scholarship. Alessio Lanna is funded by an University College London "bench-to-bedside" PhD scholarship. Christopher Bricogne is funded by an University College London MB-PhD scholarship. The Structural Genomics Consortium Oxfod is a registered UK charity (number 1097737) that receives funds from the Canadian Institutes of Health Research, The Canadian Foundation for Innovation, Genome Canada through the Ontario Genomics Insitute, GlaxoSmithKline, Karolinska Institutet, the Knut and Alice Wallenberg Foundations, the Ontario Innovation Trust, the Ontario Ministry for Research and Innovation, Merck & Co., Inc., the Novartis Research Foundation, the Swedish Foundation for Strategic Research and the Wellcome Trust. Karine Breckpot is funded by the Fund for Scientific Research- Flandes. David Escors is funded by an Arthritis Research UK Career Development Fellowship (18433).

Author details

Ines Dufait[1], Therese Liechtenstein[2], Alessio Lanna[2], Roberta Laranga[2], Antonella Padella[2], Christopher Bricogne[3], Frederick Arce[3], Grazyna Kochan[4], Karine Breckpot[1] and David Escors[2*]

*Address all correspondence to: rekades@ucl.ac.uk

1 Department of Physiology–Immunology, Medical School, Free University of Brussels, Belgium

2 Division of Infection and Immunity, Rayne Institute, University College London, United Kingdom

3 UCL Cancer Institute, University College London, United Kingdom

4 Structural Genomics Consortium Oxford, University of Oxford, Old Road Campus Research Building, United Kingdom

References

[1] Escors, D., & Breckpot, K. (2010). Lentiviral Vectors in Gene Therapy: Their Current Status and Future Potential. *Arch Immunol Ther Exp*, 58(2), 107-119.

[2] Vogt, V. M., & Simon, M. N. (1999). Mass determination of rous sarcoma virus virions by scanning transmission electron microscopy. *J Virol*, 73(8), 7050-7055.

[3] Katz, R. A., & Skalka, A. M. (1994). The retroviral enzymes. *Annual review of biochemistry*, 63, 133-173.

[4] Herschhorn, A., & Hizi, A. (2010). Retroviral reverse transcriptases. *Cell Mol Life Sci*, 67(16), 2717-2747.

[5] Charneau, P., Alizon, M., & Clavel, F. (1992). A second origin of DNA plus-strand synthesis is required for optimal human immunodeficiency virus replication. *J Virol*, 66(5), 2814-20.

[6] Naldini, L., Blomer, U., Gage, F. H., Trono, D., & Verma, I. M. (1996). Efficient transfer, integration, and sustained long-term expression of the transgene in adult rat brains injected with a lentiviral vector. *Proc Natl Acad Sci U S A*, 93(21), 11382-11388.

[7] Naldini, L., Blomer, U., Gallay, P., Ory, D., Mulligan, R., Gage, F. H., Verma, I. M., & Trono, D. (1996). In vivo gene delivery and stable transduction of nondividing cells by a lentiviral vector. *Science*, 272(5259), 263-267.

[8] Yee, J. K., Friedmann, T., & Burns, J. C. (1994). Generation of high-titer pseudotyped retroviral vectors with very broad host range. *Methods in cell biology*, 43, Pt A, 99-112.

[9] Breckpot, K., Escors, D., Arce, F., Lopes, L., Karwacz, K., Van Lint, S., Keyaerts, M., & Collins, M. (2010). HIV-1 lentiviral vector immunogenicity is mediated by Toll-like receptor 3 (TLR3) and TLR7. *J. Virol.*, 84, 5627-5636.

[10] Liechtenstein, T., Dufait, I., Lanna, A., Breckpot, K., & Escors, D. (2012). Modulating co-stimulation during antigen presentation to enhance cancer immunotherapy. *Immun., Endoc. & Metab. Agents in Med. Chem.*, 12, 00.

[11] Steinman, R. M., & Bancherau, J. (2007). Taking dendritic cells into medicine. *Nature*, 449(7161), 419-26.

[12] Janeway, C. A., Jr., & Bottomly, K. (1994). Signals and signs for lymphocyte responses. *Cell*, 76(2), 275-85.

[13] Curtsinger, J. M., Johnson, C. M., & Mescher, M. F. (2003). CD8 T cell clonal expansion and development of effector function require prolonged exposure to antigen, costimulation, and signal 3 cytokine. *Journal of immunology*, 171(10), 5165-71.

[14] Curtsinger, J. M., Lins, D. C., & Mescher, M. F. (2003). Signal 3 determines tolerance versus full activation of naive CD8 T cells: dissociating proliferation and development of effector function. *The Journal of experimental medicine*, 197(9), 1141-51.

[15] Curtsinger, J., Lins, D., & Mescher, M. (2003). Signal 3 determines tolerance versus full activation of naive CD8 T cells: dissociating proliferation and development of effector function. *Journal of experimental medicine*, 197, 1141-1151.

[16] Nurieva, R., Thomas, S., Nguyen, T., Martin-Orozco, N., Wang, Y., Kaja, M. K., Yu, X. Z., & Dong, C. (2006). T-cell tolerance or function is determined by combinatorial costimulatory signals. *Embo J.*, 25(11), 2623-2633.

[17] Karwacz, K., Bricogne, C., Macdonald, D., Arce, F., Bennett, C. L., Collins, M., & Escors, D. (2011). PD-L1 co-stimulation contributes to ligand-induced T cell receptor down-modulation on CD8(+) T cells. *EMBO molecular medicine*, 3(10), 581-92.

[18] Curtsinger, J. M., Schmidt, C. S., Mondino, A., Lins, D. C., Kedl, R. M., Jenkins, M. K., & Mescher, M. F. (1999). Inflammatory cytokines provide a third signal for activation of naive CD4+ and CD8+ T cells. *Journal of immunology*, 162(6), 3256-62.

[19] Copreni, E., Castellani, S., Palmieri, L., Penzo, M., & Conese, M. (2008). Involvement of glycosaminoglycans in vesicular stomatitis virus G glycoprotein pseudotyped lentiviral vector-mediated gene transfer into airway epithelial cells. *J Gene Med*, 10(12), 1294-1302.

[20] Burns, J. C., Matsubara, T., Lozinski, G., Yee, J. K., Friedmann, T., Washabaugh, C. H., & Tsonis, P. A. (1994). Pantropic retroviral vector-mediated gene transfer, integration, and expression in cultured newt limb cells. *Developmental biology*, 165(1), 285-289.

[21] Bouard, D., Alazard-Dany, D., & Cosset, F. L. (2009). Viral vectors: from virology to transgene expression. *British journal of pharmacology*, 157(2), 153-165.

[22] Strang, B. L., Ikeda, Y., Cosset, F. L., Collins, M. K., & Takeuchi, Y. (2004). Characterization of HIV-1 vectors with gammaretrovirus envelope glycoproteins produced from stable packaging cells. *Gene Ther*, 11(7), 591-598.

[23] Miller, A. D., Garcia, J. V., von, Suhr. N., Lynch, C. M., Wilson, C., & Eiden, M. V. (1991). Construction and properties of retrovirus packaging cells based on gibbon ape leukemia virus. *J Virol*, 65(5), 2220-2224.

[24] Vanden, Driessche. T., Thorrez, L., Naldini, L., Follenzi, A., Moons, L., Berneman, Z., Collen, D., & Chuah, M. K. (2002). Lentiviral vectors containing the human immunodeficiency virus type-1 central polypurine tract can efficiently transduce nondividing hepatocytes and antigen-presenting cells in vivo. *Blood*, 100(3), 813-22.

[25] Faix, P. H., Feldman, S. A., Overbaugh, J., & Eiden, M. V. (2002). Host range and receptor binding properties of vectors bearing feline leukemia virus subgroup B envelopes can be modulated by envelope sequences outside of the receptor binding domain. *J Virol*, 76(23), 12369-75.

[26] Esslinger, C., Chapatte, L., Finke, D., Miconnet, I., Guillaume, P., Levy, F., & Mac, Donald. H. R. (2003). In vivo administration of a lentiviral vaccine targets DCs and induces efficient CD8(+) T cell responses. *J Clin Invest*, 111(11), 1673-1681.

[27] Collins, M. K., & Cerundolo, V. (2004). Gene therapy meets vaccine development. *Trends Biotechnol*, 22(12), 623-626.

[28] Paludan, C., Schmid, D., Landthaler, M., Vockerodt, M., Kube, D., Tuschl, T., & Munz, C. (2005). Endogenous MHC class II processing of a viral nuclear antigen after autophagy. *Science*, 307(5709), 593-596.

[29] Gregers, T. F., Fleckenstein, B., Vartdal, F., Roepstorff, P., Bakke, O., & Sandlie, I. (2003). MHC class II loading of high or low affinity peptides directed by Ii/peide fusion constructs: implications for T cell activation. *International immunology*, 15(11), 1291-1299.

[30] Rowe, H. M., Lopes, L., Ikeda, Y., Bailey, R., Barde, I., Zenke, M., Chain, B. M., & Collins, M. K. (2006). Immunization with a lentiviral vector stimulates both CD4 and CD8 T cell responses to an ovalbumin transgene. *Mol Ther*, 13(2), 310-9.

[31] Sanderson, S., Frauwirth, K., & Shastri, N. (1995). Expression of endogenous peptide-major histocompatibility complex class II complexes derived from invariant chain-antigen fusion proteins. *Proceedings of the National Academy of Sciences of the United States of America*, 92(16), 7217-7221.

[32] Wu, T. C., Guarnieri, F. G., Staveley-O'Carroll, K. F., Viscidi, R. P., Levitsky, H. I., Hedrick, L., Cho, K. R., August, J. T., & Pardoll, D. M. (1995). Engineering an intracellular pathway for major histocompatibility complex class II presentation of antigens. *Proceedings of the National Academy of Sciences of the United States of America*, 92(25), 11671-11675.

[33] Miller, D. G., & Miller, A. D. (1994). A family of retroviruses that utilize related phosphate transporters for cell entry. *J Virol*, 68(12), 8270-8276.

[34] Lopes, L., Fletcher, K., Ikeda, Y., & Collins, M. (2006). Lentiviral vector expression of tumour antigens in dendritic cells as an immunotherapeutic strategy. *Cancer Immunol Immunother*, 55(8), 1011-1016.

[35] Palmowski, M. J., Lopes, L., Ikeda, Y., Salio, M., Cerundolo, V., & Collins, M. K. (2004). Intravenous injection of a lentiviral vector encoding NY-ESO-1 induces an effective CTL response. *J Immunol*, 172(3), 1582-7.

[36] Christodoulopoulos, I., & Cannon, P. M. (2001). Sequences in the cytoplasmic tail of the gibbon ape leukemia virus envelope protein that prevent its incorporation into lentivirus vectors. *J Virol*, 75(9), 4129-4138.

[37] Rasko, J. E., Battini, J. L., Gottschalk, R. J., Mazo, I., & Miller, A. D. (1999). The RD114/simian type D retrovirus receptor is a neutral amino acid transporter. *Proc Natl Acad Sci U S A*, 96(5), 2129-2134.

[38] Karwacz, K., Mukherjee, S., Apolonia, L., Blundell, M. P., Bouma, G., Escors, D., Collins, M. K., & Thrasher, A. J. (2009). Nonintegrating lentivector vaccines stimulate prolonged T-cell and antibody responses and are effective in tumor therapy. *J Virol*, 83(7), 3094-103.

[39] Goold, H. D., Escors, D., Conlan, T. J., Chakraverty, R., & Bennett, C. L. (2011). Conventional dendritic cells are required for the activation of helper-dependent CD8 T cell responses to a model antigen after cutaneous vaccination with lentiviral vectors. J Immunol, , 186(8), 4565-4572.

[40] Escors, D., Lopes, L., Lin, R., Hiscott, J., Akira, S., Davis, R. J., & Collins, M. K. (2008). Targeting dendritic cell signalling to regulate the response to immunisation. *Blood*, 111(6), 3050-3061.

[41] Breckpot, K., & Escors, D. (2009). Dendritic Cells for Active Anti-cancer Immunotherapy: Targeting Activation Pathways Through Genetic Modification. *Endocrine, metabolic & immune disorders drug targets*, 9, 328-343.

[42] Pasare, C., & Medzhitov, R. (2005). Toll-like receptors: linking innate and adaptive immunity. *Adv Exp Med Biol*, 560, 11-18.

[43] Takeda, K., & Akira, S. (2005). Toll-like receptors in innate immunity. *Int Immunol*, 17(1), 1-14.

[44] Brown, B. D., Sitia, G., Annoni, A., Hauben, E., Sergi, Sergi. L., Zingale, A., Roncarolo, M. G., Guidotti, L. G., & Naldini, L. (2006). In vivo administration of lentiviral vectors triggers a type I interferon response that restricts hepatocyte gene transfer and promotes vector clearance. *Blood*.

[45] Rossetti, M., Gregori, S., Hauben, E., Brown, B. D., Sergi, L. S., Naldini, L., & Roncarolo, M. G. (2011). HIV-1-derived lentiviral vectors directly activate plasmacytoid dendritic cells, which in turn induce the maturation of myeloid dendritic cells. *Hum Gene Ther*, 22(2), 177-188.

[46] Harman, A. N., Wilkinson, J., Bye, C. R., Bosnjak, L., Stern, J. L., Nicholle, M., Lai, J., & Cunningham, A. L. (2006). HIV induces maturation of monocyte-derived dendritic cells and Langerhans cells. *J Immunol*, 177(10), 7103-7113.

[47] Pichlmair, A., Diebold, S. S., Gschmeissner, S., Takeuchi, Y., Ikeda, Y., Collins, M. K., & Reis e Sousa, C. (2007). Tubulovesicular structures within vesicular stomatitis virus G protein-pseudotyped lentiviral vector preparations carry DNA and stimulate antiviral responses via Toll-like receptor 9. *J Virol*, 81(2), 539-47.

[48] Bao, L., Guo, H., Huang, X., Tammana, S., Wong, M., Mc Ivor, R. S., & Zhou, X. (2009). High-titer lentiviral vectors stimulate fetal calf serum-specific human CD4 T-cell responses: implications in human gene therapy. *Gene Ther*, 16(6), 788-795.

[49] Akazawa, T., Shingai, M., Sasai, M., Ebihara, T., Inoue, N., Matsumoto, M., & Seya, T. (2007). Tumor immunotherapy using bone marrow-derived dendritic cells overexpressing Toll-like receptor adaptors. *FEBS Lett*, 581(18), 3334-3340.

[50] Bagneris, C., Ageichik, A. V., Cronin, N., Wallace, B., Collins, M., Boshoff, C., Waksman, G., & Barrett, T. (2008). Crystal structure of a vFlip-IKKgamma complex: insights into viral activation of the IKK signalosome. *Molecular cell*, 30(5), 620-31.

[51] Efklidou, S., Bailey, R., Field, N., Noursadeghi, M., & Collins, M. K. (2008). vFLIP
      from KSHV inhibits anoikis of primary endothelial cells. *J Cell Sci*, 121, Pt 4, 450-7.

[52] Field, N., Low, W., Daniels, M., Howell, S., Daviet, L., Boshoff, C., & Collins, M.
      (2003). KSHV vFLIP binds to IKK-gamma to activate IKK. *J Cell Sci*, 116, Pt 18,
      3721-3728.

[53] Shimizu, A., Baratchian, M., Takeuchi, Y., Escors, D., Macdonald, D., Barrett, T., Bag-
      neris, C., Collins, M., & Noursadeghi, M. (2011). Kaposi's sarcoma-associated herpes-
      virus vFLIP and human T cell lymphotropic virus type 1 Tax oncogenic proteins
      activate IkappaB kinase subunit gamma by different mechanisms independent of the
      physiological cytokine-induced pathways. *J Virol*, 85(14), 7444-8.

[54] Rowe, H. M., Lopes, L., Brown, N., Efklidou, S., Smallie, T., Karrar, S., Kaye, P. M., &
      Collins, M. K. (2009). Expression of vFLIP in a lentiviral vaccine vector activates NF-
      {kappa}B, matures dendritic cells, and increases CD8+ T-cell responses. *J Virol*, 83(4),
      1555-62.

[55] Breckpot, K., Aerts-Toegaert, C., Heirman, C., Peeters, U., Beyaert, R., Aerts, J. L., &
      Thielemans, K. (2009). Attenuated expression of A20 markedly increases the efficacy
      of double-stranded RNA-activated dendritic cells as an anti-cancer vaccine. *J Immu-
      nol, 182* [2], 860-870.

[56] Song, X. T., Evel-Kabler, K., Shen, L., Rollins, L., Huang, X. F., & Chen, S. Y. (2008).
      A20 is an antigen presentation attenuator, and its inhibition overcomes regulatory T
      cell-mediated suppression. *Nat Med, 14* [3], 258-265.

[57] Koya, R. C., Kasahara, N., Favaro, P. M., Lau, R., Ta, H. Q., Weber, J. S., & Stripecke,
      R. (2003). Potent maturation of monocyte-derived dendritic cells after CD40L lentivi-
      ral gene delivery. *J Immunother*, 26(5), 451-60.

[58] Koya, R. C., Kimura, T., Ribas, A., Rozengurt, N., Lawson, G. W., Faure-Kumar, E.,
      Wang, H. J., Herschman, H., Kasahara, N., & Stripecke, R. (2007). Lentiviral vector-
      mediated autonomous differentiation of mouse bone marrow cells into immunologi-
      cally potent dendritic cell vaccines. *Mol Ther*, 15(5), 971-80.

[59] Karwacz, K., Arce, F., Bricogne, C., Kochan, G., & Escors, D. (2012). PD-L1 co-stimu-
      lation, ligand-induced TCR down-modulation and anti-tumor immunotherapy. *On-
      coimmunology*, 1(1), 86-88.

[60] Escors, D., Bricogne, C., Arce, F., Kochan, G., & Karwacz, K. (2011). On the Mecha-
      nism of T cell receptor down-modulation and its physiological significance. *The jour-
      nal of bioscience and medicine*, 1(1).

[61] He, Y., Zhang, J., Mi, Z., Robbins, P., & Falo, L. D., Jr. (2005). Immunization with len-
      tiviral vector-transduced dendritic cells induces strong and long-lasting T cell re-
      sponses and therapeutic immunity. *J Immunol*, 174(6), 3808-17.

[62] Park, T. S., Rosenberg, S. A., & Morgan, R. A. (2011). Treating cancer with genetically
      engineered T cells. *Trends Biotechnol*.

[63] Kochenderfer, J. N., Yu, Z., Frasheri, D., Restifo, N. P., & Rosenberg, S. A. (2010). Adoptive transfer of syngeneic T cells transduced with a chimeric antigen receptor that recognizes murine CD19 can eradicate lymphoma and normal B cells. *Blood*, 116(19), 3875-3886.

[64] Parkhurst, M. R., Yang, J. C., Langan, R. C., Dudley, M. E., Nathan, D. A., Feldman, S. A., Davis, J. L., Morgan, R. A., Merino, M. J., Sherry, R. M., Hughes, M. S., Kammula, U. S., Phan, G. Q., Lim, R. M., Wank, S. A., Restifo, N. P., Robbins, P. F., Laurencot, C. M., & Rosenberg, S. A. (2011). T cells targeting carcinoembryonic antigen can mediate regression of metastatic colorectal cancer but induce severe transient colitis. *Mol Ther*, 19(3), 620-626.

[65] Pule, M. A., Savoldo, B., Myers, G. D., Rossig, C., Russell, H. V., Dotti, G., Huls, M. H., Liu, E., Gee, A. P., Mei, Z., Yvon, E., Weiss, H. L., Liu, H., Rooney, C. M., Heslop, H. E., & Brenner, M. K. (2008). Virus-specific T cells engineered to coexpress tumor-specific receptors: persistence and antitumor activity in individuals with neuroblastoma. *Nat Med*, 14(11), 1264-1270.

[66] Till, B. G., Jensen, M. C., Wang, J., Chen, E. Y., Wood, B. L., Greisman, H. A., Qian, X., James, S. E., Raubitschek, A., Forman, S. J., Gopal, A. K., Pagel, J. M., Lindgren, C. G., Greenberg, P. D., Riddell, S. R., & Press, O. W. (2008). Adoptive immunotherapy for indolent non-Hodgkin lymphoma and mantle cell lymphoma using genetically modified autologous CD 20-specific T cells. *Blood*, 112(6), 2261-2271.

[67] Perro, M., Tsang, J., Xue, S. A., Escors, D., Cesco-Gaspere, M., Pospori, C., Gao, L., Hart, D., Collins, M., Stauss, H., & Morris, E. C. (2010). Generation of multi-functional antigen-specific human T-cells by lentiviral TCR gene transfer. *Gene Ther*, 17, 721-732.

[68] Cavalieri, S., Cazzaniga, S., Geuna, M., Magnani, Z., Bordignon, C., Naldini, L., & Bonini, C. (2003). Human T lymphocytes transduced by lentiviral vectors in the absence of TCR activation maintain an intact immune competence. *Blood*, 102(2), 497-505.

[69] Ducrey-Rundquist, O., Guyader, M., & Trono, D. (2002). Modalities of interleukin-7-induced human immunodeficiency virus permissiveness in quiescent T lymphocytes. *J Virol*, 76(18), 9103-9111.

[70] Morgan, R. A., Dudley, M. E., Wunderlich, J. R., Hughes, M. S., Yang, J. C., Sherry, R. M., Royal, R. E., Topalian, S. L., Kammula, U. S., Restifo, N. P., Zheng, Z., Nahvi, A., de Vries, C. R., Rogers-Freezer, L. J., Mavroukakis, S. A., & Rosenberg, S. A. (2006). Cancer regression in patients after transfer of genetically engineered lymphocytes. *Science* , 314(5796), 126-129.

[71] Frecha, C., Costa, C., Negre, D., Gauthier, E., Russell, S. J., Cosset, F. L., & Verhoeyen, E. (2008). Stable transduction of quiescent T cells without induction of cycle progression by a novel lentiviral vector pseudotyped with measles virus glycoproteins. *Blood*, 112(13), 4843-4852.

[72] Frecha, C., Costa, C., Levy, C., Negre, D., Russell, S. J., Maisner, A., Salles, G., Peng, K. W., Cosset, F. L., & Verhoeyen, E. (2009). Efficient and stable transduction of resting B lymphocytes and primary chronic lymphocyte leukemia cells using measles virus gp displaying lentiviral vectors. *Blood*, 114(15), 3173-3180.

[73] Frecha, C., Levy, C., Cosset, F. L., & Verhoeyen, E. (2010). Advances in the field of lentivector-based transduction of T and B lymphocytes for gene therapy. *Mol Ther*, 18(10), 1748-1757.

[74] Griesemer, A. D., Sorenson, E. C., & Hardy, M. A. (2010). The role of the thymus in tolerance. . Transplantation , 90(5), 465-474.

[75] Hori, S., Nomura, T., & Sakaguchi, S. (2003). Control of regulatory T cell development by the transcription factor Foxp3. *Science*, 299(5609), 1057-1061.

[76] Sakaguchi, S. (2003). The origin of FOXP 3-expressing CD4+ regulatory T cells: thymus or periphery. *J Clin Invest*, 112(9), 1310-1312.

[77] Sakaguchi, S., Yamaguchi, T., Nomura, T., & Ono, M. (2008). Regulatory T cells and immune tolerance. *Cell*, 133(5), 775-787.

[78] Arce, F., Breckpot, K., Stephenson, H., Karwacz, K., Ehrenstein, M. R., Collins, M., & Escors, D. (2011). Selective ERK activation differentiates mouse and human tolerogenic dendritic cells, expands antigen-specific regulatory T cells, and suppresses experimental inflammatory arthritis. *Arthritis and rheumatism*, 63, 84-95.

[79] Mahnke, K., Qian, Y., Knop, J., & Enk, A. H. (2003). Induction of CD4+/CD25+ regulatory T cells by targeting of antigens to immature dendritic cells. *Blood*, 101(12), 4862-9.

[80] O'Garra, A., & Vieira, P. (2004). Regulatory T cells and mechanisms of immune system control. *Nat Med*, 10(8), 801-5.

[81] O'Garra, A., Vieira, P. L., Vieira, P., & Goldfeld, A. E. (2004). IL-10-producing and naturally occurring CD4+ Tregs: limiting collateral damage. *J Clin Invest*, 114(10), 1372-1378.

[82] Peng, Y., Laouar, Y., Li, M. O., Green, E. A., & Flavell, R. A. (2004). TGF-beta regulates in vivo expansion of Foxp3-expressing CD4+CD25+ regulatory T cells responsible for protection against diabetes. *Proc Natl Acad Sci U S A*, 101(13), 4572-4577.

[83] Bonifaz, L., Bonnyay, D., Mahnke, K., Rivera, M., Nussenzweig, M. C., & Steinman, R. M. (2002). Efficient targeting of protein antigen to the dendritic cell receptor DEC-205 in the steady state leads to antigen presentation on major histocompatibility complex class I products and peripheral CD8+ T cell tolerance. *J Exp Med*, 196(12), 1627-38.

[84] Dhodapkar, M. V., & Steinman, R. M. (2002). Antigen-bearing immature dendritic cells induce peptide-specific CD8(+) regulatory T cells in vivo in humans. *Blood*, 100(1), 174-177.

[85] Hawiger, D., Inaba, K., Dorsett, Y., Guo, M., Mahnke, K., Rivera, M., Ravetch, J. V., Steinman, R. M., & Nussenzweig, M. C. (2001). Dendritic cells induce peripheral T cell unresponsiveness under steady state conditions in vivo. *J Exp Med*, 194(6), 769-779.

[86] Kretschmer, K., Apostolou, I., Hawiger, D., Khazaie, K., Nussenzweig, M. C., & von Boehmer, H. (2005). Inducing and expanding regulatory T cell populations by foreign antigen. *Nat Immunol*, 6(12), 1219-27.

[87] Rutella, S., Danese, S., & Leone, G. (2006). Tolerogenic dendritic cells: cytokine modulation comes of age. *Blood*, 108(5), 1435-40.

[88] Manicassamy, S., Ravindran, R., Deng, J., Oluoch, H., Denning, T. L., Kasturi, S. P., Rosenthal, K. M., Evavold, B. D., & Pulendran, B. (2009). Toll-like receptor 2-dependent induction of vitamin A-metabolizing enzymes in dendritic cells promotes T regulatory responses and inhibits autoimmunity. *Nat Med*, 15(4), 401-409.

[89] Ilarregui, J. M., Croci, D. O., Bianco, G. A., Toscano, M. A., Salatino, M., Vermeulen, M. E., Geffner, J. R., & Rabinovich, G. A. (2009). Tolerogenic signals delivered by dendritic cells to T cells through a galectin-1-driven immunoregulatory circuit involving interleukin 27 and interleukin 10. . Nat Immunol , 10(9), 981-991.

[90] Dillon, S., Agrawal, S., Banerjee, K., Letterio, J., Denning, T. L., Oswald-Richter, K., Kasprowicz, D. J., Kellar, K., Pare, J., van Dyke, T., Ziegler, S., Unutmaz, D., & Pulendran, B. (2006). Yeast zymosan, a stimulus for TLR2 and dectin-1, induces regulatory antigen-presenting cells and immunological tolerance. *J Clin Invest*, 116(4), 916-928.

[91] Corinti, S., Albanesi, C., la Sala, A., Pastore, S., & Girolomoni, G. (2001). Regulatory activity of autocrine IL-10 on dendritic cell functions. *J Immunol*, 166(7), 4312-8.

[92] Ghiringhelli, F., Puig, P. E., Roux, S., Parcellier, A., Schmitt, E., Solary, E., Kroemer, G., Martin, F., Chauffert, B., & Zitvogel, L. (2005). Tumor cells convert immature myeloid dendritic cells into TGF-beta-secreting cells inducing CD4+CD25+ regulatory T cell proliferation. *J Exp Med*, 202(7), 919-929.

[93] Saraiva, M., & O'Garra, A. (2010). The regulation of IL-10 production by immune cells. *Nature reviews*, 10(3), 170-181.

[94] Kuhn, R., Lohler, J., Rennick, D., Rajewsky, K., & Muller, W. (1993). Interleukin-10-deficient mice develop chronic enterocolitis. *Cell*, 75(2), 263-274.

[95] Takayama, T., Nishioka, Y., Lu, L., Lotze, M. T., Tahara, H., & Thomson, A. W. (1998). Retroviral delivery of viral interleukin-10 into myeloid dendritic cells markedly inhibits their allostimulatory activity and promotes the induction of T-cell hyporesponsiveness. *Transplantation*, 66(12), 1567-74.

[96] Sakuishi, K., Apetoh, L., Sullivan, J. M., Blazar, B. R., Kuchroo, V. K., & Anderson, A. C. (2010). Targeting Tim-3 and PD-1 pathways to reverse T cell exhaustion and restore anti-tumor immunity. *J Exp Med*, 207(10), 2187-2194.

[97]   Wang, L., Pino-Lagos, K., de Vries, V. C., Guleria, I., Sayegh, M. H., & Noelle, R. J. (2008). Programmed death 1 ligand signaling regulates the generation of adaptive Foxp3+CD4+ regulatory T cells. *Proc Natl Acad Sci U S A*, 105(27), 9331-9336.

[98]   Sica, G. L., Choi, I. H., Zhu, G., Tamada, K., Wang, S. D., Tamura, H., Chapoval, A. I., Flies, D. B., Bajorath, J., & Chen, L. (2003). B7-H4, a molecule of the B7 family, negatively regulates T cell immunity. *Immunity*, 18(6), 849-861.

[99]   Belladonna, M. L., Orabona, C., Grohmann, U., & Puccetti, P. (2009). TGF-beta and kynurenines as the key to infectious tolerance. *Trends in molecular medicine*, 15(2), 41-9.

[100]   Cobbold, S. P., Adams, E., Farquhar, C. A., Nolan, K. F., Howie, D., Lui, K. O., Fairchild, P. J., Mellor, A. L., Ron, D., & Waldmann, H. (2009). Infectious tolerance via the consumption of essential amino acids and mTOR signaling. *Proc Natl Acad Sci U S A*, 106(29), 12055-12060.

[101]   Fallarino, F., Vacca, C., Orabona, C., Belladonna, M. L., Bianchi, R., Marshall, B., Keskin, D. B., Mellor, A. L., Fioretti, M. C., Grohmann, U., & Puccetti, P. (2002). Functional expression of indoleamine 2,3-dioxygenase by murine CD8 alpha(+) dendritic cells. *Int Immunol*, 14(1), 65-68.

[102]   Mellor, A. L., & Munn, D. H. (2004). IDO expression by dendritic cells: tolerance and tryptophan catabolism. *Nature reviews*, 4(10), 762-74.

[103]   Munder, M. (2009). Arginase: an emerging key player in the mammalian immune system. *British journal of pharmacology*, 158(3), 638-651.

[104]   Norian, L. A., Rodriguez, P. C., O'Mara, L. A., Zabaleta, J., Ochoa, A. C., Cella, M., & Allen, P. M. (2009). Tumor-infiltrating regulatory dendritic cells inhibit CD8+ T cell function via L-arginine metabolism. *Cancer Res*, 69(7), 3086-3094.

[105]   Lee, W. C., Zhong, C., Qian, S., Wan, Y., Gauldie, J., Mi, Z., Robbins, P. D., Thomson, A. W., & Lu, L. (1998). Phenotype, function, and in vivo migration and survival of allogeneic dendritic cell progenitors genetically engineered to express TGF-beta. *Transplantation*, 66(12), 1810-1817.

[106]   Morita, Y., Yang, J., Gupta, R., Shimizu, K., Shelden, E. A., Endres, J., Mule, J. J., Mc Donagh, K. T., & Fox, D. A. (2001). Dendritic cells genetically engineered to express IL-4 inhibit murine collagen-induced arthritis. *J Clin Invest*, 107(10), 1275-1284.

[107]   Henry, E., Desmet, C. J., Garze, V., Fievez, L., Bedoret, D., Heirman, C., Faisca, P., Jaspar, F. J., Gosset, P., Jacquet, A. P., Desmecht, D., Thielemans, K., Lekeux, P., Moser, M., & Bureau, F. (2008). Dendritic cells genetically engineered to express IL-10 induce long-lasting antigen-specific tolerance in experimental asthma. *J Immunol*, 181(10), 7230-7242.

[108]   Delgado, M., Toscano, M. G., Benabdellah, K., Cobo, M., O'Valle, F., Gonzalez-Rey, E., & Martin, F. (2008). In vivo delivery of lentiviral vectors expressing vasoactive in-

testinal peptide complementary DNA as gene therapy for collagen-induced arthritis. *Arthritis and rheumatism*, 58(4), 1026-1037.

[109] Toscano, M. G., Delgado, M., Kong, W., Martin, F., Skarica, M., & Ganea, D. (2010). Dendritic cells transduced with lentiviral vectors expressing VIP differentiate into VIP-secreting tolerogenic-like DCs. *Mol Ther*, , 18(5), 1035-1045.

[110] Agrawal, A., Dillon, S., Denning, T. L., & Pulendran, B. (2006). ERK1-/- mice exhibit Th1 cell polarization and increased susceptibility to experimental autoimmune encephalomyelitis. *J Immunol*, 176(10), 5788-5796.

[111] Anastasaki, C., Estep, A. L., Marais, R., Rauen, K. A., & Patton, E. E. (2009). Kinase-activating and kinase-impaired cardio-facio-cutaneous syndrome alleles have activity during zebrafish development and are sensitive to small molecule inhibitors. *Human molecular genetics*, 18(14), 2543-2554.

[112] Caparros, E., Munoz, P., Sierra-Filardi, E., Serrano-Gomez, D., Puig-Kroger, A., Rodriguez-Fernandez, J. L., Mellado, M., Sancho, J., Zubiaur, M., & Corbi, A. L. (2006). DC-SIGN ligation on dendritic cells results in ERK and PI3K activation and modulates cytokine production. *Blood*, 107(10), 3950-3958.

[113] Pages, G., Brunet, A., L'Allemain, G., & Pouyssegur, J. (1994). Constitutive mutant and putative regulatory serine phosphorylation site of mammalian MAP kinase kinase (MEK1). *Embo J*, 13(13), 3003-3010.

[114] Raingeaud, J., Whitmarsh, A. J., Barrett, T., Derijard, B., & Davis, R. J. (1996). MKK3- and MKK6-regulated gene expression is mediated by the 38 mitogen-activated protein kinase signal transduction pathway. *Mol Cell Biol*, 16(3), 1247-1255.

[115] Li, Y., Chu, N., Rostami, A., & Zhang, G. X. (2006). Dendritic cells transduced with SOCS-3 exhibit a tolerogenic/DC2 phenotype that directs type 2 Th cell differentiation in vitro and in vivo. *J Immunol*, 177(3), 1679-88.

[116] Zhang, Y., Yang, H., Xiao, B., Wu, M., Zhou, W., Li, J., Li, G., & Christadoss, P. (2009). Dendritic cells transduced with lentiviral-mediated RelB-specific ShRNAs inhibit the development of experimental autoimmune myasthenia gravis. *Molecular immunology*, 46(4), 657-667.

[117] Yang, M., Sun, L., Wang, S., Ko, K. H., Xu, H., Zheng, B. J., Cao, X., & Lu, L. (2010). Novel function of B cell-activating factor in the induction of IL-10-producing regulatory B cells. . J Immunol , 184(7), 3321-3325.

[118] Batten, M., Groom, J., Cachero, T. G., Qian, F., Schneider, P., Tschopp, J., Browning, J. L., & Mackay, F. (2000). BAFF mediates survival of peripheral immature B lymphocytes. *J Exp Med*, 192(10), 1453-1466.

[119] Lai, Kwan., Lam, Q., King, Hung., Ko, O., Zheng, B. J., & Lu, L. (2008). Local BAFF gene silencing suppresses Th17-cell generation and ameliorates autoimmune arthritis. *Proc Natl Acad Sci U S A*, 105(39), 14993-14998.

Chapter 7

Targeted Lentiviral Vectors: Current Applications and Future Potential

Cleo Goyvaerts, Therese Liechtenstein,
Christopher Bricogne, David Escors and
Karine Breckpot

Additional information is available at the end of the chapter

1. Introduction

About two decades ago recombinant human immunodeficiency virus type 1 (HIV-1) was proposed as a blueprint for the development of lentiviral vectors (LVs) (Naldini, Blomer et al. 1996). Lentiviral vectors exhibit several characteristics that make them favorable tools for gene therapy, including sustained gene delivery through vector integration, transduction of both dividing and non-dividing cells, applicability to different target cell types, absence of expression of viral proteins after transduction, delivery of complex genetic elements, low genotoxicity and the relative ease of vector manipulation and production (Cattoglio, Facchini et al. 2007; Bauer, Dao et al. 2008). This is reflected in the numerous applications such as: transgene (tg) overexpression (Lopez-Ornelas, Mejia-Castillo et al. 2011), persistent gene silencing (Wang, Hu et al. 2012), immunization (Breckpot, Emeagi et al. 2008), generation of transgenic animals (Baup, Fraga et al. 2010), *in vivo* imaging (Roet, Eggers et al. 2012), induction of pluripotent cells, stem cell modification (Sanchez-Danes, Consiglio et al. 2012), lineage tracking and site-directed gene editing (Lombardo, Genovese et al. 2007) as well as many applications targeting cancer cells (Petrigliano, Virk et al. 2009).

Recombinant LVs can be derived from primate as well as non-primate lentiviruses such as HIV-1 and simian immunodeficiency virus (SIV) next to the equine infectious anemia virus, caprine arthritis-encephalitis virus, maedi-visna virus, feline immunodeficiency virus (FIV) and bovine immunodeficiency virus respectively (Escors and Breckpot 2010). They are all members of the *Retroviridae* family with 'retro' referring to their capacity to retro-transcribe their diploid single stranded (ss) RNA genome into a double stranded (ds) DNA copy that is integrated in the genome of the infected host cell (Figure 1A). Since LVs are most often derived from HIV-1, the generation of recombinant LVs has been accompanied by several safety concerns such as the generation of replication-competent lentiviruses (RCLs). Another potential biosafety concern is the induction of insertional mutagenesis, a major genotoxic problem that emerged in gene therapy clinical trials using their γ-retroviral counterparts (Manilla, Rebello et al. 2005). Generally, LVs are produced by transiently transfecting HEK 293 or 293T cells with plasmids encoding structural and functional sequences, imperative for proper LV particle generation. Over the last decades, vector development has largely focused on the design of these plasmids. Firstly, only critical viral structural and functional sequences are provided and secondly, these sequences are divided over a certain number of individual plasmids either in *cis* (encoded by the LV) or *trans* (packaged as a protein within the LV particle), with a minimal overlap between viral sequences. This led to a LV production procedure where at least three different plasmids are used: (1) a packaging plasmid which provides all viral structural and enzymatic sequences (encoded by *gag* and *pol*) in *trans* to generate a functional particle, (2) a transfer plasmid providing the expression cassette in *cis*, cloned into the non-coding remains of the original lentiviral genome (Figure 1B, adapted from (Delenda 2004)) including a packaging signal and the two long terminal repeats (LTRs) of which the promoter activity has been deleted from the 3' LTR and (3) an envelope plasmid encoding an envelope glycoprotein (gp) consisting of a transmembranary domain (TM) and a receptor-binding domain (SU) that determines the LVs' tropism (Figure 1A).

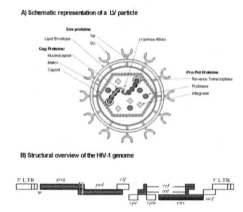

Figure 1. Schematic representation of an HIV-1 particle (A) and its genome (B). The diploid ssRNA genome of HIV-1 is stabilized by structural nucleocapsid proteins and together with the enzymatic proteins reverse transcriptase, protease and integrase packaged in a nucleocapsid structure, which in turn is enclosed by capsid proteins. This nucleocapsid is surrounded by a matrix protein layer and a producer cell derived phospholipid bilayer in which the envelope proteins consisting of an SU and TM part, are embedded (A). All proviral genes (*gag, pol, pro, vif, vpr, vpu, ref, tat, env* en *nef*) are flanked by two identical LTRs that consist of three regions: U3, R and U5. Within the U3 region, all proviral transcriptional control elements are situated such as the promoter and several enhancer sequences. Ψ represents the packaging signal. At the 3' end of the pol gene the central polypurine tract (red) and central termination sequence (green) are located. Both ensure the formation of a triple stranded DNA flap, crucial for nuclear entry of the pre-integration complex in non-dividing cells (B).

Besides this division over different plasmids, other important construct optimization steps have been implemented. While in the first generation LV packaging plasmids the entire *gag* and pol genes were encoded together with all accessory regulatory and virulence genes, the second generation was multiply attenuated by removal of the four virulence genes, but not the regulatory genes *tat* and *rev* (Zufferey, Nagy et al. 1997). In the third generation, the *rev* gene is expressed from a separate plasmid and the *tat* gene is removed by insertion of a strong constitutive promoter replacing the U3 region in the 5' LTR of the transfer plasmid (Dull, Zufferey et al. 1998). A major improvement was achieved with the development of SIN or self-inactivating LVs where a deletion in the U3 region of the 3' LTR of the transfer plasmid abolished the production of full-length vector RNA in transduced cells. This not only minimizes the risk for RCLs, but also reduces the chance that the viral LTR enhancers interfere with the expression cassette, which minimizes aberrant expression of adjacent cellular coding regions. Subsequently these and many other optimization steps paved the way towards a more effective and safer version of the lentiviral gene delivery vehicle (Romano, Claudio et al. 2003).

In addition to packaging and transfer plasmid optimization, also the envelope plasmid was modified by replacing the natural HIV-1 envelope gp with an alternative gp gene, most often the gp of vesicular stomatitis virus (VSV.G). This concept is called pseudotyping and VSV.G endowed the LV particle with an increased stability and broad cellular tropism (to most if not all mammalian cells). However, it became clear that for numerous *in vivo* applications, a broad tropism may not be desirable. First, the tg that is encoded could be toxic to many cell types, *e.g.* pro-apoptotic or suicide genes, so a stringent control over the induction of tg expression in time and/or place is a necessity (Uch, Gerolami et al. 2003; Seo, Kim et al. 2009). A second point of concern is the risk for insertional mutagenesis; the more cells get infected, the higher this risk becomes. Although it has been demonstrated that LVs intrinsically exhibit low genotoxicity, clonal expansion and dominance of transduced hematopoietic progenitors have been reported in a clinical trial in which hematopoietic stem cells were genetically modified with a LV that expressed the β-globin gene for treatment of β-thalassemia (Fehse and Roeder 2008; Cavazzana-Calvo, Payen et al. 2010). Thirdly, while a broad tropism LV is favorable in antitumor immunotherapy to efficiently transduce antigen-presenting cells (APCs) which can induce an antigen specific immune response (Palmowski, Lopes et al. 2004), this is not desirable when a genetic disorder has to be restored as in this case the tg may not become an immunological target (Annoni, Battaglia et al. 2007). Finally, during production of pantropic viruses encoding oncogenes, narrow tropism vectors would be more valuable due to biosafety level handling requirements and safety issues (Barrilleaux and Knoepfler 2011). Therefore, in view of safety as well as applicability aspects, four main targeting strategies can be brought forward: targeted gene expression or transcriptional targeting, targeted gene translation or microRNA based (de)targeting, targeted infection or transductional targeting, and targeted integration of the proviral DNA.

2. Transcriptional targeting

Most often a strong constitutive promoter with or without enhancer sequences is used to drive the LV encoded tg. These include the cytomegalovirus (CMV), spleen focus forming virus (SFFV), human polypeptide chain elongation factor-1alpha (EF-1alpha), phosphogly-cerate kinase (PGK) and ubiquitin C promoters (Kim, Kim et al. 2007; Gilham, Lie et al. 2010; Li, Husic et al. 2010). Although these promoters generally induce strong and ubiquitous expression of the tg, they present some disadvantages. A first drawback is that they are more prone to promoter inactivation than cell-specific promoters. In addition, they are more potent in terms of activating the host-cell defense machinery and increasing the long-distance effects of insertional mutagenesis caused by their enhancer sequences (Liu, Wang et al. 2004; Stein, Ott et al. 2010; Singhal, Deng et al. 2011). These downsides resulted in the development of various strategies to allow cell-specific tg expression by incorporating cell type specific regulatory elements and/or promoter(s) in the expression cassette of the LV. Because of the availability of a large number of endogenous cellular promoters, targeted expression can be achieved to potentially any cell type or tissue. In addition, its advantage over unselective expression has been demonstrated in numerous studies (Di Nunzio, Maruggi et al. 2008; Kerns, Ryu et al. 2010; Cao, Sodhi et al. 2011). This is exemplified by a study where LV encoding iduronidase under the control of the hepatocyte specific albumin gene promoter was injected intravenously to treat mucopolysaccharidosis type I. While the same LV with a CMV promoter resulted in the induction of an immune response that diminished the tg expression over time, the albumin gene promoter enabled stable and prolonged tg expression with a partial correction of the pathology (Di Domenico, Di Napoli et al. 2006). In addition to hepatocyte specific targeting, an ever-growing list of cell-type specific promoters has been used for the specific expression in tissues such as the erythroid lineage, endothelial cells, myocardial cells, retinal cells, B cells, epidermal, hematopoietic stem cells, *etcetera* (Hanawa, Persons et al. 2002; De Palma, Venneri et al. 2003; Semple-Rowland, Eccles et al. 2007; Di Nunzio, Maruggi et al. 2008; Leuci, Gammaitoni et al. 2009; Kerns, Ryu et al. 2010; Semple-Rowland, Coggin et al. 2010; Cao, Sodhi et al. 2011; Lee, Fan et al. 2011; Friedrich, Nopora et al. 2012).

Besides the advantage of increased and prolonged expression levels when expressed in the target cell of choice, targeted expression can also be a necessity when the tg causes undesirable damage in non-target cells. For the treatment of Mpl-deficient aplastic anemia, for example, targeted transfer to hematopoietic stem cells is inevitable since ectopic Mpl expression causes lethal adverse reactions (Heckl, Wicke et al. 2011). The same holds true for toxin, pro-apoptotic or suicide gene encoding LVs used in anti-tumor therapy (Zheng, Chen et al. 2003; Hsieh, Chen et al. 2011). LVs are excellent candidates to modulate the tumor and its environment since they transduce both dividing cells such as most cancer cells but also non- or very slowly dividing cells such as cancer stem cells. Furthermore LVs are able to integrate in the genome of transduced cells, potentially generating clonal populations of genetically modi-fied cancer cells, which may then spread throughout the tumor mass (Steffens, Tebbets et al. 2004). Vector targeting can be attempted by local vector delivery, although this raises practical concerns for non-solid and metastatic tumor cells. Consequently, systemic delivery of a targeted LVs and subsequent exclusive tg expression in cancer cells is the ultimate goal. Metastatic prostate cancer, for example, has been transcriptionally targeted in various ways (1) using a prostate-specific antigen (PSA) promoter to drive the expression of diphtheria toxin A, (2) using the prostate-stem cell antigen (PSCA) promoter to drive the expression of the Herpes Simplex Virus thymidine kinase (HSV-TK) suicide gene, or (3) combining the prostate-specific promoter ARR2PB and a short DNA sequence in the 5'-untranslated region that is recognized by the translation initiation factor eIF4E, often overexpressed in malignant cells, to drive the expression of the HSV-TK suicide gene (Yu, Chen et al. 2001; Zheng, Chen et al. 2003; Yu, Scott et al. 2006; Kimura, Koya et al. 2007; Petrigliano, Virk et al. 2009). Additionally, the tumor vasculature has been transcriptionally targeted using the endothelial specific Tie2 promoter to drive the conditionally toxic nitroreductase and subsequently diminish tumor growth (De Palma, Venneri et al. 2003). Another cancer cell type specific targeting strategy to limit tg expression to hepatocarcinoma was applied by Uch et al. They constructed a LV expressing HSV-TK under the control of the rat alpha-fetoprotein promoter elements (Uch, Gerolami et al. 2003). Besides cancer cell type specific strategies, also more generalized cancer targeting strategies have been developed. For example, as the human telomerase reverse transcriptase (hTERT) is expressed in most malignant tumors, its promoter has been used to drive the expression of the cytosine deaminase gene together with a green fluorescent protein (GFP) reporter gene. It was demonstrated that hTERT-positive tumors could be visualized after intratumoral injection of the LV in tumor-bearing nude mice and, more importantly, that significant tumor growth suppression was observed after delivery of the pro-drug 5-fluorocytosine (Yu, Li et al. 2011). Besides avoidance of toxic tg expression in a non-tumor cell, tumor specific gene therapy is also interesting for targeted imaging. For example, the use of the chimeric promoter EIIAPA containing the alpha-fetoprotein promoter and hepatitis B virus enhancer II was used to control the downstream expression of luciferase genes to subsequently assay the selective transcriptional activity by bioluminescence imaging (Hsieh, Chen et al. 2011).

As LVs efficiently infect non-dividing cells, they provide suitable platforms for tg delivery to multiple mammalian neuronal cell types. It has been shown that stereotactic injection of LVs in the brain parenchyma leads to transduction of the striatum, hippocampus and thalamus (Watson, Kobinger et al. 2002). Moreover, transcriptional targeting has proven to be a reliable technique to unravel the complexity of the nervous system by neuron and brain specific assessment of the effects of therapeutic proteins and RNA interference, or to investigate neuronal gene expression (Hioki, Kameda et al. 2007; Gascon, Paez-Gomez et al. 2008; Kuroda, Kutner et al. 2008; Peviani, Kurosaki et al. 2012). Regulatory sequences of rat neuron specific enolase, human glial fibrillary acidic protein and myelin basic protein have already been exploited to obtain LV-mediated selective gene targeting of neurons, astrocytes and oligodendrocytes, respectively (Jakobsson, Ericson et al. 2003; McIver, Lee et al. 2005). This has led to applications like subregional tg expression in the hippocampus using the hybrid hEF1alfa/HTLV promoter or neuron specific synapsin I promoter or targeting the central serotonergic neurons using a two-step transcriptional amplification strategy co-expressing the tryptophan hydroxylase-2 gene promoter with the chimeric enhancer GAL4/p65 (Kuroda, Kutner et al. 2008; Benzekhroufa, Liu et al. 2009). Next to the central nervous system, Bendotti et al. recently focused on selective tg expression in mouse spinal cord motor neurons using motor neuron specific regulatory sequences derived from the promoter of the homeobox gene Hb9 (Benzekhroufa, Liu et al. 2009; Peviani, Kurosaki et al. 2012). However, neuron specific gene expression is not always very efficient and therefore several groups have attempted to improve the endogenous promoters using extra enhancers or artificial transcriptional activators such as the bidirectional promoter. For the latter, Liu et al. based their bidirectional promoter on the transcriptional activity of the human synapsin-1 promoter and the compact glial fibrillary acidic protein (GfaABC1D) promoter. In the opposite orientation, a minimal core promoter of 65 basepairs (bp) derived from the CMV promoter was joined upstream of both promoters, which were flanked with two gene expression cassettes. The 5′ cassette transcribed the artificial transcriptional activator while the downstream cassette drove the expression of the gene of interest (Liu, Paton et al. 2008).

To fulfill the high expectations of gene therapy, both efficient delivery and sustained expression of the therapeutic gene are essential requirements. However, one of the major barriers to stable gene transfer by LVs is the development of innate and adaptive immune responses to the delivery vector and the transferred therapeutic tg. It became clear that *in vivo* administered broad tropism LVs efficiently transduce APCs and that these play a major role in the induction of tg specific immune responses (Annoni, Battaglia et al. 2007; Vandendriessche, Thorrez et al. 2007). Consequently transcriptional targeting can be applied to avoid tg expression in APCs. Brown et al. demonstrated stable GFP production by modified cells *in vivo* when tg expression was prevented in APCs (Brown, Venneri et al. 2006). Another study combined the hepatocyte specific enhanced transthyretin promoter with an APC-detargeting microRNA strategy, and showed the induction of GFP-specific regulatory T cells and the promotion of immunological tolerance (Annoni, Brown et al. 2009). Moreover, Matrai et al. demonstrated that hepatocyte-targeted expression by an integrase-defective LV (IDLV) induced tolerance to coagulation factor IX with prevention of the induction of neutralizing antibodies in mice (Matrai, Cantore et al. 2011). In contrast to gene therapy, immunotherapy pursuits the induction of a tg-specific immune response where APC-specific transduction is imperative. Therefore, LVs that drive tg expression *via* an APC-specific promoter have been developed. For instance Cui et al. used the HLA-DR promoter to target human MHC class II+ cells like dendritic cells (DCs, CD83+) and macrophages (CD14+). They demonstrated the induction of an allogeneic T cell response *in vitro* (Cui, Golob et al. 2002). The dectin-2 promoter was used to target the expression of the human melanoma antigen NY-ESO-1 to murine APCs. After intravenous injection of the targeted LVs, selective tg expression in dectin-2+ splenic myeloid and plasmacytoid DCs as well as in F4/80+ macrophages was reported. Furthermore CD11c+ draining lymph node residing DCs were targeted after subcutaneous injection which resulted in strong NY-ESO-1 specific CD8+ and CD4+ T cell responses (Lopes, Dewannieux et al. 2008). On the other hand, DC-induced tg specific tolerance has also been achieved after the use of a DC-specific promoter. When LVs carrying a CD11c promoter were used to make DC-specific transgenic mice by injecting the purified virus into the perivitelline space of single-cell embryos, the tg became an autologous antigen to which immunological tolerance was induced. Furthermore, this tg was only expressed in CD11c⁺ cells derived from the spleen, lymph nodes as well as the thymus (Zhang, Zou et al. 2009). Dresch et al. made use of the DC-STAMP promoter to engineer bone marrow-targeted LVs. Therefore, *ex vivo* transduced hematopoietic stem cells (HSC) were injected in lethally irradiated mice to make HSC chimeric animals (Dresch, Edelmann et al. 2008). When GFP expression was analyzed in the leukocyte population isolated from the spleen, the main DC subpopulations such as CD11b⁻CD8⁺ DCs, CD11b⁺CD8⁻ DCs, and plasmacytoid DCs were GFP positive next to a small percentage of CD11c⁻CD11b⁺ monocytes. Furthermore, tg expression could only be detected in CD11c⁺ cells in the thymus. While the previous two tolerance inducing studies could be explained by the fact that undifferentiated DC precursors were transduced, Kimura et al. intravenously injected LVs encoding Trp2 driven by the MHCII promoter and also observed persistent tg expression selectively in the CD11c, CD11b and CD19⁺ MHCII⁺ cells of the spleen without CD8⁺ T cell responses against Trp2 in contrast to a CMV carrying construct (Kimura, Koya et al. 2007; Dresch, Edelmann et al. 2008). The induction of tolerance in this study might be explained by the activation status of the transduced APCs. Induction of tg specific effector T cells requires fully activated APCs. Since, DC activation by LVs was shown to be dose-dependent, the LV titers used in these studies could explain the tolerogenic instead of stimulatory outcome (Breckpot, Emeagi et al. 2007; Breckpot, Escors et al. 2010).

Finally, also controllable or inducible tg expression can be a prerequisite. Reasons to use tg regulation are: to maintain appropriate levels of a gene product within the therapeutic range, to modulate, stop or resume tg expression in response to disease evolution, or in response to an endogenous molecule as *e.g.* the secretion of insulin induced by hyperglycemia. For human gene therapy, several ligand dependent transcription regulatory systems have been developed. For clinical applications, such systems need to be safe, specific, highly inducible, reversible and only show dose dependent activation with low basal activity while their ligands need to be bioavailable and low in immunogenicity (Toniatti, Bujard et al. 2004). One of the first and most widely used ligands is Tetracylin (Tet) or its more potent analog Doxycycline (Dox) (Efrat, Fusco-DeMane et al. 1995; Reiser, Lai et al. 2000). In contrast to the bacterial lac repressor/operator or the Cre-loxP recombinase system, it is applicable *in vivo* and reversible (Deuschle, Hipskind et al. 1990; Lakso, Sauer et al. 1992). The original bacterial Tet system is based on a Tet repressor protein (TetR) that inhibits the expression of the bacterial Tet resistance genes by binding to cognate operator sequences (TetO) in their regulatory regions. Upon the addition of Tet, the repressor is inactivated by allosteric change, allowing gene transcription (Gossen and Bujard 1992). The artificial Tet-off system is based on the generation of a hybrid transactivator (tTA) by fusion of the TetR to the transcription activation domain of the HSV VP16 protein. This fusion product will bind and activate transcription at promoters that include TetO while the presence of Dox impairs this binding, resulting in the shut off of gene expression (Furth, St Onge et al. 1994) (Figure 2A, adapted from (Ramezani and Hawley 2002). In contrast, the reverse Tet transactivator (rtTA), generated by random mutagenesis of tTA, requires Dox to bind to cognate operator sequences and activate transcription resulting in the inducible Tet-on system (Figure 2B).

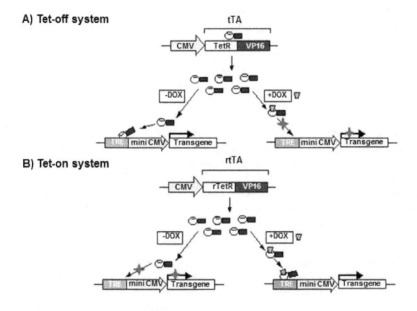

Figure 2. Representation of the artificial Tet-off (A) and Tet-on system (B). While the Dox binding transactivator (tTA) binds to the tetracycline-responsive promoter element (TRE) and stimulates tg transcription in the absence of Dox(A), the mutant reverse Tet-controlled transactivator (rtTA) binds to the TRE in the presence of Dox and stimulates transcription(B).

However, the *in vivo* applicability of the Tet system remained limited due to leakiness and insufficient induction levels. Therefore the Tet-on system has been optimized *e.g.* by isolating novel rtTA variants and incorporating a Dox-dependent trans-silencer called tTS which consists of the KRAB (Kruppel-Associated Box) trans-repressing domain of the human Kid-1 protein fused to the wild type TetR. This tTS has been used by the group of Szulc et al. to develop a LV-based conditional gene expression system for drug-controllable expression of inhibitory short hairpin RNAs (shRNAs), and reported on a robust and versatile system that governed the tight control over the tg expression both *in vitro* as well as *in vivo* among others to generate transgenic mice (Szulc, Wiznerowicz et al. 2006). Moreover, Dox is orally bioavailable, has a half-life of 14-22 hrs and has an excellent tissue penetration. Therefore numerous groups have used both the Tet-on and Tet-off system within LV-based gene reporter and therapeutic applications (Blomer, Naldini et al. 1997; Bahi, Boyer et al. 2004; Blesch, Conner et al. 2005; Liu, Wang et al. 2008; Hioki, Kuramoto et al. 2009; Adriani, Boyer et al. 2010). This is exemplified by a study of Seo et al. who developed an oncolytic LV-mediated Tet-on inducible system based on co-transduction of two LVs to drive the expression of a pro-apoptotic gene by the promoter of matrix-metalloproteinase-2 (MMP-2), which is highly expressed in several cancer cell lines. The first LV expressed a rtTA under the control of the MMP-2 promoter, whereas the second LV expressed the pro-apoptotic gene Bax, under the control of the tetracycline-responsive element (Seo, Kim et al. 2009). While most Dox inducible systems are based on the co-transduction of two LVs, all-in-one vectors have also been described recently (Ogueta, Yao et al. 2001; Barde, Zanta-Boussif et al. 2006; Herold, van den Brandt et al. 2008; Wiederschain, Wee et al. 2009; Benabdellah, Cobo et al. 2011). Furthermore, an extra Dox-regulated system based on the original TetR protein was developed in 1998. It serves as an alternative to the tTA- and rtTA-based systems because the latter were accompanied by secondary effects due to expression of the transactivator domains. Benabdellah et al. made use of the Dox-responsive cassette driving the expression of eGFP and the SFFV promoter expressing high amounts of the TetR protein in an all-in one vector system. This LV efficiently produced Dox-regulated cell lines, including primary human fibroblasts and human mesenchymal stem cells. However, a major concern using Dox remains the possibility to develop resistance to the antibioticum Tet, and although it seems a non-immunogenic system in several mouse strains, studies with intramuscularly delivered Tet-on activators in non-human primates did elicit a cellular and humoral response (Latta-Mahieu, Rolland et al. 2002).

Besides the Tet on/off systems, a plethora of inducible systems has been examined both *in vitro* and *in vivo*. An interesting strategy is based on the use of small molecules with distinct binding surfaces for two different polypeptides to modulate the activity of dimerizer-regulated systems. The prototype molecule is rapamycin, which mediates the heterodimer formation between two molecules (FK506-binding protein and FKBP rapamycin binding) that are coupled to a DNA binding domain (DBD) and transcription activation domain (AD) respectively (Pollock, Issner et al. 2000). The rapamycin inducible system has low basal activity because of the physical separation of the DBD and AD molecules, the ligand has a short half-life of about 4.5 hrs although the induced gene expression lasts for days due to the strong stability of the DBD-AD assembled complex (Toniatti, Bujard et al. 2004). Tian et al. used a variant of this system to engineer LVs that produce a fusion protein between the furin-cleavable proinsulin and the self-dimerization mutant of FK506-binding protein to yield bioactive insulin in keratinocytes. Epidermal keratinocytes in culture, in stratified bioengineered epidermis as well as implanted in diabetic athymic mice released insulin within maximally 1 hr after addition of rapamycin. Secretion slowed or stopped within 2-3 hrs after removal of the inducing agent. Even in diabetic animals with severe hyperglycemia, decreased serum glucose levels to normal levels were reported (Tian, Lei et al. 2008). The major disadvantage of this technique is the immunosuppressing activity of rapamycin and the only partial oral availability, which renders this system impractical for clinical applications.

Another strategy is based on the fact that heterologous proteins can be made hormone responsive by fusing them with the hormone-binding domain of steroid receptors. The best-characterized system is regulated by mifepristone or RU486, a synthetic progesterone antagonist. Prototypically the RU486-binding chimera known as GeneSwitch® consists of the

GAL4 DBD from *Saccharomyces cerevisiae* fused to the ligand-binding domain of a mutant progesterone receptor and the activation domain of the p65 subunit of human NF-κB (Abruzzese, Godin et al. 2000; Sirin and Park 2003). Upon ligand binding the GeneSwitch® protein binds to GAL4 upstream activating sequences in the promoter driving the expression of the tg of interest. An advantage of the GeneSwitch® system is that the majority of its components are modified human proteins with no impact on cell viability. Furthermore, usage of a mifepristone-inducible (auto-inducible) promoter to regulate expression of the chimeric transactivator dramatically reduced basal expression of the tg in the absence of the inducer, thereby improving the dynamic range of *in vivo* tg regulation (Shinoda, Hieda et al. 2009). In addition, although mifepristone has anti-progesterone and -glucocorticoid activities, the concentration needed for ligand-inducible transactivation of the target gene is much lower than the concentration producing an anti-progesterone effect in humans. However, it is thought that the lower dosage may still affect the ovarian cycle and exert a contraceptive activity. Therefore the search for other inducers that are unable to interact with endogenous progesterone would be more appropriate for clinical use (Sarkar 2002). As an alternative steroid-receptor based inducible system, the glucocorticosteroid responsive element (GRE5) was cloned into a LV (LV-GRE-IL10) encoding interleukin-10 (IL-10). Expression of IL-10 by LV-GRE-IL-10 appeared rapidly, was sustained and inducible in both ovine and human corneas in the presence of dexamethasone (Parker, Brereton et al. 2009). Another alternative can be the steroid hormone ecdysone, which plays a fundamental role during insect molting and metamorphosis. Ecdysteroids are considered safe because they are found in large amounts as phytoecdysteroids in vegetables, present in the human diet without detrimental effects. Mouse hematopoietic progenitors transduced with LVs containing an ecdysone-regulated GFP expression cassette efficiently turned GFP expression on and off in transplanted animals with low basal activity (Xu, Mizuguchi et al. 2003; Galimi, Saez et al. 2005). Possibly, several other systems will be developed to control tg expression after LV transduction. Potential systems could be based on the cell-cell communication quorum sensing process (Neddermann, Gargioli et al. 2003) or the naturally evolved mechanisms of antibiotic resistance to pristinamycin, a composite streptogramin antibiotic or erythromycin, a member of the macrolide antibiotics (Fussenegger, Morris et al. 2000; Roberts 2002).

3. microRNA detargeting

Recently, the concept of microRNA (miRNA) mediated post-transcriptional tg regulation was introduced in LV-based targeting. miRNAs are 21-22 nucleotide long non-coding fragments which are partially or extensively complementary to an endogenous mRNA molecule (Lai 2002). In mammals, over 400 different miRNAs have been identified so far, most of which are well conserved among species ranging from plants, worms, insects to humans (Brown and Naldini 2009). Some of these miRNAs are expressed ubiquitously whereas others are only expressed at certain developmental stages or in a certain cell type. Upon binding of a miRNA molecule to its complementary target sequence, repression of translation or direct destruction of the mRNA is induced. The detailed mechanisms involved in this post-transcriptional regulation process, do not lie within the scope of this book chapter but are reviewed elsewhere (Nelson, Kiriakidou et al. 2003; Bartel 2004). A brief description together with a schematic representation is depicted in Figure 3 (adapted from http://www.micro-rna.ic.cz/mirna4.html).

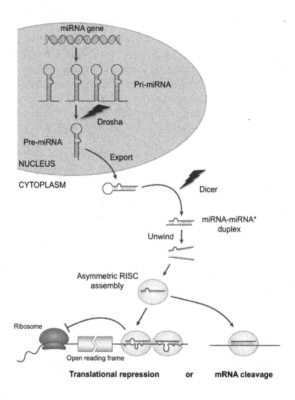

Figure 3. miRNA-based post-transcriptional gene silencing. Briefly, endogenous miRNA genes are transcribed by RNA polymerase II to pri-miRNA precursor molecules in the nucleus. These are processed to pre-miRNA by a specialized enzymatic pathway called Pasha/Drosha and will release the pre-miRNA in short hairpin RNA (shRNA). Then, these pre-miRNAs are exported to the cytoplasm where Dicer degrades most of the shRNA, leaving a miRNA duplex which is loaded onto the AGO complex (Argonaut), forming the preRISC (RNA Interference Silencing Complex). Subsequently the miRNA strand is degraded, leaving its complementary miRNA intact within the RISC complex. Then, this complex scans mRNAs and when complementation is found, the mRNA is degraded or the poly-A tail is removed, leading to mRNA destabilization or stalled mRNA translation.

In order to limit undesired vector tg expression, LVs encoding target sequences of endogenous miRNAs have been developed. By incorporating at the 3 'UTR region of the expression cassette one or more copies of a sequence that is perfectly complementary to a miRNA (miRNA tagging), the transgenic mRNA will be degraded or repressed in cells where the complementary miRNA is expressed. This new way of controlling tg expression at the level of the mRNA product came as a complementary strategy to transcriptional targeting since the latter is associated with some disadvantages such as: (1) difficulty to identify and faithfully reconstitute a gene's promoter; (2) for integrating LVs, promoters and enhancers can be trapped, leading to aberrant expression (De Palma, Montini et al. 2005), (3) transcription can be promiscuous and (4) only few genes have truly cell-specific transcriptional patterns while several promoters are active in many different cell types or states. Moreover, as miRNAs regulate expression at the post-transcriptional level, copy number and vector integration site have no appreciable effect on their regulation, which ensures consistent control throughout the transduced cell population.

Successful outcomes of LV-based gene therapy have long been precluded by the development of tg-specific immunity as a consequence of the direct expression of the tg product by professional APCs. Therefore Brown et al. challenged mice with LVs encoding a target sequence for miRNA-142-3p, a microRNA specifically expressed in the hematopoietic lineages. Upon injection, they demonstrated a 100-fold suppression of reporter gene expression in intravascular and extravascular hematopoietic lineages, including APCs (Brown, Venneri et al. 2006). One year later, its usefulness was evidenced by the miRNA-142-3p regulated LV mediated stable correction of hemophilia B in mice (Brown, Cantore et al. 2007). Its expression leads to reduced tg expression in APCs and subsequently lower anti-tg immune responses. Moreover it was demonstrated that *in vivo* delivery of this post-transcriptionally regulated LV induced tg-specific Foxp3$^+$ regulatory CD4$^+$ T cells, which promoted immunologic tolerance (Annoni, Brown et al. 2009). Curiously, they also reported the necessity of a hepatocyte specific promoter for this immunological tolerance. So, these studies showed the impressive potential of miRNA-based detargeting to overcome a major hurdle for clinical gene therapy, however also other factors than tg expression in APCs seem to influence the immunological outcome of a gene transfer procedure. Examples are the type of vector used, the tissue targeted and the presence of inflammation (Brown and Lillicrap 2002; Cao, Furlan-Freguia et al. 2007).

Another reason to pursue stringent tg regulation, is to express the tg in a specific developmental state. Brown et al. showed that multiple endogenous miRNAs can be used to achieve tg expression patterns that rapidly adjust and sharply discriminate among the myeloid and lymphoid lineage in therapeutically relevant HSCs and their progeny with miRNA-223, or among immature and mature APCs using miRNA-155 (Brown, Gentner et al. 2007). Another example is provided by Gentner et al. who used the miRNA-126 target sequence to detarget tg expression from stem cells and progenitors from the hematopoietic cell lineage in order to avoid expression of the highly toxic GALC in these stages, while inducing GALC expression in mature cells from the hematopoietic lineage to correct globoid cell leukodystrophy (Gentner, Visigalli et al. 2010). Furthermore the group of Sachdeva et al. used miRNA-292 regulated LVs to visualize and segregate differentiating neural progenitors in pluripotent cultures and demonstrated that miRNA-regulated vectors allow a potentially broad use on stem cell applications (Sachdeva, Jonsson et al. 2010). Finally, Sadelain et al. used LVs that encode antigen specific receptors together with target sites for miRNA-181a to suppress the expression of the receptor in late thymocytes. This avoided clonal deletion of antigen specific T cells in

the thymus and subsequent challenge with antigen expressing tumors did not result in tumor growth (Papapetrou, Kovalovsky et al. 2009).

Furthermore this technology is useful as a mechanism to increase vector safety and efficacy
by limiting the expression of a toxic or pro-apoptotic tg to certain target cells. For example
Lachmann et al. used the miRNA-150 target sequence to suppress GFP expression in lymphocytes and thereby prevented tg-induced lymphotoxicity (Lachmann, Jagielska et al.
2011). On the other hand unrestrained growth of transduced cells could also be avoided using miRNA-based detargeting when growth-promoting gens are replaced (Hawley, Fong et
al. 1998). Moreover, miRNA-based regulation could be desirable when targeted gene expression is needed to assess the contribution of a particular cell type to physiological processes
or for the development of new therapeutic strategies. This is exemplified by the work of Colin et al. who segregated tg expression between neurons and astrocytes following injection
into the brain by exploiting the activity of miRNA-124 (Colin, Faideau et al. 2009). Another
miRNA-based targeting strategy developed a few years ago was the concept of miRNA
sponges, decoys, erasers, antagomirs or knockdowns (Ebert, Neilson et al. 2007; Scherr, Venturini et al. 2007; Gentner, Schira et al. 2009). Therefore vectors expressing miRNA target
sites can effectively saturate an endogenous miRNA and prevent it from regulating its natural targets. This technology enables a new way of investigating miRNA biology and has already been used to study the role of miRNAs in cancer, cardiac function and hematopoiesis
(Scherr, Venturini et al. 2007; Bonci, Coppola et al. 2008; Kumar, Erkeland et al. 2008; Sayed,
Rane et al. 2008; Gentner, Schira et al. 2009; Valastyan, Reinhardt et al. 2009).

A possible concern of miRNA-based detargeting is whether sufficient target knockdown can
be achieved for specific applications without escape mutants arising (Kelly, Hadac et al.
2008). In addition, it is highly likely that overexpression of the synthetic target sites will saturate their corresponding endogenous miRNAs and deregulate expression of natural targets
with deleterious consequences. However, the latter has not been reported so far (Brown,
Gentner et al. 2007). Moreover, miRNA-based regulation is a very robust system since at low
copy vector number miRNA regulation of tg expression remains effective. Apparently,
when a threshold miRNA concentration is present, the tg will be suppressed. This robustness can probably be explained by the perfect complementarity of the target sequence and
the endogenous miRNA sequence. Indeed, when imperfectly complementary sites were
used, this did result in a detectable decrease in target suppression, although only at very
high vector copy numbers. So, although it should be recognized that the knowledge regarding miRNA biology and function is still limited, this strategy holds great potential to carefully move towards clinical translation (Brown and Naldini 2009)

4. Transductional targeting

Although the strategies described above demonstrate cell-specific gene expression, they often require broad tropism LVs which does not reduce the risk for RCL formation or insertional mutagenesis. Therefore transductional targeting of LVs seems a more interesting

strategy to tackle both safety and efficacy concerns. The concept of swapping the viral envelope proteins of different viral species is called pseudotyping. Already in 1979, the envelope
glycoprotein of the avian retrovirus was used to pseudotype VSV virions in order to selectively enrich for VSV temperature-sensitive mutants of VSV.G biosynthesis (Lodish and
Weiss 1979). Later it was shown that wild type HIV-1 particles which were produced in cells
that were infected with another virus, *e.g.* murine leukemia virus (MLV) or VSV, led to the
generation of phenotypically mixed virions with an expanded host range (Canivet, Hoffman
et al. 1990; Zhu, Chen et al. 1990). These observations introduced the concept of pseudotyping and in the early 90's the gp160 sequence of a replication defective HIV-1 derived LV was
replaced by a MLV gp (Page, Landau et al. 1990). Later on the natural envelope gp from an
MLV-based vector was replaced with the viral attachment protein of VSV (Emi, Friedmann
et al. 1991; Burns, Friedmann et al. 1993). Today, most synthetic LVs are pseudotyped with a
heterologous envelope protein to increase their stability, infectivity and safety. Notably, the
first LVs were not pseudotyped but displayed the native HIV-1 envelope protein at their
surface. This limited their tropism to CD4-expressing cells (Dropulic 2011). Interestingly,
VSV.G pseudotyped vectors are more stable than their natural counterparts. This allows
concentration to higher titers by ultracentrifugation and confers broad tropism, as VSV.G
binds to a still unknown ubiquitous membrane component (Cronin, Zhang et al. 2005). This
superior transduction efficiency comes in handy for the treatment of genetic disorders such
as β-thalassemia and X-linked adenoleukodystrophy (Cartier, Hacein-Bey-Abina et al. 2009;
Cavazzana-Calvo, Payen et al. 2010). Nonetheless, VSV.G pseudotyped LVs also present
several downsides. Firstly, the VSV gp is cytotoxic when expressed constitutively at high
concentrations, which impedes the production of stable packaging cell lines (Lopes, Dewannieux et al. 2011). In addition, cytotoxicity associated with VSV.G pseudotyped LVs has
been observed when *in vivo* administered at high concentration, in comparison with other
pseudotypes (Watson, Kobinger et al. 2002). Another critical hurdle for systemic delivery using VSV.G pseudotyped LVs is their susceptibility to neutralization by human serum complement, although this can be bypassed by polyethylene glycol-modification (PEGylation) of
the virions (DePolo, Reed et al. 2000; Croyle, Callahan et al. 2004).

An ever-growing list of alternative pantropic as well as ecotropic naturally occurring gps
has been evaluated for LV pseudotyping. These vary in origin, tropism, titer, stability, efficiency of packaging, inactivation by complement, efficiency of cell transduction and induction of an immune response (Cronin, Zhang et al. 2005). They can be of retroviral origin such
as those from T-lymphotropic virus, maedi-visna virus, MLV, feline endogenous retrovirus
and gibbon ape leukemia virus (GALV) (Rasko, Battini et al. 1999; Stitz, Buchholz et al. 2000;
Zeilfelder and Bosch 2001; Strang, Ikeda et al. 2004; Sakuma, De Ravin et al. 2010). In general, LVs pseudotyped with a γ-retroviral envelope transduce CD34[+] hematopoetic precursors,
a property that has been used for the correction of X-linked severe combined immunodeficiency (SCID) using the GALV or MLV-A envelopes (Cavazzana-Calvo, Hacein-Bey et al.
2000; Gaspar, Parsley et al. 2004). Nonetheless, envelope gps of numerous non-retroviral
families have been used as well to pseudotype LVs. A first example is provided by the *Toga-
viridae* family, where their envelope gps (from alphaviruses such as the Ross River virus)
equips the LV with a mouse and human DC-specific tropism when injected intravenously

(Strang, Takeuchi et al. 2005), and with an astrocyte and oligodendrocyte specific tropism when injected into the mouse brain (Kang, Stein et al. 2002). Another example is provided by the family of the *Baculoviridae* where the gp64 gp ensures high particle stability in addition to a hepatocyte specific tropism (Matsui, Hegadorn et al. 2011). LVs pseudotyped with the lymphocytic choriomeningitis virus (LCMV) envelope from the *Arenaviridae* preferentially transduce cells from the central nervous system such as neural stem cells and progenitor cells, and also to glioma cells and insulin secreting β-cells (Kobinger, Deng et al. 2004; Miletic, Fischer et al. 2004; Stein, Martins et al. 2005). As there is an increasing interest in the development of gene therapeutic strategies for malignant gliomas, the most frequent primary brain tumors with very poor prognosis, several groups report on the use of LCMV gp pseudotyped LVs to target almost exclusively astrocytes, the main source of malignant glioma cells (Beyer, Westphal et al. 2002; Miletic, Fischer et al. 2004; Steffens, Tebbets et al. 2004). The H and F envelope proteins from the *Paramyxoviridae* family, such as those derived from measles viruses, provide LVs with the capacity to bind to SLAM and CD46, which confers efficient virus entry, nuclear transport and integration in non-activated B and T lymphocytes. This property is particularly important, since primary unstimulated B and T cells are generally difficult to transduce if not pre-treated to induce progression through the cell cycle (*e.g.* through stimulation with anti-CD3/anti-CD28 antibodies or cytokines) (Frecha, Levy et al. 2010; Frecha, Levy et al. 2011). To transduce airway epithelial cells efficiently, envelope proteins from several viruses that infect respiratory tissues or cells have been evaluated. For efficient transduction of unconditioned airway epithelial cells from the apical side, envelopes derived from the ebola virus (*Filoviridae*), members of the *Paramyxoviridae* such as the respiratory syncytial (RSV) and sendai viruses, and members of the *Orthomyxoviridae* such as the influenza and fowl plaque viruses have been evaluated (Kobinger, Weiner et al. 2001; Nefkens, Garcia et al. 2007; Mitomo, Griesenbach et al. 2010). Surprisingly, it has been reported that the S protein of the severe acute respiratory syndrome-associated coronavirus (*Coronaviridae*) mediates entry into hepatoma cell lines (Hofmann, Hattermann et al. 2004). Finally, although the vesicular stomatitis, mokola and rabies virus are all derived from the *Rhabdoviridae* family, only LVs pseudotyped with the rabies-G envelope enable retrograde transport to motoneurons of the spinal cord upon intramuscular injection or to the thalamus upon striatal injection. In contrast, VSV.G displaying LVs transduce cells only locally while mokola-pseudotyped LVs preferentially target non-neuronal glial cells (Mazarakis, Azzouz et al. 2001; Azzouz, Ralph et al. 2004; Wong, Azzouz et al. 2004; Colin, Faideau et al. 2009; Calame, Cachafeiro et al. 2011).

Although the use of an existing viral envelope gp seems the most straightforward way to pseudotype LVs, a natural variant with the desired delivery properties is not available for every therapeutic application. Moreover, natural gps can come with limitations such as sensitivity to neutralization by the host immune response, lack of specificity and/or insufficient transduction efficiency. Also their production and purification can be inefficient (Schaffer, Koerber et al. 2008). Therefore, the development of LVs with customized, user-defined gene delivery properties by molecular engineering of the envelope gps is an alternative strategy to retarget the LV to specific cell-surface receptors. This molecular engineering has become a collective term for many different strategies, which will be described below.

A first strategy to alter the tropism of a virally derived gp is by rational point and domain mutagenesis. This is exemplified by the DC-specific targeting strategy from Yang et al. Certain subsets of DCs carry the DC-SIGN protein (also known as CD209) on their surface, which is a C-type lectin-like receptor that potentiates rapid binding and endocytosis of materials. The sindbis virus envelope gp consists of two integral membrane gps that form a heterodimer and function as one unit. The fusogenic monomer is E1 and needs binding *via* E2 to mediate low pH-dependent fusion. The latter binds to the DC-SIGN receptor, next to the canonical viral receptor heparin sulfate, expressed by many cell types. Since both protein binding sites are physically separated, selective mutation at the E2 monomer is possible, abrogating the heparin sulfate binding part while leaving the DC-SIGN binding part intact. By pseudotyping a LV with this mutated sindbis virus derived envelope gp, targeted infection of DCs *in vivo* after direct subcutaneous administration was achieved. Moreover, this elicited a strong antigen-specific immune response (Yang, Yang et al. 2008; Hu, Dai et al. 2010). Another example is the substitution of the V3-loop region of the SIV envelope gp with the corresponding region of a T cell tropic HIV-1 to create a T-cell targeted MLV vector, pseudotyped with this engineered SIV gp (Steidl, Stitz et al. 2002). A final example is provided by Dylla et al. who diminished the alfa-dystroglycan affinity of the LCMV WE45 strain envelope gp by a point mutation. When a FIV derived LV was pseudotyped with this point mutated LCMV gp, their intravenous injection in adult mice yielded low transduction efficiencies in hepatocytes in contrast to abundant liver and cardiomyocyte transduction with the wild type LCMV gp pseudotyped FIVs (Dylla, Xie et al. 2011).

Apart from genetic alterations, chemical modifications can also alter LV tropism. PEGylation of VSV.G pseudotyped LVs is one such example where the LVs' tropism is not altered. Nevertheless, chemical modifications can lead to targeted gene delivery vehicles, for example by tagging the MLV vector with galactose to selectively transduce human hepatoma cell lines expressing asialo-gp receptors specific for oligosaccharides with terminal galactose residues (Neda, Wu et al. 1991). Furthermore, Morizono et al. reported the production of LVs pseudotyped with sindbis virus gps in the presence of deoxymannojirimycin. This modification altered the structures of N-glycans from complex to high mannose structures as it inhibits mannosidase. This led to DC-SIGN specific binding although the gps were genetically modified to prevent interaction with DC-SIGN (Morizono, Ku et al. 2010). Furthermore it was demonstrated that binding of sindbis virus gp to DCs is directly related to the amount of high-mannose structures on the gp (Tai, Froelich et al. 2011). Unfortunately, the effectiveness of the chemically modified particles strongly depends on the reaction conditions of the applied modifications.

Other chimeric envelope gps can be generated by covalently fusing a short peptide, a ligand or an antibody to an envelope gp. The advantages of short peptides are that they don't severely disrupt the original envelope gps' function and that *via* high-throughput library approaches, targeted peptides with strong binding affinity and unlimited specificity within the context of a particular gp can be generated (Schaffer, Koerber et al. 2008). However, they can hinder multimerisation of capsid monomers, create fusion products with lower thermostability and hinder proper intracellular trafficking of the gp during viral production. The latter is exemplified by the blockage in trafficking in the producer cells to the plasma membrane of VSV.G when linked to a collagen-binding motif (Guibinga, Hall et al. 2004). Different kinds of ligands such as cytokines and growth factors have been linked to the amino-terminal region or receptor-binding domain of the envelope gp, most often derived of MLV. This is amongst others exemplified by fusion of the MLV gp to hepatocyte growth factor to target the LV to hepatocytes (Nguyen, Pages et al. 1998), or to the insulin-like growth factor (IGF-I) (Chadwick, Morling et al. 1999). Interestingly, these ligands can elevate the transduction efficiency by altering the targets' physiological state. When the fusion product of the MLV gp and IL-2 is used to pseudotype LVs, a 34-fold higher infection efficiency was observed of quiescent IL-2 receptor expressing cells compared to LVs pseudotyped with the wild type MLV gp. This was explained by IL-2 induced activation of the cell cycle from the otherwise barely transducible quiescent cells (Maurice, Mazur et al. 1999). However, a very low to unobservable transduction profile is often reported which can be attributed to sequestration of the LV particles at the target cell surface, directing the viral particle to a degradation pathway after endocytosis and/or inability of the fusion product to trigger a conformational change essential for viral fusion and subsequent infection (Lavillette, Russell et al. 2001; Katane, Takao et al. 2002). In addition to peptides and ligands, also antibodies and their derivatives can be used. In general, single chain variable fragments or scFvs offer higher specificity than short peptides but as they are larger in size, the chance that they disrupt the process of conformational changes of the gp to mediate membrane fusion increases. Therefore scFvs are most often linked to a spacer peptide that permits proper conformation of both the scFv domain and the envelope gp as exemplified by the fusion of the MLV gp to a scFv against MHC class I (Karavanas, Marin et al. 2002). For LV targeting to APCs, several attempts have been made to couple an anti-MHC class II scFv to an ecotropic gp such as MLV or VSV.G (Dreja and Piechaczyk 2006; Gennari, Lopes et al. 2009). Recently, the use of DARPins or designed ankyrin repeat proteins has been reported. These can be fused to the H protein of measles virus for example and then be co-displayed with the fusogenic F protein on the surface of the LV. The advantage is that DARPins can be selected to become high-affinity binders to any kind of target molecule thus this seems a promising alternative to scFvs for retargeting LVs (Munch, Muhlebach et al. 2011). So, in general, the use of chimeric envelope proteins for LV targeting has proven to offer tremendous opportunities but at the same time to be a challenge as the function of chimeric gps is often severely compromised which leads to a very inefficient transduction profile (Fielding, Maurice et al. 1998; Dreja and Piechaczyk 2006; Waehler, Russell et al. 2007; Buchholz, Duerner et al. 2008).

Several solutions have been created to circumvent the problems associated with the formation of conformational dysfunctional fusion products. One solution is the inclusion of a protease cleavable peptide between the gp and the ligand. This is certainly an interesting strategy for the targeting of tumor cells, as they secrete MMP, which degrade the extracellular matrix to metastasize. By linking a proline-rich hinge and an MMP cleavage site to the fusion product of a scFv recognizing carcinoembryonic antigen (CEA) and the MLV gp, selective targeting of CEA-positive cells after *in vivo* injection of producer cells at the tumor site was observed (Chowdhury, Chester et al. 2004). Taking this hinge region idea one step further, the concept of 'molecular bridges' was introduced where a bispecific linker molecule recognizes both the viral gp as well as the molecular determinant on the target cell. This concept is based on a bridging system that was introduced more than 20 years ago and where three different linker molecules were involved: two biotinylated antibodies that bound the MLV gp and MHC class I or II proteins on the target cells respectively, and a bridging streptavidin molecule linking both antibodies. This led to the generation of a MLV that was capable of transducing MHC class I and II expressing cells (Roux, Jeanteur et al. 1989). Subsequently, two-protein molecular bridges have been exploited based on the avidin-biotin system. A recent example is provided by O'Leary et al. who used a detoxified recombinant form of the full-length botulinum neurotoxin, fused to core streptavidin that for its part was coupled to a biotinylated LV. This envelope gp construct endowed the LV particle with considerable neuron selectivity *in vitro* as well as *in vivo* after injection into the trachea (O'Leary, Ovsepian et al. 2011). Nowadays, alternative linkers such as ligand-receptor, chemical conjugations and monoclonal antibodies have been exploited to retarget LVs as well (Roux, Jeanteur et al. 1989; Boerger, Snitkovsky et al. 1999). For the latter, the E2 protein of the sindbis gp has been modified to contain the Fc-binding domain (ZZ domain) of protein A, making it possible to bind to a monoclonal antibody specific for a target molecule *via* its Fab antigen recognition end (Morizono, Xie et al. 2005). However, doubts are raised about the affinity of the adaptor-virus complex, as this may not be sufficient to prevent dissociation within the patient's blood. Moreover, complexity ascends as both the virion as the adaptor must be produced, purified and fully characterized for clinical approval. Another alternative possibility is to co-display a chimeric envelope gp together with a wild type gp such as VSV.G to enhance the transduction efficiency (Maurice, Verhoeyen et al. 2002; Verhoeyen, Dardalhon et al. 2003; Verhoeyen, Wiznerowicz et al. 2005). However, this had also limited success due to partial loss of targeting specificity. Therefore, a final alternative is the usage of a mutated fusogenic but binding-defective envelope gp to mediate fusion upon binding by the chimeric gp. The group of Lin et al. co-expressed the MLV gp fused to soluble Fms-like tyrosine kinase 3 (Flt3)-ligand together with a binding-defective influenza hemagglutinin protein from the fowl plague virus rostock 34 (HAmu). When LVs were pseudotyped with both of these gps, Flt3-targeted transduction was enhanced when compared to LVs without HAmu and could be competed away by the addition of soluble Flt3-ligand (Lin, Kasahara et al. 2001). Another more straightforward strategy is the use of the E1/E2 heterodimer gp of sindbis virus as the fusion and binding functions are already separated over two different monomers. By mutating the binding E2 monomer, its binding property can be completely abolished. Therefore, this binding defective E2 protein forms an ideal scaffold for cell-specific antibody conjugation to confer specific tropism to an endless list of cell types such as P-gp-expressing melanoma progenitor cells and endothelial cells (Morizono, Xie et al. 2005; Pariente, Mao et al. 2008). A drawback is that they only induce fusion upon low pH. Therefore alternatives were explored such as the H and F protein of the measles virus, which induce fusion without the need for endocytosis (Earp, Delos et al. 2005; Funke, Schneider et al. 2009). This is exemplified by a study were a binding defective form of the H protein was fused to a CD20 specific scFv to pseudotype LVs. When these LVs were used to kill cells in culture, they selectively killed the CD20+ human lymphocytes in co-culture with CD20- cells. This demonstrated the ability of these LVs to exclusively transfer a potentially hazardous therapeutic protein into targeted cell populations with virtual absence of background transduction in non-target cells (Funke, Maisner et al. 2008). Meanwhile, a broad variety of surface antigens has been successfully targeted using this strategy (Blechacz and Russell 2008)

A fourth strategy to target LVs is based on two concepts: (1) the separation of binding and fusion functions over two distinct envelope molecules and (2) the ability of LVs to incorporate host cell proteins into their envelope as they bud from the plasmamembrane of their producer cells (Chandrashekran, Gordon et al. 2004; Kueng, Leb et al. 2007). Chandrashekran et al. reported on efficient and specific targeting to human cells expressing stem cell factor (SCF) receptor (c-kit) by an ecotropic gp pseudotyped LV which also displayed surface SCF. Another example is the overexpression of the HIV-1 derived primary receptor CD4 and fusogenic co-receptor CXCR4 or CCR5 on the membrane of producer cells. From these cells, LVs were generated that infect HIV-1 envelope gp expressing cells next to cells infected with HIV-1, enabling the development of novel antiviral therapy approaches (Somia, Miyoshi et al. 2000). Since the transduction efficiency was relatively low, LV co-enveloped with the HIV-1 cellular receptor CD4 and the E2 protein from sindbis virus were created. These turned out to have a higher infectivity level than in the former strategy (Lee, Dang et al. 2011). In another study the binding defective but fusogenic E1/E2 heterodimer was used to be co-displayed with a separate membrane bound anti-CD20 antibody in order to transduce exclusively CD20+ B cells (Lei, Joo et al. 2009). Today, numerous examples are found that apply this principle to target the following: immunoglobulin-expressing B cells, CD3+ T cells and CD117+ HSCs (Ziegler, Yang et al. 2008; Froelich, Ziegler et al. 2009; Yang, Joo et al. 2009). However, clinical applications with LVs displaying scFvs are hampered by lack of stability, size and immunogenicity leading to the development of neutralizing antibodies. To solve these problems, we developed the Nanobody (Nb) display technology (Goyvaerts, De Groeve et al. 2012). In this strategy, a fusogenic but binding-defective form of VSV.G (VSV.GS) (Zhang, Kutner et al. 2010) is co-displayed with a surface bound form of a cell-specific Nb to confer target binding (Figure 4). Some twenty years ago, Hamers-Casterman et al. discovered that part of the humoral response of Camelids is based on a unique repertoire of antibodies, which only consisted of two heavy chains (Hamers-Casterman, Atarhouch et al. 1993). The antigen binding part of these antibodies is composed of only one single variable region, termed VHH or Nb. These Nbs have unique characteristics and offer many advantages over scFvs to target LVs to specific cell types. These include (1) they are highly soluble, (2) they can refold after denaturation whilst retaining their binding capacity, (3) cloning and selection of antigen-specific Nbs obviate the need for construction and screening of large libraries, (4) as Nbs can be fused to other proteins, it is possible to present them on the cell membrane of a producer cell line, thus generating LVs that incorporate a cell-specific Nb in their envelope during budding. Using the Nb display technology, we demonstrated production of stable Nb pseudotyped LV stocks at high titers with a DC subtype specific transduction profile both *in vitro* as well as *in vivo* (Goyvaerts, De Groeve et al. 2012). As ligand specific Nbs can be generated to potentially every cell surface molecule, this technology will be applicable to target LVs to every cell type for which cell specific surface molecules are characterized (Gainkam, Huang et al. 2008; Vaneycken, Devoogdt et al. 2011).

The downside of the use of the above-described strategies is that they rely on the fusogenic capacity of a gp that is derived from viruses infectious to humans such as VSV, measles virus, sindbis virus and MLV. Their exposure to the complement or immune system, leading to anti-gp antibodies, might limit their clinical applicability. To surmount these obstacles, Frecha et al. pseudotyped LVs with a mutant fusogenic gp derived from an endogenous feline virus, named RD114. The mutant RD114 gp is an attractive candidate for in *vivo* use as it is resistant to degradation by the human complement. By co-displaying the early-acting-cytokine SCF together with mutant RD114 gp, human CD34+ HSCs could be targeted *in vivo* (Frecha, Fusil et al. 2011; Frecha, Costa et al. 2012). SCF was responsible for a slight and transient stimulation of the HSCs while preserving the 'stemness' of the targeted HSCs. In that way, the need for CD3/CD28 or cytokine pretreatment was obviated. Springfeld et al. recently pseudotyped LVs with the H and F gps of the *Tupaia paramyxovirus* (TPMV), an animal virus without close human pathogenic relatives. Moreover, as this virus does not infect human cells, detargeting the H protein from its natural receptors is unnecessary. When LVs were pseudotyped with the TPMV envelope protein linked to an anti-CD20 single chain antibody, selective transduction of CD20+ cells, including quiescent primary human B cells, was reported (Enkirch, Kneissl et al. 2012).

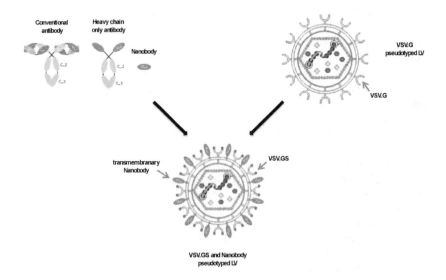

Figure 4. Principle of the Nb display technology. The Nb display technology is based on the fact that LVs need to bind and fuse with the membrane of a target cell for proper infection. While VSV.G accounts for both of these functions, we propose to separate these functions over two different molecules: (1) binding via a membrane bound Nb against the target cell of choice and (2) fusion via VSV.GS, which is a binding defective truncated version of VSV.G.

Recently an innovative alternative strategy has been described by Mannell et al. for site specific vascular gene delivery. In this case, the LVs were first coupled to magnetic nanoparticles, which were in turn coupled to lipid microbubbles. LVs coupled to magnetic nanoparticles to target them to specific cell types *in vitro* using an external magnetic field has been described before. However, when these LV-nanoparticle constructs are considered for *in vivo* use, a sufficient magnetic moment is needed as the particles are subject to flow velocity within the blood vessels. As the magnetic moment is proportional to particle size, Mannell et al. coated the LV-nanoparticle constructs with magnetic microbubbles for enlargement. Upon intravenous delivery, the LV magnetic microbubbles were first trapped at the site of interest. Next ultrasound mediated destruction of the microbubbles resulted in fast release of the LVs at the site of interest with high transduction efficiency without the cost of higher cytotoxicity (Mannell, Pircher et al. 2012).

In conclusion, there seem to be some general prerequisites for successful transductional targeting of LVs: (1) use envelope gps with defined receptor binding sites, (2) abolish the natural recognition sites of the attachment gp, (3) separate fusion and attachment functions over two different molecules, (4) avoid the construction of large fusion constructs since their fusogenic capacities can be severely compromised and (5) avoid the use of immunogenic gps (Buchholz, Muhlebach et al. 2009).

5. Genomic targeting

Nowadays, LVs have become valuable tools for the treatment of several monogenic disorders such as hemophilia B, β-thalassemia and X-linked adrenoleukodystrophy (Cartier, Hacein-Bey-Abina et al. 2012; Payen, Colomb et al. 2012). However, the use of viral vectors that integrate their cargo into the genome of the host cell can trigger oncogenesis by insertional mutagenesis. This is exemplified by the incident where two out of 11 patients treated with a γ-retroviral vector to correct X-linked SCID, developed leukemia. This was caused by the γ-retroviral construct's tendency to insert into active genes, in this case the LMO-2 oncogene (Marshall 2002). Later on, using the same vector type to treat chronic granulomatous disease, genomic instability and myelodysplasia was observed (Stein, Ott et al. 2010). These incidents prompted substantial research into design, safety testing and optimization of integrating vectors. Thus far several measures have been taken to pose a reduced risk on insertional mutagenesis such as the development of SIN LVs containing a moderate cellular promoter (Modlich and Baum 2009; Montini, Cesana et al. 2009). Furthermore LVs are intrinsically less genotoxic than their retroviral counterparts (Montini, Cesana et al. 2006). Nevertheless, LVs have a higher transduction efficiency, which could counterbalance the reduced risk of mutagenic vector integration into the patient's genome. In addition, accumulating studies report the concept of LV-induced clonal dominance related to growth and/or survival advantage *e.g.* induced by vector integration and subsequent formation of aberrantly spliced mRNA forms (Fehse and Roeder 2008; Cavazzana-Calvo, Payen et al. 2010; Cesana, Sgualdino et al. 2012; Moiani, Paleari et al. 2012). In an extensive analysis to explore the effect of promoter-enhancer selection on efficacy and safety of LVs, no clear underlying mechanism could be provided for the observed. They concluded that other ill-defined risk factors must be involved for oncogenesis, including replicative stress (Ginn, Liao et al. 2010).

Finally, next to transcriptional activation of neighboring genes, also transcriptional shut off of the tg has been reported. This was due to chromatin remodeling at the site of insertion and cessation of the therapeutic effect (Stein, Ott et al. 2010).

Therefore additional strategies have been considered to reduce the side effects related to random insertion. The most straightforward strategy is to prevent integration of the proviral cargo by the use of IDLVs. These IDLVs are produced with a mutated integrase, which results in prevention of proviral integration and generation of increased levels of circular vector episomes within the infected cells. They appear to be safer with only a 0,1 to 2,3% chance that the episomal transcript gets integrated without a marked loss in effectiveness in terms of immune stimulatory potential of the IDLV-based vaccines (Vargas, Gusella et al. 2004; Philippe, Sarkis et al. 2006; Karwacz, Mukherjee et al. 2009; Wanisch and Yanez-Munoz 2009). However, as the lentiviral episomes lack replication signals, they are gradually lost by dilution in dividing cells and only stable in quiescent cells, which is undesirable for permanent correction of any genetic disorder. Furthermore also lower tg expression levels have been reported compared to integrative vectors (Bayer, Kantor et al. 2008). Therefore several alternative strategies have been brought forward to target the integrative process to a specific 'safe' genomic site.

In a first attempt, several groups tried to fuse a heterologous DNA binding domain directly to the integrase. Bushman et al. were the first to evaluate the activity of a hybrid, composed of the HIV-1 integrase and the lambda repressor. They reported on integration primarily near the lambda operator sites on the same face of the β-DNA helix (Bushman 1994). Later a model system was used were the integrase, derived from the avian sarcoma virus or HIV-1 respectively was fused to the *Escherichia coli* LexA repressor protein DNA binding domain (Katz, Merkel et al. 1996; Holmes-Son and Chow 2000). When this construct was packaged into the virion in *trans* either by replacing the original integrase gene or by cloning it adjacent to the HIV-1 accessory protein Vpr, they observed that this enhanced the use of integration sites adjacent to the *lex*A operators. In another study, the HIV-1 derived integrase was fused to a synthetic polydactyl zinc finger protein E2C, which binds specifically to a contiguous 18 bp E2C recognition site (Tan, Dong et al. 2006). Although in all studies clearly a higher preference for integration near the target sequence of choice was observed, this also implicated reduced DNA-binding specificity of the fusion protein with associated decrease of integration frequency of about 80 percent compared to viruses containing wild type integrase. Furthermore this strategy is also limited by the difficulty to incorporate the fusion protein into infectious virions (Michel, Yu et al. 2010).

Another strategy is targeting the integration away from genes using tethering domains linked to the host cell-encoded transcriptional co-activator lens epithelium-derived growth factor/p75 (LEDGF/p75), a cellular integrase binding protein. For example the LEDGF/p75 chromatin interaction-binding domain has been replaced with CBX1, which binds histone H3 di- or trimethylated on K9. Subsequently proviral integration was directed to pericentric heterochromatin and intergenic regions (Llano, Vanegas et al. 2006; Ferris, Wu et al. 2010; Gijsbers, Ronen et al. 2010; Silvers, Smith et al. 2010). As this requires engineering of a host cell protein, it is not feasible for clinical applications at the present stage (Izmiryan, Basmaciogullari et al. 2011). Site-specific proviral integration can also be mediated by the use of site-specific recombinases. The best known are derived from the lambda integrase family of enzymes and include the bacteriophage P1 Cre recombinase, bacteriophage lambda integrase, the yeast Flp recombinase and bacterial XerCD recombinase. They catalyze site specific recombination by a transient DNA-protein covalent linkage that brings two specific DNA repeats together (Van Duyne 2001). Depending on the orientation of the DNA repeats, the DNA segment will either be excised or inverted when in the same or opposite orientation respectively (Figure 5A, adapted from http://www.ruf.rice.edu/~rur/issue1_files/ norman.html). The Cre-loxP system has been developed for gene studies to conditionally knock out a target gene in a cell- or tissue specific manner to overcome embryonic lethality due to permanent inactivation of the target gene in an early developmental stage (Ray, Fagan et al. 2000). This system is based on two palindromic loxP sites of 34 bp that flank the gene of interest. Although these loxP sites are prevalent in the genomes of bacteriophages, they are absent in the mouse genome where they have to be introduced by targeted mutagenesis (Kos 2004). Throughout the human genome, however, loxP-like sequences or pseudo-loxP sites are present that can be recognized by either wild-type Cre or Cre variants. This last feature enables site-specific insertion of a gene in a defined loxP site in the human genome if a Cre recombinase is provided in cis or trans. Michel et al. evaluated the feasibility of combining the Cre-loxP system for gene targeting with the versatile gene delivery system of LVs for site-specific gene insertion in human cell lines. They transduced a loxP site containing cell line with a LV containing Cre recombinase in trans as a fusion protein to the HIV accessory protein Vpr. Moreover the LV contained a cassette containing a loxP site followed by the neomycin resistant gene, inserted in the U3 region of the 3'LTR. Upon reverse transcription, the loxP-neo sequence would appear in both LTRs, thereby providing a substrate for recombination that could be catalyzed by the virion-associated Vpr-Cre. Upon this recombination step, a circular product was produced that was on his turn inserted into the loxP site of the cell line, again catalyzed by virion-associated Vpr-Cre. Another example is provided by the group of Jiang et al. who demonstrated a selective inhibitory effect on the lens epithelial cells and not the retinal pigment epithelial cells (Jiang, Lu et al. 2011). Therefore they used an enhanced Cre/loxP system with a LV expressing Cre under the control of the lens-specific promoter LEP503 in combination with another LV that contained a stiffer sequence encoding eGFP with a functional polyadenylation signal between two loxP sites, followed by the HSV-TK gene, both under the control of the human phosphoglycerate kinase promoter. Expression of the downstream HSV-TK was activated by co-expression of Cre under the control of the lens-specific promoter LEP503. Although this technology allows site-specific tg insertion, there are only a limited amount of pseudo-loxP sites in the human genome and even none in the mouse genome, which makes this technique unusable for fundamental research in laboratory animals. Furthermore, two recombination events are required which has a major impact on its efficiency.

A recent strategy makes use of site-specific endonucleases to target the tg to neutral 'safe harbor' genome regions or stimulate the process of homologous recombination for gene repair (Fischer, Hacein-Bey-Abina et al. 2011). Endonucleases induce site-specific ds breaks that can be repaired by homology-directed repair, a form of homologous recombination that uses a copy of the genetic information from the broken DNA molecule. When the latter is provided by the same or another LV, this copy will be used to repair the ds break (Urnov, Miller et al. 2005; O'Driscoll and Jeggo 2006). The advantage of gene repair/correction is that both function and expression of the affected gene are restored while the risk associated with random vector integration is avoided. Besides the advantage of the reduced risk for insertional mutagenesis, this strategy is also used to target genes in order to knock them down or replace them with another gene by homologous recombination. The disadvantage is that the nuclease coding sequences are expressed for several days, which is not optimal for translation to the clinic due to the background off-target generation of dsDNA breaks.

One possibility is the use of the zinc finger nuclease strategy. For this, the Cys2His2 class of zinc finger DNA binding domains is engineered to recognize a DNA sequence of interest, fused to the nuclease domain of the FokI type II restriction endonuclease to yield a highly specific zinc finger (Figure 5 B, adapted from http://biol1020-2011-2.blogspot.be/2011/09/zinc-finger-nucleases-zfn-emerging.html) (Kim, Cha et al. 1996; Pabo, Peisach et al. 2001). When two different zinc fingers are designed to bind the same sequence of interest in the opposite orientation, this will allow dimerization of the FokI domains which leads to a zinc finger induced dsDNA break (Bitinaite, Wah et al. 1998). Various strategies have been developed to engineer the Cys2His2 zinc fingers in order to bind a specific sequence either by modular assembly or by selection strategies using phage display or a cellular selection system. Naldini et al. evaluated the use of zinc finger nucleases in combination with an IDLV for gene editing. Therefore they co-transduced several cell lines with three different IDLVs, one encoding the donor sequence and two encoding the two zinc fingers (Lombardo, Genovese et al. 2007). A few years later they also used this strategy to assess zinc finger specificity genome-wide by comprehensively mapping the locations of the IDLV integration sites in cells co-transduced with GFP and zinc finger encoding LVs (Gabriel, Lombardo et al. 2011). They observed a very high efficiency and specificity, yet a measurable rate of vector integration at unidentified sites occurred with this approach, which is the sum of zinc finger mediated and background levels of IDLV integration. Moreover co-transduction with three different LVs may be a rate-limiting step in this system. Therefore the use of a single construct to express the zinc fingers and deliver the donor tg must be evaluated, especially for less permissive cells such as hematopoietic progenitors.

Another way to target the proviral genome is by the provision of a vector-associated meganuclease encoded by a separate vector or supplied as a protein within the viral particle. (Izmiryan, Basmaciogullari et al. 2011). For the latter, Ismiryan et al. fused the prototypic meganuclease I-SceI from yeast to Vpr. This avoided the potentially toxic sustained expression of the introduced endonuclease. IDLVs encoding the donor sequence and containing the meganuclease-SceI fusion construct were tested in reporter cells in which targeting events were scored by the repair of a puromycin resistance gene. They reported a two-fold higher frequency of the expected recombination event when the nuclease was delivered as a protein rather than encoded by a separate vector and therefore improved both the safety and efficacy of this LV-based gene targeting system. In conclusion, although the field of genomic targeting is relatively new for LV-based gene therapy, it opens a tremendous amount

of new possibilities.

A) Cre loxP recombination

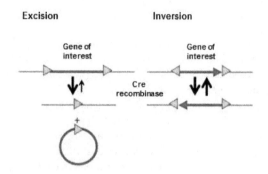

B) The zinc finger nuclease complex

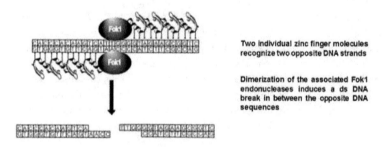

Two individual zinc finger molecules recognize two opposite DNA strands

Dimerization of the associated Fok1 endonucleases induces a ds DNA break in between the opposite DNA sequences

Figure 5. Schematic representation of targeted genome modification by the Cre-loxP system (A) or by the zinc-finger nuclease complex (B). Cre recombinases recognize specific loxP sites in the genome, bind them en bring them together. Depending on their orientation this leads to excision (same orientation) or inversion (opposite orientation) of the sequence flanked by the two loxP sites(A). Two individual zinc finger molecules each recognize a 9 to 18 bp DNA sequence using between three and six individual zinc finger repeats that bind the major groove of DNA. The DNA sequences are non-palindromic DNA sites located respectively up -and downstream of the intended cleavage site, which is mostly about 5-7 bp long. If the zinc finger domains are perfectly specific for their intended target site then even a pair of three-finger ZFNs that recognize a total of 18 bp can theoretically target a single locus in a mammalian genome. Next, the associated Fok1 nucleases dimerize and induce a double stranded break which can be restored by either non-homologous end-joining or homology-directed repair, which faithfully restores the original sequence by copying it from the sister chromatid or using the homologous sequence provided by a LV(B).

6. Concluding remarks

LVs have proven to be efficient vehicles to deliver one or more tgs to any cell type of choice, which has led to a promising list of therapeutic applications. As the demand for experimentation in gene delivery to specific cell types increases, technologies that precisely target LV-based gene expression will become more important for research and clinical applications. Four main groups of strategies with their own possibilities as well as difficulties have been developed so far. Self-evidently, further optimization and fine-tuning of these strategies is a necessity to fulfill the expectations for targeted LV delivery *in vivo*. In addition to extra optimization steps, combinations of two or more of these strategies can also lead to an overall more selective, efficient and most importantly, safe LV system. Several attempts to combine the different strategies have been reported (Brown, Cantore et al. 2007; Pariente, Morizono et al. 2007; Escors and Breckpot 2011). Pariente et al. for example, reported on a LV that was transductionally targeted to prostate cancer bone metastases by a modified sindbis virus envelope that interacts with PSCA and transcriptionally targeted with a prostate cell specific promoter. This dual-targeted LV enhanced specificity to prostate cancer bone metastases after systemic delivery with respect to individual transcriptional or transductional targeting. As the developed targeting strategies already resulted in a major step forward for LV-based gene therapy, their potential will most likely be more exploited in the future, paving the way towards an all-embracing LV-based tg vehicle for the gene therapeutic field.

Author details

Cleo Goyvaerts[1], Therese Liechtenstein[2], Christopher Bricogne[2], David Escors[2] and Karine Breckpot[1]

1 Laboratory of Molecular and Cellular Therapy, Department of Immunology-Physiology, Vrije Universiteit Brussel, Jette, Belgium

2 Division of Infection and Immunity, Rayne Institute, University College London, London, UK

References

[1] Abruzzese, R. V., D. Godin, et al. (2000). "Ligand-dependent regulation of vascular endothelial growth factor and erythropoietin expression by a plasmid-based autoinducible GeneSwitch system." Mol Ther 2(3): 276-87.

[2] Adriani, W., F. Boyer, et al. (2010). "Social withdrawal and gambling-like profile after lentiviral manipulation of DAT expression in the rat accumbens." Int J Neuropsychopharmacol 13(10): 1329-42.

[3] Annoni, A., M. Battaglia, et al. (2007). "The immune response to lentiviral-delivered transgene is modulated in vivo by transgene-expressing antigen-presenting cells but not by CD4+CD25+ regulatory T cells." Blood 110(6): 1788-96.

[4] Annoni, A., B. D. Brown, et al. (2009). "In vivo delivery of a microRNA-regulated transgene induces antigen-specific regulatory T cells and promotes immunologic tolerance." Blood 114(25): 5152-61.

[5] Azzouz, M., G. S. Ralph, et al. (2004). "VEGF delivery with retrogradely transported lentivector prolongs survival in a mouse ALS model." Nature 429(6990): 413-7.

[6] Bahi, A., F. Boyer, et al. (2004). "CD81-induced behavioural changes during chronic cocaine administration: in vivo gene delivery with regulatable lentivirus." Eur J Neurosci 19(6): 1621-33.

[7] Barde, I., M. A. Zanta-Boussif, et al. (2006). "Efficient control of gene expression in the hematopoietic system using a single Tet-on inducible lentiviral vector." Mol Ther 13(2): 382-90.

[8] Barrilleaux, B. and P. Knoepfler (2011). "Transduction of human cells with polymer-complexed ecotropic lentivirus for enhanced biosafety." J Vis Exp 2011(53).

[9] Bartel, D. P. (2004). "MicroRNAs: genomics, biogenesis, mechanism, and function." Cell 116(2): 281-97.

[10] Bauer, G., M. A. Dao, et al. (2008). "In vivo biosafety model to assess the risk of adverse events from retroviral and lentiviral vectors." Mol Ther 16(7): 1308-15.

[11] Baup, D., L. Fraga, et al. (2010). "Variegation and silencing in a lentiviral-based murine transgenic model." Transgenic Res 19(3): 399-414.

[12] Bayer, M., B. Kantor, et al. (2008). "A large U3 deletion causes increased in vivo expression from a nonintegrating lentiviral vector." Mol Ther 16(12): 1968-76.

[13] Benabdellah, K., M. Cobo, et al. (2011). "Development of an all-in-one lentiviral vector system based on the original TetR for the easy generation of Tet-ON cell lines." PLoS One 6(8): e23734.

[14] Benzekhroufa, K., B. H. Liu, et al. (2009). "Targeting central serotonergic neurons with lentiviral vectors based on a transcriptional amplification strategy." Gene Ther 16(5): 681-8.

[15] Beyer, W. R., M. Westphal, et al. (2002). "Oncoretrovirus and lentivirus vectors pseudotyped with lymphocytic choriomeningitis virus glycoprotein: generation, concentration, and broad host range." J Virol 76(3): 1488-95.

[16] Bitinaite, J., D. A. Wah, et al. (1998). "FokI dimerization is required for DNA cleavage." Proc Natl Acad Sci U S A 95(18): 10570-5.

[17] Blechacz, B. and S. J. Russell (2008). "Measles virus as an oncolytic vector platform." Curr Gene Ther 8(3): 162-75.

[18] Blesch, A., J. Conner, et al. (2005). "Regulated lentiviral NGF gene transfer controls rescue of medial septal cholinergic neurons." Mol Ther 11(6): 916-25.

[19] Blomer, U., L. Naldini, et al. (1997). "Highly efficient and sustained gene transfer in adult neurons with a lentivirus vector." J Virol 71(9): 6641-9.

[20] Boerger, A. L., S. Snitkovsky, et al. (1999). "Retroviral vectors preloaded with a viral receptor-ligand bridge protein are targeted to specific cell types." Proc Natl Acad Sci U S A 96(17): 9867-72.

[21] Bonci, D., V. Coppola, et al. (2008). "The miR-15a-miR-16-1 cluster controls prostate cancer by targeting multiple oncogenic activities." Nat Med 14(11): 1271-7.

[22] Breckpot, K., P. Emeagi, et al. (2007). "Activation of immature monocyte-derived dendritic cells after transduction with high doses of lentiviral vectors." Hum Gene Ther 18(6): 536-46.

[23] Breckpot, K., P. U. Emeagi, et al. (2008). "Lentiviral vectors for anti-tumor immuno-therapy." Curr Gene Ther 8(6): 438-48.

[24] Breckpot, K., D. Escors, et al. (2010). "HIV-1 lentiviral vector immunogenicity is mediated by Toll-like receptor 3 (TLR3) and TLR7." J Virol 84(11): 5627-36.

[25] Brown, B. D., A. Cantore, et al. (2007). "A microRNA-regulated lentiviral vector me-diates stable correction of hemophilia B mice." Blood 110(13): 4144-52.

[26] Brown, B. D., B. Gentner, et al. (2007). "Endogenous microRNA can be broadly ex-ploited to regulate transgene expression according to tissue, lineage and differentia-tion state." Nat Biotechnol 25(12): 1457-67.

[27] Brown, B. D. and D. Lillicrap (2002). "Dangerous liaisons: the role of "danger" signals in the immune response to gene therapy." Blood 100(4): 1133-40.

[28] Brown, B. D. and L. Naldini (2009). "Exploiting and antagonizing microRNA regula-tion for therapeutic and experimental applications." Nat Rev Genet 10(8): 578-85.

[29] Brown, B. D., M. A. Venneri, et al. (2006). "Endogenous microRNA regulation sup-presses transgene expression in hematopoietic lineages and enables stable gene transfer." Nat Med 12(5): 585-91.

[30] Buchholz, C. J., L. J. Duerner, et al. (2008). "Retroviral display and high throughput screening." Comb Chem High Throughput Screen 11(2): 99-110.

[31] Buchholz, C. J., M. D. Muhlebach, et al. (2009). "Lentiviral vectors with measles virus glycoproteins - dream team for gene transfer?" Trends Biotechnol 27(5): 259-65.

[32] Burns, J. C., T. Friedmann, et al. (1993). "Vesicular stomatitis virus G glycoprotein pseudotyped retroviral vectors: concentration to very high titer and efficient gene transfer into mammalian and nonmammalian cells." Proc Natl Acad Sci U S A 90(17): 8033-7.

[33] Bushman, F. D. (1994). "Tethering human immunodeficiency virus 1 integrase to a DNA site directs integration to nearby sequences." Proc Natl Acad Sci U S A 91(20): 9233-7.

[34] Calame, M., M. Cachafeiro, et al. (2011). "Retinal degeneration progression changes lentiviral vector cell targeting in the retina." PLoS One 6(8): e23782.

[35] Canivet, M., A. D. Hoffman, et al. (1990). "Replication of HIV-1 in a wide variety of animal cells following phenotypic mixing with murine retroviruses." Virology 178(2): 543-51.

[36] Cao, J., K. Sodhi, et al. (2011). "Lentiviral-human heme oxygenase targeting endothelium improved vascular function in angiotensin II animal model of hypertension." Hum Gene Ther 22(3): 271-82.

[37] Cao, O., C. Furlan-Freguia, et al. (2007). "Emerging role of regulatory T cells in gene transfer." Curr Gene Ther 7(5): 381-90.

[38] Cartier, N., S. Hacein-Bey-Abina, et al. (2012). "Lentiviral hematopoietic cell gene therapy for X-linked adrenoleukodystrophy." Methods Enzymol 507: 187-98.

[39] Cartier, N., S. Hacein-Bey-Abina, et al. (2009). "Hematopoietic stem cell gene therapy with a lentiviral vector in X-linked adrenoleukodystrophy." Science 326(5954): 818-23.

[40] Cattoglio, C., G. Facchini, et al. (2007). "Hot spots of retroviral integration in human CD34+ hematopoietic cells." Blood 110(6): 1770-8.

[41] Cavazzana-Calvo, M., S. Hacein-Bey, et al. (2000). "Gene therapy of human severe combined immunodeficiency (SCID)-X1 disease." Science 288(5466): 669-72.

[42] Cavazzana-Calvo, M., E. Payen, et al. (2010). "Transfusion independence and HMGA2 activation after gene therapy of human beta-thalassaemia." Nature 467(7313): 318-22.

[43] Cesana, D., J. Sgualdino, et al. (2012). "Whole transcriptome characterization of aberrant splicing events induced by lentiviral vector integrations." J Clin Invest 122(5): 1667-76.

[44] Chadwick, M. P., F. J. Morling, et al. (1999). "Modification of retroviral tropism by display of IGF-I." J Mol Biol 285(2): 485-94.

[45] Chandrashekran, A., M. Y. Gordon, et al. (2004). "Targeted retroviral transduction of c-kit+ hematopoietic cells using novel ligand display technology." Blood 104(9): 2697-703.

[46] Chowdhury, S., K. A. Chester, et al. (2004). "Efficient retroviral vector targeting of carcinoembryonic antigen-positive tumors." Mol Ther 9(1): 85-92.

[47] Colin, A., M. Faideau, et al. (2009). "Engineered lentiviral vector targeting astrocytes in vivo." Glia 57(6): 667-79.

[48] Cronin, J., X. Y. Zhang, et al. (2005). "Altering the tropism of lentiviral vectors through pseudotyping." Curr Gene Ther 5(4): 387-98.

[49] Croyle, M. A., S. M. Callahan, et al. (2004). "PEGylation of a vesicular stomatitis virus G pseudotyped lentivirus vector prevents inactivation in serum." J Virol 78(2): 912-21.

[50] Cui, Y., J. Golob, et al. (2002). "Targeting transgene expression to antigen-presenting cells derived from lentivirus-transduced engrafting human hematopoietic stem/progenitor cells." Blood 99(2): 399-408.

[51] De Palma, M., E. Montini, et al. (2005). "Promoter trapping reveals significant differences in integration site selection between MLV and HIV vectors in primary hematopoietic cells." Blood 105(6): 2307-15.

[52] De Palma, M., M. A. Venneri, et al. (2003). "In vivo targeting of tumor endothelial cells by systemic delivery of lentiviral vectors." Hum Gene Ther 14(12): 1193-206.

[53] Delenda, C. (2004). "Lentiviral vectors: optimization of packaging, transduction and gene expression." J Gene Med 6 Suppl 1: S125-38.

[54] DePolo, N. J., J. D. Reed, et al. (2000). "VSV-G pseudotyped lentiviral vector particles produced in human cells are inactivated by human serum." Mol Ther 2(3): 218-22.

[55] Deuschle, U., R. A. Hipskind, et al. (1990). "RNA polymerase II transcription blocked by Escherichia coli lac repressor." Science 248(4954): 480-3.

[56] Di Domenico, C., D. Di Napoli, et al. (2006). "Limited transgene immune response and long-term expression of human alpha-L-iduronidase in young adult mice with mucopolysaccharidosis type I by liver-directed gene therapy." Hum Gene Ther 17(11): 1112-21.

[57] Di Nunzio, F., G. Maruggi, et al. (2008). "Correction of laminin-5 deficiency in human epidermal stem cells by transcriptionally targeted lentiviral vectors." Mol Ther 16(12): 1977-85.

[58] Dreja, H. and M. Piechaczyk (2006). "The effects of N-terminal insertion into VSV-G of an scFv peptide." Virol J 3: 69.

[59] Dresch, C., S. L. Edelmann, et al. (2008). "Lentiviral-mediated transcriptional targeting of dendritic cells for induction of T cell tolerance in vivo." J Immunol 181(7): 4495-506.

[60] Dropulic, B. (2011). "Lentiviral vectors: their molecular design, safety, and use in laboratory and preclinical research." Hum Gene Ther 22(6): 649-57.

[61] Dull, T., R. Zufferey, et al. (1998). "A third-generation lentivirus vector with a conditional packaging system." J Virol 72(11): 8463-71.

[62] Dylla, D. E., L. Xie, et al. (2011). "Altering alpha-dystroglycan receptor affinity of LCMV pseudotyped lentivirus yields unique cell and tissue tropism." Genet Vaccines Ther 9: 8.

[63] Earp, L. J., S. E. Delos, et al. (2005). "The many mechanisms of viral membrane fusion proteins." Curr Top Microbiol Immunol 285: 25-66.

[64] Ebert, M. S., J. R. Neilson, et al. (2007). "MicroRNA sponges: competitive inhibitors of small RNAs in mammalian cells." Nat Methods 4(9): 721-6.

[65] Efrat, S., D. Fusco-DeMane, et al. (1995). "Conditional transformation of a pancreatic beta-cell line derived from transgenic mice expressing a tetracycline-regulated onco-gene." Proc Natl Acad Sci U S A 92(8): 3576-80.

[66] Emi, N., T. Friedmann, et al. (1991). "Pseudotype formation of murine leukemia virus with the G protein of vesicular stomatitis virus." J Virol 65(3): 1202-7.

[67] Enkirch, T., S. Kneissl, et al. (2012). "Targeted lentiviral vectors pseudotyped with the Tupaia paramyxovirus glycoproteins." Gene Ther.

[68] Escors, D. and K. Breckpot (2010). "Lentiviral vectors in gene therapy: their current status and future potential." Arch Immunol Ther Exp (Warsz) 58(2): 107-19.

[69] Escors, D. and K. Breckpot (2011). "Lentiviral vectors in gene therapy: their current status and future potential." Arch Immunol Ther Exp (Warsz) 58(2): 107-19.

[70] Fehse, B. and I. Roeder (2008). "Insertional mutagenesis and clonal dominance: bio-logical and statistical considerations." Gene Ther 15(2): 143-53.

[71] Ferris, A. L., X. Wu, et al. (2010). "Lens epithelium-derived growth factor fusion pro-teins redirect HIV-1 DNA integration." Proc Natl Acad Sci U S A 107(7): 3135-40.

[72] Fielding, A. K., M. Maurice, et al. (1998). "Inverse targeting of retroviral vectors: se-lective gene transfer in a mixed population of hematopoietic and nonhematopoietic cells." Blood 91(5): 1802-9.

[73] Fischer, A., S. Hacein-Bey-Abina, et al. (2011). "Gene therapy for primary adaptive immune deficiencies." J Allergy Clin Immunol 127(6): 1356-9.

[74] Frecha, C., C. Costa, et al. (2012). "A novel lentiviral vector targets gene transfer into human hematopoietic stem cells in marrow from patients with bone marrow failure syndrome and in vivo in humanized mice." Blood 119(5): 1139-50.

[75] Frecha, C., F. Fusil, et al. (2011). "In vivo gene delivery into hCD34+ cells in a human-ized mouse model." Methods Mol Biol 737: 367-90.

[76] Frecha, C., C. Levy, et al. (2010). "Advances in the field of lentivector-based transduc-tion of T and B lymphocytes for gene therapy." Mol Ther 18(10): 1748-57.

[77] Frecha, C., C. Levy, et al. (2011). "Measles virus glycoprotein-pseudotyped lentiviral vector-mediated gene transfer into quiescent lymphocytes requires binding to both SLAM and CD46 entry receptors." J Virol 85(12): 5975-85.

[78] Friedrich, R. I., K. Nopora, et al. (2012). "Transcriptional targeting of B cells with viral vectors." European Journal of Cell Biology 91(1): 86-96.

[79] Froelich, S., L. Ziegler, et al. (2009). "Targeted gene delivery to CD117-expressing cells in vivo with lentiviral vectors co-displaying stem cell factor and a fusogenic molecule." Biotechnol Bioeng 104(1): 206-15.

[80] Funke, S., A. Maisner, et al. (2008). "Targeted cell entry of lentiviral vectors." Mol Ther 16(8): 1427-36.

[81] Funke, S., I. C. Schneider, et al. (2009). "Pseudotyping lentiviral vectors with the wild-type measles virus glycoproteins improves titer and selectivity." Gene Ther 16(5): 700-5.

[82] Furth, P. A., L. St Onge, et al. (1994). "Temporal control of gene expression in transgenic mice by a tetracycline-responsive promoter." Proc Natl Acad Sci U S A 91(20): 9302-6.

[83] Fussenegger, M., R. P. Morris, et al. (2000). "Streptogramin-based gene regulation systems for mammalian cells." Nat Biotechnol 18(11): 1203-8.

[84] Gabriel, R., A. Lombardo, et al. (2011). "An unbiased genome-wide analysis of zinc-finger nuclease specificity." Nat Biotechnol 29(9): 816-23.

[85] Gainkam, L. O., L. Huang, et al. (2008). "Comparison of the biodistribution and tumor targeting of two 99mTc-labeled anti-EGFR nanobodies in mice, using pinhole SPECT/micro-CT." J Nucl Med 49(5): 788-95.

[86] Galimi, F., E. Saez, et al. (2005). "Development of ecdysone-regulated lentiviral vectors." Mol Ther 11(1): 142-8.

[87] Gascon, S., J. A. Paez-Gomez, et al. (2008). "Dual-promoter lentiviral vectors for constitutive and regulated gene expression in neurons." J Neurosci Methods 168(1): 104-12.

[88] Gaspar, H. B., K. L. Parsley, et al. (2004). "Gene therapy of X-linked severe combined immunodeficiency by use of a pseudotyped gammaretroviral vector." Lancet 364(9452): 2181-7.

[89] Gennari, F., L. Lopes, et al. (2009). "Single-chain antibodies that target lentiviral vectors to MHC class II on antigen-presenting cells." Hum Gene Ther 20(6): 554-62.

[90] Gentner, B., G. Schira, et al. (2009). "Stable knockdown of microRNA in vivo by lentiviral vectors." Nat Methods 6(1): 63-6.

[91] Gentner, B., I. Visigalli, et al. (2010). "Identification of hematopoietic stem cell-specific miRNAs enables gene therapy of globoid cell leukodystrophy." Sci Transl Med 2(58): 58ra84.

[92] Gijsbers, R., K. Ronen, et al. (2010). "LEDGF hybrids efficiently retarget lentiviral integration into heterochromatin." Mol Ther 18(3): 552-60.

[93] Gilham, D. E., A. L. M. Lie, et al. (2010). "Cytokine stimulation and the choice of pro-
      moter are critical factors for the efficient transduction of mouse T cells with HIV-1
      vectors." J Gene Med 12(2): 129-36.

[94] Ginn, S. L., S. H. Liao, et al. (2010). "Lymphomagenesis in SCID-X1 mice following
      lentivirus-mediated phenotype correction independent of insertional mutagenesis
      and gammac overexpression." Mol Ther 18(5): 965-76.

[95] Gossen, M. and H. Bujard (1992). "Tight control of gene expression in mammalian
      cells by tetracycline-responsive promoters." Proc Natl Acad Sci U S A 89(12): 5547-51.

[96] Goyvaerts, C., K. De Groeve, et al. (2012). "Development of the Nanobody display
      technology to target lentiviral vectors to antigen-presenting cells." Gene Ther.

[97] Guibinga, G. H., F. L. Hall, et al. (2004). "Ligand-modified vesicular stomatitis virus
      glycoprotein displays a temperature-sensitive intracellular trafficking and virus as-
      sembly phenotype." Mol Ther 9(1): 76-84.

[98] Hamers-Casterman, C., T. Atarhouch, et al. (1993). "Naturally occurring antibodies
      devoid of light chains." Nature 363(6428): 446-8.

[99] Hanawa, H., D. A. Persons, et al. (2002). "High-level erythroid lineage-directed gene
      expression using globin gene regulatory elements after lentiviral vector-mediated
      gene transfer into primitive human and murine hematopoietic cells." Hum Gene
      Ther 13(17): 2007-16.

[100] Hawley, T. S., A. Z. Fong, et al. (1998). "Leukemic predisposition of mice transplant-
      ed with gene-modified hematopoietic precursors expressing flt3 ligand." Blood 92(6):
      2003-11.

[101] Heckl, D., D. C. Wicke, et al. (2011). "Lentiviral gene transfer regenerates hemato-
      poietic stem cells in a mouse model for Mpl-deficient aplastic anemia." Blood 117(14):
      3737-47.

[102] Herold, M. J., J. van den Brandt, et al. (2008). "Inducible and reversible gene silencing
      by stable integration of an shRNA-encoding lentivirus in transgenic rats." Proc Natl
      Acad Sci U S A 105(47): 18507-12.

[103] Hioki, H., H. Kameda, et al. (2007). "Efficient gene transduction of neurons by lentivi-
      rus with enhanced neuron-specific promoters." Gene Ther 14(11): 872-82.

[104] Hioki, H., E. Kuramoto, et al. (2009). "High-level transgene expression in neurons by
      lentivirus with Tet-Off system." Neurosci Res 63(2): 149-54.

[105] Hofmann, H., K. Hattermann, et al. (2004). "S protein of severe acute respiratory syn-
      drome-associated coronavirus mediates entry into hepatoma cell lines and is targeted
      by neutralizing antibodies in infected patients." J Virol 78(12): 6134-42.

[106] Holmes-Son, M. L. and S. A. Chow (2000). "Integrase-lexA fusion proteins incorpo-
      rated into human immunodeficiency virus type 1 that contains a catalytically inactive
      integrase gene are functional to mediate integration." J Virol 74(24): 11548-56.

[107] Hsieh, Y. J., F. D. Chen, et al. (2011). "The EIIAPA Chimeric Promoter for Tumor Specific Gene Therapy of Hepatoma." Mol Imaging Biol.

[108] Hu, B., B. Dai, et al. (2010). "Vaccines delivered by integration-deficient lentiviral vectors targeting dendritic cells induces strong antigen-specific immunity." Vaccine 28(41): 6675-83.

[109] Izmiryan, A., S. Basmaciogullari, et al. (2011). "Efficient gene targeting mediated by a lentiviral vector-associated meganuclease." Nucleic Acids Res 39(17): 7610-9.

[110] Jakobsson, J., C. Ericson, et al. (2003). "Targeted transgene expression in rat brain using lentiviral vectors." J Neurosci Res 73(6): 876-85.

[111] Jiang, Y. X., Y. Lu, et al. (2011). "Using HSV-TK/GCV suicide gene therapy to inhibit lens epithelial cell proliferation for treatment of posterior capsular opacification." Mol Vis 17: 291-9.

[112] Kang, Y., C. S. Stein, et al. (2002). "In vivo gene transfer using a nonprimate lentiviral vector pseudotyped with Ross River Virus glycoproteins." J Virol 76(18): 9378-88.

[113] Karavanas, G., M. Marin, et al. (2002). "The insertion of an anti-MHC I ScFv into the N-terminus of an ecotropic MLV glycoprotein does not alter its fusiogenic potential on murine cells." Virus Res 83(1-2): 57-69.

[114] Karwacz, K., S. Mukherjee, et al. (2009). "Nonintegrating lentivector vaccines stimulate prolonged T-cell and antibody responses and are effective in tumor therapy." J Virol 83(7): 3094-103.

[115] Katane, M., E. Takao, et al. (2002). "Factors affecting the direct targeting of murine leukemia virus vectors containing peptide ligands in the envelope protein." EMBO Rep 3(9): 899-904.

[116] Katz, R. A., G. Merkel, et al. (1996). "Targeting of retroviral integrase by fusion to a heterologous DNA binding domain: in vitro activities and incorporation of a fusion protein into viral particles." Virology 217(1): 178-90.

[117] Kelly, E. J., E. M. Hadac, et al. (2008). "Engineering microRNA responsiveness to decrease virus pathogenicity." Nat Med 14(11): 1278-83.

[118] Kerns, H. M., B. Y. Ryu, et al. (2010). "B cell-specific lentiviral gene therapy leads to sustained B-cell functional recovery in a murine model of X-linked agammaglobulinemia." Blood 115(11): 2146-55.

[119] Kim, S., G. J. Kim, et al. (2007). "Efficiency of the elongation factor-1alpha promoter in mammalian embryonic stem cells using lentiviral gene delivery systems." Stem Cells Dev 16(4): 537-45.

[120] Kim, Y. G., J. Cha, et al. (1996). "Hybrid restriction enzymes: zinc finger fusions to Fok I cleavage domain." Proc Natl Acad Sci U S A 93(3): 1156-60.

[121] Kimura, T., R. C. Koya, et al. (2007). "Lentiviral vectors with CMV or MHCII promoters administered in vivo: immune reactivity versus persistence of expression." Mol Ther 15(7): 1390-9.

[122] Kobinger, G. P., S. Deng, et al. (2004). "Transduction of human islets with pseudotyped lentiviral vectors." Hum Gene Ther 15(2): 211-9.

[123] Kobinger, G. P., D. J. Weiner, et al. (2001). "Filovirus-pseudotyped lentiviral vector can efficiently and stably transduce airway epithelia in vivo." Nat Biotechnol 19(3): 225-30.

[124] Kos, C. H. (2004). "Cre/loxP system for generating tissue-specific knockout mouse models." Nutr Rev 62(6 Pt 1): 243-6.

[125] Kueng, H. J., V. M. Leb, et al. (2007). "General strategy for decoration of enveloped viruses with functionally active lipid-modified cytokines." J Virol 81(16): 8666-76.

[126] Kumar, M. S., S. J. Erkeland, et al. (2008). "Suppression of non-small cell lung tumor development by the let-7 microRNA family." Proc Natl Acad Sci U S A 105(10): 3903-8.

[127] Kuroda, H., R. H. Kutner, et al. (2008). "A comparative analysis of constitutive and cell-specific promoters in the adult mouse hippocampus using lentivirus vector-mediated gene transfer." J Gene Med 10(11): 1163-75.

[128] Lachmann, N., J. Jagielska, et al. (2011). "MicroRNA-150-regulated vectors allow lymphocyte-sparing transgene expression in hematopoietic gene therapy." Gene Ther.

[129] Lai, E. C. (2002). "Micro RNAs are complementary to 3' UTR sequence motifs that mediate negative post-transcriptional regulation." Nat Genet 30(4): 363-4.

[130] Lakso, M., B. Sauer, et al. (1992). "Targeted oncogene activation by site-specific recombination in transgenic mice." Proc Natl Acad Sci U S A 89(14): 6232-6.

[131] Latta-Mahieu, M., M. Rolland, et al. (2002). "Gene transfer of a chimeric trans-activator is immunogenic and results in short-lived transgene expression." Hum Gene Ther 13(13): 1611-20.

[132] Lavillette, D., S. J. Russell, et al. (2001). "Retargeting gene delivery using surface-engineered retroviral vector particles." Curr Opin Biotechnol 12(5): 461-6.

[133] Lee, C. J., X. Fan, et al. (2011). "Promoter-specific lentivectors for long-term, cardiac-directed therapy of Fabry disease." J Cardiol 57(1): 115-22.

[134] Lee, C. L., J. Dang, et al. (2011). "Engineered lentiviral vectors pseudotyped with a CD4 receptor and a fusogenic protein can target cells expressing HIV-1 envelope proteins." Virus Res 160(1-2): 340-50.

[135] Lei, Y., K. I. Joo, et al. (2009). "Engineering fusogenic molecules to achieve targeted transduction of enveloped lentiviral vectors." J Biol Eng 3: 8.

[136] Leuci, V., L. Gammaitoni, et al. (2009). "Efficient transcriptional targeting of human hematopoietic stem cells and blood cell lineages by lentiviral vectors containing the regulatory element of the Wiskott-Aldrich syndrome gene." Stem Cells 27(11): 2815-23.

[137] Li, M., N. Husic, et al. (2010). "Optimal promoter usage for lentiviral vector-mediated transduction of cultured central nervous system cells." J Neurosci Methods 189(1): 56-64.

[138] Lin, A. H., N. Kasahara, et al. (2001). "Receptor-specific targeting mediated by the co-expression of a targeted murine leukemia virus envelope protein and a binding-defective influenza hemagglutinin protein." Hum Gene Ther 12(4): 323-32.

[139] Liu, B., J. F. Paton, et al. (2008). "Viral vectors based on bidirectional cell-specific mammalian promoters and transcriptional amplification strategy for use in vitro and in vivo." BMC Biotechnol 8: 49.

[140] Liu, B., S. Wang, et al. (2008). "Enhancement of cell-specific transgene expression from a Tet-Off regulatory system using a transcriptional amplification strategy in the rat brain." J Gene Med 10(5): 583-92.

[141] Liu, B. H., X. Wang, et al. (2004). "CMV enhancer/human PDGF-beta promoter for neuron-specific transgene expression." Gene Ther 11(1): 52-60.

[142] Llano, M., M. Vanegas, et al. (2006). "Identification and characterization of the chromatin-binding domains of the HIV-1 integrase interactor LEDGF/p75." J Mol Biol 360(4): 760-73.

[143] Lodish, H. F. and R. A. Weiss (1979). "Selective isolation of mutants of vesicular stomatitis virus defective in production of the viral glycoprotein." J Virol 30(1): 177-89.

[144] Lombardo, A., P. Genovese, et al. (2007). "Gene editing in human stem cells using zinc finger nucleases and integrase-defective lentiviral vector delivery." Nat Biotechnol 25(11): 1298-306.

[145] Lopes, L., M. Dewannieux, et al. (2008). "Immunization with a lentivector that targets tumor antigen expression to dendritic cells induces potent CD8+ and CD4+ T-cell responses." J Virol 82(1): 86-95.

[146] Lopes, L., M. Dewannieux, et al. (2011). "A lentiviral vector pseudotype suitable for vaccine development." J Gene Med 13(3): 181-7.

[147] Lopez-Ornelas, A., T. Mejia-Castillo, et al. (2011). "Lentiviral transfer of an inducible transgene expressing a soluble form of Gas1 causes glioma cell arrest, apoptosis and inhibits tumor growth." Cancer Gene Ther 18(2): 87-99.

[148] Manilla, P., T. Rebello, et al. (2005). "Regulatory considerations for novel gene therapy products: a review of the process leading to the first clinical lentiviral vector." Hum Gene Ther 16(1): 17-25.

[149] Mannell, H., J. Pircher, et al. (2012). "Targeted endothelial gene delivery by ultrasonic destruction of magnetic microbubbles carrying lentiviral vectors." Pharm Res 29(5): 1282-94.

[150] Marshall, E. (2002). "Gene therapy. What to do when clear success comes with an unclear risk?" Science 298(5593): 510-1.

[151] Matrai, J., A. Cantore, et al. (2011). "Hepatocyte-targeted expression by integrase-defective lentiviral vectors induces antigen-specific tolerance in mice with low genotoxic risk." Hepatology 53(5): 1696-707.

[152] Matsui, H., C. Hegadorn, et al. (2011). "A microRNA-regulated and GP64-pseudotyped lentiviral vector mediates stable expression of FVIII in a murine model of Hemophilia A." Mol Ther 19(4): 723-30.

[153] Maurice, M., S. Mazur, et al. (1999). "Efficient gene delivery to quiescent interleukin-2 (IL-2)-dependent cells by murine leukemia virus-derived vectors harboring IL-2 chimeric envelope glycoproteins." Blood 94(2): 401-10.

[154] Maurice, M., E. Verhoeyen, et al. (2002). "Efficient gene transfer into human primary blood lymphocytes by surface-engineered lentiviral vectors that display a T cell-activating polypeptide." Blood 99(7): 2342-50.

[155] Mazarakis, N. D., M. Azzouz, et al. (2001). "Rabies virus glycoprotein pseudotyping of lentiviral vectors enables retrograde axonal transport and access to the nervous system after peripheral delivery." Hum Mol Genet 10(19): 2109-21.

[156] McIver, S. R., C. S. Lee, et al. (2005). "Lentiviral transduction of murine oligodendrocytes in vivo." J Neurosci Res 82(3): 397-403.

[157] Michel, G., Y. Yu, et al. (2010). "Site-specific gene insertion mediated by a Cre-loxP-carrying lentiviral vector." Mol Ther 18(10): 1814-21.

[158] Miletic, H., Y. H. Fischer, et al. (2004). "Selective transduction of malignant glioma by lentiviral vectors pseudotyped with lymphocytic choriomeningitis virus glycoproteins." Hum Gene Ther 15(11): 1091-100.

[159] Mitomo, K., U. Griesenbach, et al. (2010). "Toward gene therapy for cystic fibrosis using a lentivirus pseudotyped with Sendai virus envelopes." Mol Ther 18(6): 1173-82.

[160] Modlich, U. and C. Baum (2009). "Preventing and exploiting the oncogenic potential of integrating gene vectors." J Clin Invest 119(4): 755-8.

[161] Moiani, A., Y. Paleari, et al. (2012). "Lentiviral vector integration in the human genome induces alternative splicing and generates aberrant transcripts." J Clin Invest 122(5): 1653-66.

[162] Montini, E., D. Cesana, et al. (2009). "The genotoxic potential of retroviral vectors is strongly modulated by vector design and integration site selection in a mouse model of HSC gene therapy." J Clin Invest 119(4): 964-75.

[163] Montini, E., D. Cesana, et al. (2006). "Hematopoietic stem cell gene transfer in a tu-mor-prone mouse model uncovers low genotoxicity of lentiviral vector integration." Nat Biotechnol 24(6): 687-96.

[164] Morizono, K., A. Ku, et al. (2010). "Redirecting lentiviral vectors pseudotyped with Sindbis virus-derived envelope proteins to DC-SIGN by modification of N-linked glycans of envelope proteins." J Virol 84(14): 6923-34.

[165] Morizono, K., Y. Xie, et al. (2005). "Lentiviral vector retargeting to P-glycoprotein on metastatic melanoma through intravenous injection." Nat Med 11(3): 346-52.

[166] Munch, R. C., M. D. Muhlebach, et al. (2011). "DARPins: an efficient targeting do-main for lentiviral vectors." Mol Ther 19(4): 686-93.

[167] Naldini, L., U. Blomer, et al. (1996). "In vivo gene delivery and stable transduction of nondividing cells by a lentiviral vector." Science 272(5259): 263-7.

[168] Neda, H., C. H. Wu, et al. (1991). "Chemical modification of an ecotropic murine leu-kemia virus results in redirection of its target cell specificity." J Biol Chem 266(22): 14143-6.

[169] Neddermann, P., C. Gargioli, et al. (2003). "A novel, inducible, eukaryotic gene ex-pression system based on the quorum-sensing transcription factor TraR." EMBO Rep 4(2): 159-65.

[170] Nefkens, I., J. M. Garcia, et al. (2007). "Hemagglutinin pseudotyped lentiviral parti-cles: characterization of a new method for avian H5N1 influenza sero-diagnosis." J Clin Virol 39(1): 27-33.

[171] Nelson, P., M. Kiriakidou, et al. (2003). "The microRNA world: small is mighty." Trends Biochem Sci 28(10): 534-40.

[172] Nguyen, T. H., J. C. Pages, et al. (1998). "Amphotropic retroviral vectors displaying hepatocyte growth factor-envelope fusion proteins improve transduction efficiency of primary hepatocytes." Hum Gene Ther 9(17): 2469-79.

[173] O'Driscoll, M. and P. A. Jeggo (2006). "The role of double-strand break repair - in-sights from human genetics." Nat Rev Genet 7(1): 45-54.

[174] O'Leary, V. B., S. V. Ovsepian, et al. (2011). "Innocuous full-length botulinum neuro-toxin targets and promotes the expression of lentiviral vectors in central and auto-nomic neurons." Gene Ther 18(7): 656-65.

[175] Ogueta, S. B., F. Yao, et al. (2001). "Design and in vitro characterization of a single regulatory module for efficient control of gene expression in both plasmid DNA and a self-inactivating lentiviral vector." Mol Med 7(8): 569-79.

[176] Pabo, C. O., E. Peisach, et al. (2001). "Design and selection of novel Cys2His2 zinc fin-ger proteins." Annu Rev Biochem 70: 313-40.

[177] Page, K. A., N. R. Landau, et al. (1990). "Construction and use of a human immunodeficiency virus vector for analysis of virus infectivity." J Virol 64(11): 5270-6.

[178] Palmowski, M. J., L. Lopes, et al. (2004). "Intravenous injection of a lentiviral vector encoding NY-ESO-1 induces an effective CTL response." J Immunol 172(3): 1582-7.

[179] Papapetrou, E. P., D. Kovalovsky, et al. (2009). "Harnessing endogenous miR-181a to segregate transgenic antigen receptor expression in developing versus post-thymic T cells in murine hematopoietic chimeras." J Clin Invest 119(1): 157-68.

[180] Pariente, N., S. H. Mao, et al. (2008). "Efficient targeted transduction of primary human endothelial cells with dual-targeted lentiviral vectors." J Gene Med 10(3): 242-8.

[181] Pariente, N., K. Morizono, et al. (2007). "A novel dual-targeted lentiviral vector leads to specific transduction of prostate cancer bone metastases in vivo after systemic administration." Mol Ther 15(11): 1973-81.

[182] Parker, D. G., H. M. Brereton, et al. (2009). "A steroid-inducible promoter for the cornea." Br J Ophthalmol 93(9): 1255-9.

[183] Payen, E., C. Colomb, et al. (2012). "Lentivirus vectors in beta-thalassemia." Methods Enzymol 507: 109-24.

[184] Petrigliano, F. A., M. S. Virk, et al. (2009). "Targeting of prostate cancer cells by a cytotoxic lentiviral vector containing a prostate stem cell antigen (PSCA) promoter." Prostate 69(13): 1422-34.

[185] Peviani, M., M. Kurosaki, et al. (2012). "Lentiviral vectors carrying enhancer elements of Hb9 promoter drive selective transgene expression in mouse spinal cord motor neurons." J Neurosci Methods 205(1): 139-47.

[186] Philippe, S., C. Sarkis, et al. (2006). "Lentiviral vectors with a defective integrase allow efficient and sustained transgene expression in vitro and in vivo." Proc Natl Acad Sci U S A 103(47): 17684-9.

[187] Pollock, R., R. Issner, et al. (2000). "Delivery of a stringent dimerizer-regulated gene expression system in a single retroviral vector." Proc Natl Acad Sci U S A 97(24): 13221-6.

[188] Ramezani, A. and R. G. Hawley (2002). "Overview of the HIV-1 Lentiviral Vector System." Curr Protoc Mol Biol Chapter 16: Unit 16 21.

[189] Rasko, J. E., J. L. Battini, et al. (1999). "The RD114/simian type D retrovirus receptor is a neutral amino acid transporter." Proc Natl Acad Sci U S A 96(5): 2129-34.

[190] Ray, M. K., S. P. Fagan, et al. (2000). "The Cre-loxP system: a versatile tool for targeting genes in a cell- and stage-specific manner." Cell Transplant 9(6): 805-15.

[191] Reiser, J., Z. Lai, et al. (2000). "Development of multigene and regulated lentivirus vectors." J Virol 74(22): 10589-99.

[192] Roberts, M. C. (2002). "Resistance to tetracycline, macrolide-lincosamide-streptogramin, trimethoprim, and sulfonamide drug classes." Mol Biotechnol 20(3): 261-83.

[193] Roet, K. C., R. Eggers, et al. (2012). "Non-invasive bioluminescence imaging of olfactory ensheathing glia and Schwann cells following transplantation into the lesioned rat spinal cord." Cell Transplant.

[194] Romano, G., P. P. Claudio, et al. (2003). "Human immunodeficiency virus type 1 (HIV-1) derived vectors: safety considerations and controversy over therapeutic applications." Eur J Dermatol 13(5): 424-9.

[195] Roux, P., P. Jeanteur, et al. (1989). "A versatile and potentially general approach to the targeting of specific cell types by retroviruses: application to the infection of human cells by means of major histocompatibility complex class I and class II antigens by mouse ecotropic murine leukemia virus-derived viruses." Proc Natl Acad Sci U S A 86(23): 9079-83.

[196] Sachdeva, R., M. E. Jonsson, et al. (2010). "Tracking differentiating neural progenitors in pluripotent cultures using microRNA-regulated lentiviral vectors." Proc Natl Acad Sci U S A 107(25): 11602-7.

[197] Sakuma, T., S. S. De Ravin, et al. (2010). "Characterization of retroviral and lentiviral vectors pseudotyped with xenotropic murine leukemia virus-related virus envelope glycoprotein." Hum Gene Ther 21(12): 1665-73.

[198] Sanchez-Danes, A., A. Consiglio, et al. (2012). "Efficient generation of A9 midbrain dopaminergic neurons by lentiviral delivery of LMX1A in human embryonic stem cells and induced pluripotent stem cells." Hum Gene Ther 23(1): 56-69.

[199] Sarkar, N. N. (2002). "Mifepristone: bioavailability, pharmacokinetics and use-effectiveness." Eur J Obstet Gynecol Reprod Biol 101(2): 113-20.

[200] Sayed, D., S. Rane, et al. (2008). "MicroRNA-21 targets Sprouty2 and promotes cellular outgrowths." Mol Biol Cell 19(8): 3272-82.

[201] Schaffer, D. V., J. T. Koerber, et al. (2008). "Molecular engineering of viral gene delivery vehicles." Annu Rev Biomed Eng 10: 169-94.

[202] Scherr, M., L. Venturini, et al. (2007). "Lentivirus-mediated antagomir expression for specific inhibition of miRNA function." Nucleic Acids Res 35(22): e149.

[203] Semple-Rowland, S. L., W. E. Coggin, et al. (2010). "Expression characteristics of dual-promoter lentiviral vectors targeting retinal photoreceptors and Muller cells." Mol Vis 16: 916-34.

[204] Semple-Rowland, S. L., K. S. Eccles, et al. (2007). "Targeted expression of two proteins in neural retina using self-inactivating, insulated lentiviral vectors carrying two internal independent promoters." Mol Vis 13: 2001-11.

[205] Seo, E., S. Kim, et al. (2009). "Induction of cancer cell-specific death via MMP2 promoterdependent Bax expression." BMB Rep 42(4): 217-22.

[206] Shinoda, Y., K. Hieda, et al. (2009). "Efficient transduction of cytotoxic and anti-HIV-1 genes by a gene-regulatable lentiviral vector." Virus Genes 39(2): 165-75.

[207] Silvers, R. M., J. A. Smith, et al. (2010). "Modification of integration site preferences of an HIV-1-based vector by expression of a novel synthetic protein." Hum Gene Ther 21(3): 337-49.

[208] Singhal, R., X. Deng, et al. (2011). "Long-distance effects of insertional mutagenesis." PLoS One 6(1): e15832.

[209] Sirin, O. and F. Park (2003). "Regulating gene expression using self-inactivating lentiviral vectors containing the mifepristone-inducible system." Gene 323: 67-77.

[210] Somia, N. V., H. Miyoshi, et al. (2000). "Retroviral vector targeting to human immunodeficiency virus type 1-infected cells by receptor pseudotyping." J Virol 74(9): 4420-4.

[211] Steffens, S., J. Tebbets, et al. (2004). "Transduction of human glial and neuronal tumor cells with different lentivirus vector pseudotypes." J Neurooncol 70(3): 281-8.

[212] Steidl, S., J. Stitz, et al. (2002). "Coreceptor Switch of [MLV(SIVagm)] pseudotype vectors by V3-loop exchange." Virology 300(2): 205-16.

[213] Stein, C. S., I. Martins, et al. (2005). "The lymphocytic choriomeningitis virus envelope glycoprotein targets lentiviral gene transfer vector to neural progenitors in the murine brain." Mol Ther 11(3): 382-9.

[214] Stein, S., M. G. Ott, et al. (2010). "Genomic instability and myelodysplasia with monosomy 7 consequent to EVI1 activation after gene therapy for chronic granulomatous disease." Nat Med 16(2): 198-204.

[215] Stitz, J., C. J. Buchholz, et al. (2000). "Lentiviral vectors pseudotyped with envelope glycoproteins derived from gibbon ape leukemia virus and murine leukemia virus 10A1." Virology 273(1): 16-20.

[216] Strang, B. L., Y. Ikeda, et al. (2004). "Characterization of HIV-1 vectors with gammaretrovirus envelope glycoproteins produced from stable packaging cells." Gene Ther 11(7): 591-8.

[217] Strang, B. L., Y. Takeuchi, et al. (2005). "Human immunodeficiency virus type 1 vectors with alphavirus envelope glycoproteins produced from stable packaging cells." J Virol 79(3): 1765-71.

[218] Szulc, J., M. Wiznerowicz, et al. (2006). "A versatile tool for conditional gene expression and knockdown." Nat Methods 3(2): 109-16.

[219] Tai, A., S. Froelich, et al. (2011). "Production of lentiviral vectors with enhanced efficiency to target dendritic cells by attenuating mannosidase activity of mammalian cells." J Biol Eng 5(1): 1.

[220] Tan, W., Z. Dong, et al. (2006). "Human immunodeficiency virus type 1 incorporated with fusion proteins consisting of integrase and the designed polydactyl zinc finger

protein E2C can bias integration of viral DNA into a predetermined chromosomal region in human cells." J Virol 80(4): 1939-48.

[221] Tian, J., P. Lei, et al. (2008). "Regulated insulin delivery from human epidermal cells reverses hyperglycemia." Mol Ther 16(6): 1146-53.

[222] Toniatti, C., H. Bujard, et al. (2004). "Gene therapy progress and prospects: transcription regulatory systems." Gene Ther 11(8): 649-57.

[223] Uch, R., R. Gerolami, et al. (2003). "Hepatoma cell-specific ganciclovir-mediated toxicity of a lentivirally transduced HSV-TkEGFP fusion protein gene placed under the control of rat alpha-fetoprotein gene regulatory sequences." Cancer Gene Ther 10(9): 689-95.

[224] Urnov, F. D., J. C. Miller, et al. (2005). "Highly efficient endogenous human gene correction using designed zinc-finger nucleases." Nature 435(7042): 646-51.

[225] Valastyan, S., F. Reinhardt, et al. (2009). "A pleiotropically acting microRNA, miR-31, inhibits breast cancer metastasis." Cell 137(6): 1032-46.

[226] Van Duyne, G. D. (2001). "A structural view of cre-loxp site-specific recombination." Annu Rev Biophys Biomol Struct 30: 87-104.

[227] Vandendriessche, T., L. Thorrez, et al. (2007). "Efficacy and safety of adeno-associated viral vectors based on serotype 8 and 9 vs. lentiviral vectors for hemophilia B gene therapy." J Thromb Haemost 5(1): 16-24.

[228] Vaneycken, I., N. Devoogdt, et al. (2011). "Preclinical screening of anti-HER2 nanobodies for molecular imaging of breast cancer." FASEB J 25(7): 2433-46.

[229] Vargas, J., Jr., G. L. Gusella, et al. (2004). "Novel integrase-defective lentiviral episomal vectors for gene transfer." Hum Gene Ther 15(4): 361-72.

[230] Verhoeyen, E., V. Dardalhon, et al. (2003). "IL-7 surface-engineered lentiviral vectors promote survival and efficient gene transfer in resting primary T lymphocytes." Blood 101(6): 2167-74.

[231] Verhoeyen, E., M. Wiznerowicz, et al. (2005). "Novel lentiviral vectors displaying "early-acting cytokines" selectively promote survival and transduction of NOD/SCID repopulating human hematopoietic stem cells." Blood 106(10): 3386-95.

[232] Waehler, R., S. J. Russell, et al. (2007). "Engineering targeted viral vectors for gene therapy." Nat Rev Genet 8(8): 573-87.

[233] Wang, Y., H. H. Hu, et al. (2012). "Lentiviral transgenic microRNA-based shRNA suppressed mouse cytochromosome P450 3A (CYP3A) expression in a dose-dependent and inheritable manner." PLoS One 7(1): e30560.

[234] Wanisch, K. and R. J. Yanez-Munoz (2009). "Integration-deficient lentiviral vectors: a slow coming of age." Mol Ther 17(8): 1316-32.

[235] Watson, D. J., G. P. Kobinger, et al. (2002). "Targeted transduction patterns in the mouse brain by lentivirus vectors pseudotyped with VSV, Ebola, Mokola, LCMV, or MuLV envelope proteins." Mol Ther 5(5 Pt 1): 528-37.

[236] Wiederschain, D., S. Wee, et al. (2009). "Single-vector inducible lentiviral RNAi system for oncology target validation." Cell Cycle 8(3): 498-504.

[237] Wong, L. F., M. Azzouz, et al. (2004). "Transduction patterns of pseudotyped lentiviral vectors in the nervous system." Mol Ther 9(1): 101-11.

[238] Xu, Z. L., H. Mizuguchi, et al. (2003). "Regulated gene expression from adenovirus vectors: a systematic comparison of various inducible systems." Gene 309(2): 145-51.

[239] Yang, H., K. I. Joo, et al. (2009). "Cell type-specific targeting with surface-engineered lentiviral vectors co-displaying OKT3 antibody and fusogenic molecule." Pharm Res 26(6): 1432-45.

[240] Yang, L., H. Yang, et al. (2008). "Engineered lentivector targeting of dendritic cells for in vivo immunization." Nat Biotechnol 26(3): 326-34.

[241] Yu, D., D. Chen, et al. (2001). "Prostate-specific targeting using PSA promoter-based lentiviral vectors." Cancer Gene Ther 8(9): 628-35.

[242] Yu, D., C. Scott, et al. (2006). "Targeting and killing of prostate cancer cells using lentiviral constructs containing a sequence recognized by translation factor eIF4E and a prostate-specific promoter." Cancer Gene Ther 13(1): 32-43.

[243] Yu, S. T., C. Li, et al. (2011). "Noninvasive and real-time monitoring of the therapeutic response of tumors in vivo with an optimized hTERT promoter." Cancer 118(7): 1884-93.

[244] Zeilfelder, U. and V. Bosch (2001). "Properties of wild-type, C-terminally truncated, and chimeric maedi-visna virus glycoprotein and putative pseudotyping of retroviral vector particles." J Virol 75(1): 548-55.

[245] Zhang, J., L. Zou, et al. (2009). "Rapid generation of dendritic cell specific transgenic mice by lentiviral vectors." Transgenic Res 18(6): 921-31.

[246] Zhang, X. Y., R. H. Kutner, et al. (2010). "Cell-specific targeting of lentiviral vectors mediated by fusion proteins derived from Sindbis virus, vesicular stomatitis virus, or avian sarcoma/leukosis virus." Retrovirology 7: 3.

[247] Zheng, J. Y., D. Chen, et al. (2003). "Regression of prostate cancer xenografts by a lentiviral vector specifically expressing diphtheria toxin A." Cancer Gene Ther 10(10): 764-70.

[248] Zhu, Z. H., S. S. Chen, et al. (1990). "Phenotypic mixing between human immunodeficiency virus and vesicular stomatitis virus or herpes simplex virus." J Acquir Immune Defic Syndr 3(3): 215-9.

[249] Ziegler, L., L. Yang, et al. (2008). "Targeting lentiviral vectors to antigen-specific immunoglobulins." Hum Gene Ther 19(9): 861-72.

[250] Zufferey, R., D. Nagy, et al. (1997). "Multiply attenuated lentiviral vector achieves efficient gene delivery in vivo." Nat Biotechnol 15(9): 871-5.

Chapter 8

Vectors for Highly Efficient and Neuron-Specific Retrograde Gene Transfer for Gene Therapy of Neurological Diseases

Shigeki Kato, Kenta Kobayashi, Ken-ichi Inoue,
Masahiko Takada and Kazuto Kobayashi

Additional information is available at the end of the chapter

1. Introduction

Viral vectors have been widely used to deliver several therapeutic genes in the clinical approach of gene therapy. The lentiviral vector permits stable and efficient gene transfer into non-dividing cells in the central nervous system of neurological and neurodegenerative diseases (Deeks, et al., 2002; Mavilo, et al., 2006; Rossi et al., 2007; Ciceri, et al., 2009; Naldini, 2011). Moreover, long-term expression of delivered gene attributed to genome integration has an advantage not only for clinical application, but also for gene therapy trials in animal models (Naldini et al., 1996; Reiser et al., 1996; Mochizuki et al., 1998; Mitrophanous et al., 1999; Wong et al., 2006; Lundberg et al., 2008). Among many lentiviral vector systems, the most familiar is the human immunodeficiency virus type-1 (HIV-1)-based vector of which molecular biological property has been extensively studied (Rabson and Martin, 1985; Joshi and Joshi, 1996; Nielsen et al., 2005; Pluta and Kacprzak, 2009).

Axonal transport in the retrograde direction, as observed in the case of some viral vectors, has a considerable advantage for transferring genes into neuronal cell bodies situated in regions remote from the injection sites of the vectors (see Fig.1). These viral vectors, for example, injected into the striatum, transfer the genes via retrograde transport into nigrostriatal dopaminergic neurons, which are the major target for gene therapy of Parkinson's disease (Zheng et al., 2005; Barkats et al., 2006). Intramuscular injection of the vectors also delivers retrogradely the genes into motor neurons that are the target for gene therapy of motor neuron diseases (Baumgartner & Shine, 1998; Perrelet et al., 2000; Mazarakis et al., 2001; Sakamoto et al., 2003; Azzouz et al., 2004).

In our previous study, we generated an HIV-1-based vector pseudotyped with a variant of rabies virus glycoprotein (RV-G) gene and tested gene transfer through retrograde axonal transport into several brain regions (Kato et al., 2007). Although this pseudotyped vector showed gene transfer through retrograde transport in the rodent and nonhuman primate brains, higher titer stocks of the vector was required for the application of gene therapy trials. To enhance the efficiency of retrograde gene transfer, we subsequently developed a novel type of lentiviral vector that shows highly efficient retrograde gene transfer (HiRet) by pseudotyping an HIV-1-based vector with fusion glycoprotein B type (FuG-B) composed of parts of RV-G and vesicular stomatitis virus glycoprotein (VSV-G) (Kato et al., 2011a,b).

More recently, we developed another vector system for neuron-specific retrograde gene transfer (NeuRet) by pseudotyping the HIV-1-based vector with fusion glycoprotein C type (FuG-C) composed of a different set of parts of RV-G and VSV-G (Kato et al., 2011c). Interestingly, the NeuRet vector shows high efficiency of retrograde gene transfer into various neuronal populations, whereas it remarkably reduces gene transduction into dividing cells including glial and nerural stem/progenitor cells around the vector injection sites. One significant issue on the therapeutic use of lentiviral vectors is transgene integration into the host genome in dividing cells, which may lead to tumorigenesis by altering the expression of proto-oncogenes adjacent to the integration sites (De Palma et al., 2005; Themis et al., 2005; Montini et al., 2006). In this context, the NeuRet vector can reduce the risk of vector transduction into dividing cells in the brain and improve the safety of future gene therapy trials for neurological and neurodegenerative disorders.

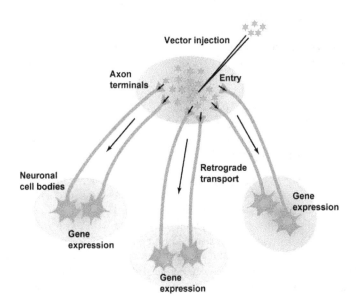

Figure 1. Gene transfer process through retrograde axonal transport.

The viral vectors enter nerve terminals and are retrogradely transported through axons into neuronal cell bodies, resulting in the induction of transgene expression.

In this chapter, we recapitulate gene transduction property of the HiRet and NeuRet vectors, and then describe the application of the NeuRet vector for retrograde gene transfer into the nigrostriatal dopamine system in nonhuman primates.

2. Gene transduction property of HiRet and NeuRet vectors

2.1. HiRet vector

The HiRet vector is a pseudotype of the HIV-1 lentiviral vector with FuG-B, which is composed of the extracellular and transmembrane domains of RV-G (challenged virus standard strain) and the cytoplasmic domain of VSV-G (Fig. 2A) (Kato et al., 2011a). When the HiRet vector encoding green fluorescent protein (GFP) was injected into the dorsal striatum of mice, we observed high efficiency of retrograde gene transfer into the brain regions innervating the striatum, including the primary motor cortex (M1), primary somatosensory cortex (S1), parafascicular nucleus (PF) in the thalamus, and substantia nigra pars compacta (SNc) in the ventral midbrain (Fig. 2B). The extent of gene transfer efficiency increased compared with that of the RV-G pseudotype, ranging from 8- to 14-folds dependent on the neural pathways. The high efficiency of gene transfer was also detected in the brain regions that project to the nucleus accumbens or medial prefrontal cortex in mice. In addition, we observed gene transduction of the HiRet vector into glial cells (~75%) and a small number of neuronal cells (~20%) in the striatum around the injection sites (Fig. 2C). Recently, we created a variant of FuG-B (termed FuG-B2), in which the extracellular and transmembrane domains of RV-G derived from the challenged virus standard strain was exchanged with the counterparts of Pasteur virus strain, and the vector pseudotyped with FuG-B2 exhibited a further increase in the retrograde gene transfer efficiency in the rodent brain (Kato et al., 2011b). More recently, Carpentier et al. (2012) reported the increased psudotyping efficiency of an HIV-1 vector by a chimeric envelope glycoprotein composed of RV-G and VSV-G domains, which corresponds to our FuG-B.

The host range of lentiviral vectors is altered by pseudotyping with different envelope glycoproteins (Cronin et al., 2005). Therefore, the possibility arises that some mutations in RV-G shift the efficiency of gene transduction or host cell specificity of the pseudotyped vector. Indeed, substitution of the cytoplasmic domain of RV-G with the corresponding part of the VSV-G enhanced the efficiency of retrograde gene transfer. The cytoplasmic domain differs in length between RV-G (44 amino acids) and VSV-G (29 amino acids), but their amino acid sequences do not show any particular homology (Rose et al., 1982). It appears that the cytoplasmic domain is involved in the mechanism underlying vector entry into synaptic terminals or the transduction level of the vector, resulting in enhanced retrograde gene transfer.

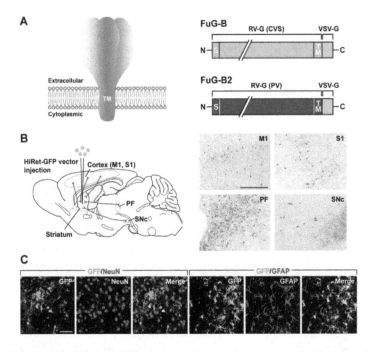

Figure 2. Gene trasnfer by HiRet vector. **(A)**Fusion envelope glycoprotein. The structure of viral envelope glycoprotein is schematically illustrated in the left panel. FuG-B is composed of the extracellular and transmembrane (TM) domains of RV-G derived from the challenge virus standard (CVS) strain fused to the cytoplasmic domain of VSV-G. In FuG-B2, the RV-G domains are exchanged by the counterparts of RV-G derived from Pasteur virus (PV) strain. S, signal peptide. **(B)** Gene transfer through retrograde transport. The HiRet vector pseudotyped with FuG-B, encoding GFP transgene was injected into the mouse striatum. Four weeks later, sections were processed for GFP immunostaining (right panel). GFP expression can be seen in the brain regions innervating the striatum, including the M1, S1, PF, and SNc. **(C)** Gene transduction around the injection sites. Sections through the striatum were stained by double immunofluorescence histochemistry for GFP/NeuN or for GFP/glial fibrillary acidic protein (GFAP). Scale bars: 50 μm. (Data from Kato et al., 2011a)

2.2. NeuRet vector

The NeuRet vector is another pseudotype of the HIV-1 lentiviral vector with FuG-C, which is composed of the N-terminal segment of the extracellular domain (439 amino acids) of RV-G and the C-terminal segment of the extracellular domain (16 amino acids) and transmembrane/cytoplasmic domains of VSV-G (Fig. 3A) (Kato et al., 2011c). After injection of the NeuRet vector encoding GFP transgene into the mouse striatum, we found enhanced retrograde gene transfer into the brain regions innervating the striatum, such as the M1, S1, PF, and SNc (Fig. 3B). The efficiency of gene transfer of the NeuRet vector was slightly different with that of the HiRet vector (FuG-B2 pseudo type), depending on the neural pathways (see a review by Kato et al. 2012). In addition, we tested gene transduction of the NeuRet vector surrounding the injection sites. Although the NeuRet vector transduced only a small number of striatal neuronal cells (~6%), its transduction level into striatal glial cells was quite low (~0.3%) (Fig. 3C). The property of gene transduction of the NeuRet vector around the injection sites was quite different from that of the HiRet vector, and in particular, the transduction of glial cells was largely declined in the NeuRet vector. Furthermore, when the NeuRet vector was injected into the subventricular zone, gene transduction of the vector into neural stem/progenitor cells was also inefficient.

FuG-C pseudotyping of the NeuRet vector enhanced the efficiency of retrograde gene transfer into various neuronal populations, whereas it caused less efficiency of gene transduction into glial and neural stem/progenitor cells. The N-terminal segment of the RV-G extracellular domain of 439 amino acids appears to be involved in the retrograde gene transfer, probably by promoting the interaction with synaptic terminals required for retrograde transport. Actually, amino acid residues essential for rabies virus virulence are reported to exist in the RV-G-derived extracellular domain used for FuG-C construction (Prehaud et al., 1988; Coulon et al., 1998). In contrast, pseudotyping with FuG-B (FuG-B2) and FuG-C generates a marked difference in gene transduction into glial and neural stem/progenitor cells around the injection areas. This difference suggests that the C-terminal part of 16 amino acids in the extracellular domain of envelope glycoproteins may be implicated in determining the host cell specificity of vector transduction, and that this C-terminal part may contribute to the interaction with glial and neural stem/progenitor cells.

For gene therapy trials with lentiviral vectors, there is a significant issue that vector insertion into the host genome may lead to tumorigenesis by altering the expression of cellular oncogenes surrounding the integration sites (De Palma et al., 2005; Themis et al., 2005; Montini et al., 2006). One useful approach to protect this issue is to restrict vector transduction to neuronal cells. The NeuRet vector system provides a useful approach for gene therapy trials for neurological diseases through enhanced retrograde gene transfer and improves the safety of gene therapy by profoundly suppressing the efficacy of gene transduction into dividing cells in the brain.

3. Retrograde gene delivery into monkey nigrostriatal pathway by NeuRet vector

The nigrostriatal dopamine system is a major target for gene therapy of Parkinson's disease. The availability of the HiRet vector for gene transfer via retrograde transport into the nigrostriatal dopamine system in nonhuman primates was described in our previous review (Kato et al., 2011d). To verify the capability of the NeuRet vector for efficient retrograde gene transfer into the nigrostriatal pathway, we injected the NeuRetvector encoding the GFP transgene into the striatum (caudate nucleus and putamen) of crab-eating monkeys (Fig. 4A). Intrastriatal injection of the NeuRet vector produced a larger number of GFP-positive neurons in the SNc (Fig. 4B). These positive signals were in register with immunostaining for tyrosine hydroxylase, a marker of dopaminergic neurons (Fig. 4C), indicating the transgene expression in the nigrostriatal dopaminergic neurons. In addition, we assessed the property of gene transduction with the NeuRet vector around the injection sites in the monkey striatum. The vector displayed a low level of gene transfer into neuronal cell bodies (~13%), and the level of vector transduction into glial cells was also quite low in the monkey striatum (~0.6%) (Fig. 4D).The pattern of gene transduction around the injection sites was similar to that obtained from the analysis of the mouse brain sections. Therefore, the NeuRet vector mediates enhanced retrograde gene transfer, whereas it reduces the gene transfer into glial cells around the injection areas in both rodent and monkey brains.

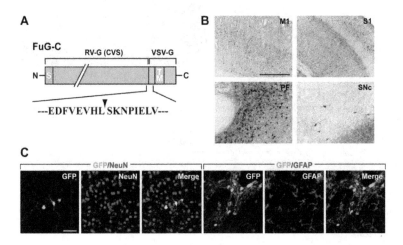

Figure 3. Gene delivery by NeuRet vector. (**A**) Structure of fusion envelope glycoprotein. FuG-C is composed of the N-terminal segment of the extracellular domain of RV-G and the C-terminal segment of the extracellular domain and the transmembrane(TM)/cytoplasmic domains of VSV-G. Amino acid sequences around the junction between the RV-G and VSV-G segments are shown. S, signal peptide. (**B**) Gene transfer through retrograde transport. The NeuRet vector encoding GFP transgene was injected into the mouse striatum, and four weeks later sections were processed for GFP immunostaining. GFP expression can be visualized in the M1, S1, PF, and SNc. (**C**) Gene transduction around the injection sites. Sections through the striatum were stained by double immunofluorescence histochemistry for GFP/NeuN or for GFP/glial fibrillary acidic protein (GFAP). Scale bars: 50 μm. (Data from Kato et al., 2011c)

The NeuRet vector system successfully achieved efficient gene transfer through retrograde transport into the nigrostriatal dopaminergic neurons in nonhuman primates. Our vector system will provide a powerful strategy for gene therapy of Parkinson's disease with enhanced retrograde gene transfer in the near future. This system will improve the safety of gene therapy by reducing the risk of gene transduction into proliferating cells (glial and neural stem/progenitor cells) in the brain.

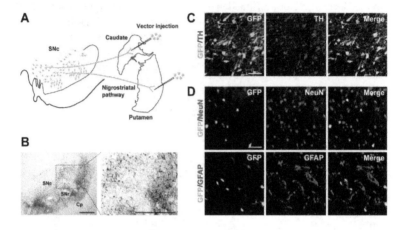

Figure 4. Transgene expression in the nigrostriatal dopamine system by NeuRet vector injection into the monkey striatum. (**A**) Gene transfer through retrograde transport after intrastriatal injection. The NeuRet vector encoding GFP transgene was stereotaxically injected into the caudate nucleus and the putamen, and histological analysis was performed on the brains fixed at the 4-week postinjection period. (**B**) GFP immunostaining in the SNc.Cp, cerebral peduncle; SNr, substantia nigra pars reticulata. (**C**) Double immunofluorescence staining for GFP and tyrosine hydroxylase (TH) in the SNc. (**D**) Double immunofluorescence staining for GFP/NeuN or GFP/glial fibrillary acidic protein (GFAP) in the striatum. Scale bars: 500 μm (**B**), and 50 μm (**C, D**). (Data from Kato et al., 2011c)

4. Conclusion

In this chapter, we mentioned the gene transduction property of the HiRet and NeuRet vectors pseudotyped with different fusion envelope glycoproteins. These two vectors showed the enhancement in gene transfer through retrograde axonal transport into various neuronal populations in both rodent and nonhuman primate brains. The HiRet vector transduced prominently glial cells around the injection sites, whereas gene transduction of the NeuRet vector into glial cells was much less efficient. The transduction level of the NeuRet vector into neural stem/progenitor cells was also low. The variation in the structure of envelope glycoproteins shifted the efficiency of retrograde gene transfer and the preference of host range. In addition, we described the application of the NeuRet vector for retrograde gene transfer into the nigrostriatal dopamine system of monkeys. The NeuRet vector, together with the HiRet vector, will offer a promising technology for gene therapy of neurological diseases through enhanced retrograde gene transfer. In particular, the NeuRet vector system will improve the safety of gene therapy by greatly suppressing the risk of gene transduction into dividing cells in the central nervous system.

Acknowledgements

This work was supported by grants-in aid from Core Research for Evolutional Science and Technology (CREST) of Japan Science and Technology Agency (JST). A part of this work was supported by "Highly Creative Animal Model Development for Brain Sciences" carried out under the Strategic Research Program for Brain Sciences by the Ministry of Education, Culture, Sports, Science and Technology of Japan. We thank St. Jude Children's Research Hospital (Dr. A. Nienhuis) and the George Washington University for providing the HIV-1-based vector system. We also grateful to M. Kikuchi, N. Sato, M. Watanabe, and T. Kobayashi for their technical support in the animal experiments.

Author details

Shigeki Kato[1], Kenta Kobayashi[2], Ken-ichi Inoue[3], Masahiko Takada[3] and Kazuto Kobayashi[1]

1 Department of Molecular Genetics, Institute of Biomedical Sciences, Fukushima Medical University School of Medicine, Fukushima, Japan

2 Section of Viral Vector Development, National Institute of Physiological Sciences, Okazaki, Japan

3 Systems Neuroscience Section, Primate Research Institute, Kyoto University, Inuyama, Japan

References

[1] Azzouz M., Ralph G. S., Storkebaum E., Walmsley L. E., Mitrophanous K. A., Kingsman S. M., Carmeliet P. & Mazarakis N. D. (2004). VEGF Delivery with Retrogradely Transported Lentivector Prolongs Survival in a Mouse ALS Model. *Nature*, Vol. 429, No. 6900, (May), pp. 413-417.

[2] Barkats M, Horellou P, Colin P, Millecamps S, Faucon-Biguet N, Mallet J. (2006). 1-Methyl-4-phenylpyridinium Neurotoxicity Is Attenuated by Adenoviral Gene Transfer of Human Cu/Zn Superoxide Dismutase. *Journal of Neuroscience Research*, (February), 83(2), pp. 233-242.

[3] Baumgartner B. J. & Shine H. D. (1998). Permanent Rescue of Lesioned Neonatal Motoneurons and Enhanced Axonal Regeneration by Adenovirus-Mediated Expression of Glial Cell Line-Derived Neurotrophic Factor. *Journal of Neuroscience Research*, Vol. 54, No. 6, (December), pp. 766-777.

[4] Carpentier D. C. J., Vevis K., Trabalza A., Georgiadis C., Ellison S. M., Asfahani R. L. & Mazarakis N. D. (2012). Enhanced Pseudotyping Efficiency of HIV-1 Lentiviral

Vectors by a Rabies/Vesicular Stomatitis Virus Chimeric Envelope Glycoprotein. *Gene Therapy*, Vol. 19, No. 7, (September), pp. 761-774.

[5] Ciceri F., Bonini C., Stanghellini M. T., Bondanza A., Traversari C., SalomoniM., Turchetto L., Colombi S., Bernardi M., Peccatori J., Pescarollo A., Servida P., Magnani Z., Perna S. K., Valtolina V., Crippa F., Callegaro L., Spoldi E., Crocchiolo R., Fleisch-hauer K., Ponzoni M., Vago L., Rossini S., Santoro A., Todisco E., Apperley J., Olavar-ria E., Slavin S., Weissinger E. M., Ganser A., Stadler M., Yannaki E., Fassas A., Anagnostopoulos A., Bregni M., Stampino C. G., Bruzzi P. & Bordignon C. (2009). In-fusion of Suicide-gene-engineered Donor Lymphocytes after Family Haploidentical Haemopoietic Stem-cell Transplantation for Leukaemia (the TK007 Trial): a Non-randomised Phase I-II Study. *The Lancet Oncology*, Vol. 10, No. 5, (May), pp. 489-500.

[6] Coulon P., Ternaux J. P., Flamand A. & Tuffereau C. (1998). An Avirulent Mutant of Rabies Virus Is Unable to Infect Motoneurons *In Vivo* and *In Vitro*. *Journal of Virology*, (January), 72(1), pp. 273-278.

[7] Cronin, J., Zhang, X. Y., & Reiser, J. (2005). Altering the Tropism of Lentiviral Vectors through Pseudotyping. *Current Gene Therapy*, (August), 5(4), 387-398.

[8] Deeks, S. G., Wagner, B., Anton, P. A., Mitsuyasu, R. T., Scadden, D. T., Huang, C., Macken, C., Richman, D. D., Christopherson, C., June, C. H., Lazar, R., Broad, D. F., Jalali, S., & Hege, K. M. (2002). A Phase II Randomized Study of HIV-specific T-cell Gene Therapy in Subjects with Undetectable Plasma Viremia on Combination Anti-retroviral Therapy. *Molecular Therapy*, (June), 5(6), 788-797.

[9] De Palma M., Montini E., Santoni de Sio F. R. S., Benedicenti F., Gentile A., Medico E. & Naldini, L. (2005). Promoter Trapping Reveals Significant Differences in Integra-tion Site Selection between MLV and HIV Vectors in Primary Hematopoietic Cells. *Blood*, (March), 105(6), pp. 2307-2315.

[10] Joshi S. & Joshi R. L. (1996). Molecular Biology of Human Immunodeficiency Virus Type-1. *Transfusion Science*, Vol. 17, No. 3, (September), pp. 351-378.

[11] Kato S., Inoue K., Kobayashi K., Yasoshima Y., Miyachi S., Inoue S., Hanawa H., Shi-mada T., Takada M. & Kobayashi K. (2007). Efficient Gene Transfer via Retrograde Transport in Rodent and Primate Brains Using a Human Immunodeficiency Virus Type 1-Based Vector Pseudotyped with Rabies Virus Glycoprotein. *Human Gene Therapy*, Vol. 18, No. 11, (November), pp. 1141-1151.

[12] Kato S., Kobayashi K., Inoue K., Kuramochi M., OkadaT., Yaginuma H., Morimoto K., Shimada T., Takada M. & Kobayashi K. (2011a). A Lentiviral Strategy for Highly Efficient Retrograde Gene Transfer by Pseudotyping with Fusion Envelope Glyco-protein. *Human Gene Therapy*, Vol. 22, No. 2, (February), pp. 197-206.

[13] Kato S., Kuramochi M., Kobayashi K., Fukabori R., Okada K., Uchigashima M., Wata-nabe M., Tsutsui Y. & Kobayashi K. (2011b). Selective Neural Pathway Targeting Re-veals Key Roles of Thalamostriatal Projection in the Control of Visual Discrimination. *Journal of Neuroscience*, Vol. 31, No. 47, (November), pp. 17169-17179.

[14] Kato S., Kuramochi M., Takasumi K., Kobayashi K., Inoue K., Takahara D., Hitoshi S., Ikenaka K., Shimada T., Takada M. & Kobayashi K. (2011c). Neuron-Specific Gene Transfer through Retrograde Transport of Lentiviral Vector Pseudotyped with a Novel Type of Fusion Envelope Glycoprotein. *Human Gene Therapy*, Vol. 22, No. 12, (December), pp. 1511-1523.

[15] Kato S., Kobayashi K., Kuramochi M., Inoue K., Takada M. & Kobayashi K. (2011d) Highly efficient retrograde gene transfer for genetic treatment of neurological diseases. *Viral Gene Therapy* (ed. KeXu) Chapter 17, InTech, Rijeka (Croatia), pp. 371-380.

[16] Kato, S., Kobayashi, K. & Kobayashi, K. (2012). Dissecting Circuit Mechanisms by Genetic Manipulation of Specific Neural Pathways. *Reviews in Neurosciences*, in press.

[17] Lundberg C., Björklund T., Carlsson T., Jakobsson J., Hantraye P., Déglon N. & Kirik D. (2008). Applications of Lentiviral Vectors for Biology and Gene Therapy of Neurological Disorders. *Current Gene Therapy*, Vol. 8, No. 6, (December), pp. 461-473.

[18] Mavilio F., Pellegrini G., Ferrari S., Di Nunzio F., Di Iorio E., Recchia A., Maruggi G., Ferrari G., Provasi E., Bonini C., Capurro S., Conti A., Magnoni C., Giannetti A. & De Luca M. (2006). Correction of Junctional Epidermolysis Bullosa by Transplantation of Genetically Modified Epidermal Stem Cells. *Nature Medicine*, Vol. 12, No. 12, (December), pp. 1397-1402.

[19] Mazarakis N. D., Azzouz M., Rohll J. B., Ellard F. M., Wilkes F. J., Olsen A. L., Carter E. E., Barber R. D., Baban D. F., Kingsman S. M., Kingsman A. J., O'Malley K. & Mitrophanous K. A. (2001). RabiesVirus Glycoprotein Pseudotyping of Lentiviral Vectors Enables Retrograde Axonal Transport and Access to the Nervous System after Peripheral Delivery. *Human Molecular Genetics*, Vol. 10, No. 19, (September), pp. 2109-2121.

[20] Mitrophanous K., Yoon S., Rohll J., Patil D., Wilkes F., Kim V., Kingsman S. Kingsman A. & Mazarakis N. (1999). Stable Gene Transfer to the Nervous System Using a Non-Primate Lentiviral Vector. *Gene Therapy*, Vol. 6, No. 11, (November), pp. 1808-1818.

[21] Mochizuki H., Schwartz J. P., Tanaka K., Brady R. O. & Reiser J. (1998). High-Titer Human Immunodeficiency Virus Type 1-Based Vector Systems for Gene Delivery into Nondividing Cells. *Journalof Virology*, Vol. 72, No. 11, (November), pp. 8873-8883.

[22] Montini E., Cesana D., Schmidt M., Sanvito F., Ponzoni M., Bartholomae C., Sergi L. S., Benedicenti F., Ambrosi A., Di Serio C., Doglioni C., von Kalle C. & Naldini L. (2006). Hematopoietic Stem Cell Gene Transfer in a Tumor-Prone Mouse Model Uncovers Low Genotoxicity of LentiviralVector Integration. *Nature Biotechnology*, Vol. 24, No. 6, (June), pp. 687-696.

[23] Naldini, L. (2011). *Ex Vivo* Gene Transfer and Correction for Cell-Based Therapies. *Nature Reviews Genetics*, (May), 12 (5), 301-315.

[24] Naldini L., Blömer U., Gage F. H., Trono D. & Verma, I. M. (1996). Efficient Transfer, Integration, and Sustained Long-Term Expression of the Transgene in Adult Rat Brains Injected with a Lentiviral Vector. *Proceedings of the National Academy of Sciences of the United States of America*, (October), 93(21), pp. 11382-11388.

[25] Nielsen, M.H., Pedersen, F.S. & Kjems, J. (2005). Molecular Strategy to Inhibit HIV-1 Replication. *Retrovirology*, (February), 2(10), 1-20.

[26] Perrelet D., Ferri A., MacKenzie A. E., Smith G. M., Korneluk R. G., Liston P., Sagot Y., Terrado J., Monnier D. & Kato A. C. (2000). IAP Family Proteins Delay Motoneuron Cell Death *In Vivo*. *European Journal of Neuroscience*, Vol. 12, No. 6, (June), pp. 2059-2067.

[27] Pluta, K. & Kacprzak, M. M. (2009). Use of HIV as a Gene Transfer Vector. *Acta Biochimica Polonica*, (November), 56(4), 531-595.

[28] Prehaud C., Coulon P., Lafay F., Thiers C. & Flamand A. (1988). Antigenic Site II of the Rabies Virus Glycoprotein: Structure and Role in Viral Virulence. *Journal of Virology*, Vol. 62, No. 1, (January), pp. 1-7.

[29] Rabson, A.B. & Martin, M.A. (1985). Molecular Organization of the AIDS Retrovirus. *Cell*, (March), 40(3), 477-480.

[30] Reiser J., Harmison G., Kluepfel-Stahl S., Brady R. O., Karlsson S. & Schubert M. (1996). Transduction of Nondividing Cells Using Pseudotyped Defective High-Titer HIV Type 1 Particles. *Proceedings of the National Academy of Sciences of the United States of America*, (December), 93(26), pp. 15266-15271.

[31] Rose J. K., Doolittle R. F., Anilionis A., Curtis P. J. & Wunner W. H. (1982). Homology between the Glycoproteins of Vesicular Stomatitis Virus and Rabies Virus. *Journal of Virology*, Vol. 43, No. 1, (July), pp. 361-364.

[32] Rossi, J.J., June, C.H., & Kohn, D.B. (2007). Genetic Therapies against HIV. *Nature Biotechnology*, (December), 25(12), 1444-1454.

[33] Sakamoto T., Kawagoe Y., Shen J. S., Takeda Y., Arakawa Y., Ogawa J., Oyanagi K., Ohashi T., Watanabe K., Inoue K., Eto Y. & Watabe K. (2003). Adenoviral Gene Transfer of GDNF, BDNF and TGF * * , but not CNTF, Cardiotrophin-1 or IGF1, Protects Injured Adult Motoneurons after Facial Nerve Avulsion. *Journal of Neuroscience Research*, Vol. 72, No. 1, (April), pp. 54-64.

[34] Themis M., Waddington S. N., Schmidt M., von Kalle C., Wang Y., Al-Allaf F., Gregory L. G., Nivsarkar M., Themis M., Holder M. V., Buckley S. M., Dighe N., Ruthe A. T., Mistry A., Bigger B., Rahim A., Nguyen T. H., Trono D., Thrasher A. J. & Coutelle C. (2005). Oncogenesis Following Delivery of a Nonprimate Lentiviral Gene Therapy Vector to Fetal and Neonatal Mice. *Molecular Therapy*, (October), 12(4), pp. 763-771.

[35] Wong L. F., Goodhead L., Prat C., Mitrophanous K. A., Kingsman S. M. & Mazarakis N. D. (2006). Lentivirus-Mediated Gene Transfer to the Central Nervous System:

Therapeutic and Research Applications. *Human Gene Therapy*, Vol. 17, No. 1, (January), pp. 1-9.

[36] Zheng J. S., Tang L. L., Zheng S. S., Zhan R. Y., Zhou Y. Q., Goudreau J., Kaufman D. & Chen A. F. (2005). Delayed Gene Therapy of Glial Cell Line-Derived Neurotrophic Factor is Efficacious in a Rat Model of Parkinson's Disease. *Molecular Brain Research*, Vol. 134, No. 1, (March), pp. 155-161.

Chapter 9

Efficient AAV Vector Production System: Towards Gene Therapy For Duchenne Muscular Dystrophy

Takashi Okada

Additional information is available at the end of the chapter

1. Introduction

1.1. Choice of vector

Successful gene therapy requires an adequate level of long-term transgene expression in the target tissues. While various viral vectors have been considered for the delivery of genes *in vivo*, an adeno-associated virus (AAV)-based vector is emerging as the gene transfer vehicle with the most potential for use in the neuromuscular gene therapies. The advantages of the AAV vector include the lack of disease associated with a wild-type virus, the ability to transduce non-dividing cells, and the long-term expression of the delivered transgenes.[1] Some serotypes of recombinant AAV (rAAV) exhibit a potent tropism for striated muscles.[2] Therefore, a supplementation of secretory protein can be achieved with this vector to use intramuscular injection.[3] Since a 5-kb genome is considered to be the upper limit for a single AAV virion, various truncated genes could be provided to meet size capacity, if nessessarry.[4]

Due to ingenious cloning and preparation techniques, adenovirus vectors are efficient delivery systems of episomal DNA into eukaryotic cell nuclei.[5] The utility of adenovirus vectors has been increased by capsid modifications that alter tropism, and by the generation of hybrid vectors that promote chromosomal insertion.[6] Also, gutted adenovirus vectors devoid of all adenoviral genes allow for the insertion of large transgenes, and trigger fewer cytotoxic and immunogenic effects than do those only deleted in the E1 regions of the adenovirus early genes.[7] Human artificial chromosomes (HACs) have the capacity to deliver genes in any size into host cells without integrating the gene into the host genome, thereby preventing the possibility of insertional mutagenesis and genomic instability.[8]

Long-term correction of genetic diseases requires permanent integration of therapeutic genes into chromosomes of the affected cells. However, retrovirus vector integration can trigger deregulated premalignant cell proliferation with unexpected frequency, most likely driven by retrovirus enhancer activity on the LMO2 gene promoter. [9] A goal in clinical gene therapy is to develop gene transfer vehicles that can integrate exogenous therapeutic genes at specific chromosomal loci as a safe harbor, so that insertional oncogenesis is prevented. AAV can insert its genome into a specific locus, designated AAVS1, on chromosome 19 of the human genome.[10] The AAV Rep78/68 proteins and the Rep78/68-binding sequences are the trans- and cis-acting elements needed for this reaction. A dual high-capacity adenovirus-AAV hybrid vector with full-length human dystrophin-coding sequences flanked by AAV integration-enhancing elements was tested for targeted integration.[11]

1.2. AAV biology

AAV is a small (20-26nm) non-enveloped dependent parvovirus with a single-stranded linear genome that contains two open reading frames (*rep* and *cap*).[12] The viral genome is characterized by the inverted terminal repeats (ITRs) to flank these open reading frames (Figure 1A). The genome encodes four replication proteins (Rep78, Rep68, Rep52, and Rep40) and three capsid proteins (Cap: VP1, VP2, and VP3). The large Rep (Rep78 and Rep68) proteins regulate AAV gene expression and hold nicking activity at the terminal resolution site as well as binding activity at Rep binding elements to process AAV replication (Figure 1B). The small Rep proteins (Rep52 and Rep40) are used for the accumulation of single-stranded viral genome followed by packaging within AAV capsids.

The minimum sets of regions in helper adenovirus that mediate AAV vector replication are the E1, E2A, E4, and VA.[13] A human embryonic kidney cell line 293 encodes the E1 region of the Ad5 genome.[14] The helper plasmid assembling E2A, E4, and VA regions (Ad-helper plasmid) is cotransfected into the 293 cells, along with plasmids encoding the AAV vector genome (vector plasmid) as well as *rep* and *cap* genes (AAV-helper plasmid). AAV vector is produced as efficiently as when adenovirus infection is employed as a helper virus. Furthermore, contamination of most adenovirus proteins can be avoided in AAV vector stock made by this helper virus-free method.

1.3. Vector application using various serotypes

The preparation of AAV vector for gene therapy study of neuromuscular diseases is greatly facilitated. Although AAV2 has been the serotype most extensively studied in preclinical and clinical trials, recently we have focused on the use of AAV vectors pseudotyped with capsid protein of alternative serotypes. A number of primate AAV serotypes have been characterized in the literature and are designated. There is divergence in homology and tropism for various AAV serotypes. For instance, the homology with capsid protein is only about 60% between AAV2 and AAV5[15], therefore the capsid structure could be responsible for the improved transduction efficiency.

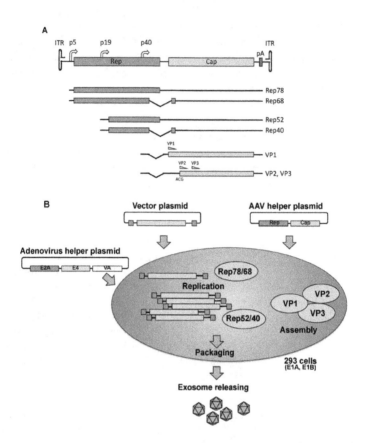

Figure 1. A) The *rep* and *cap* genes flanked by ITRs. The large Rep proteins (Rep78 and Rep68) are produced from transcripts using p5 promoter, while small Rep (Rep52 and Rep40) are produced from p19 promoter. (B) Recombinant AAV production. AAV has productive infection in the presence of adenovirus helper regions (E1, E2A, E4, and VA). This process is characterized by genome replication, assembly of the capsid proteins (VP1, VP2, and VP3), and packaging leading to virion production along with exosome releasing.

We found that choice of AAV serotypes and promoters could be quite useful for targeted transgene expression. For instance, the transgene expression of rAAV5 with the Rous sarcoma virus (RSV) promoter was preferentially found in the granular cells of the gerbil hippocampus, whereas transgene expression of rAAV2 with the RSV promoter was found in the pyramidal and granular cells.[16] Since AAV3 vector can specifically transduce cochlear inner hair cells with high efficiency *in vivo*, rAAV-mediated transduction might be promising for gene replacement strategies to correct recessive genetic hearing loss due to monogenic mutation.[17] Also, there is a significant difference in transgene expression by various AAV serotypes transduced into muscle. We observed that intramuscular injection of AAV5-IL-10 promoted a much higher serum level of secreted transgene product, as compared to AAV2-

mediated transfer.[18] We further demonstrated that AAV1 could more efficiently transduce the muscle than AAV5. Intramuscular single injection of modest doses of rAAV1 expressing IL-10 (6×10^{10} g.c. per rat) introduced therapeutic levels of the transgene expression over the long-term to treat pulmonary arterial hypertension.[3] rAAV1-mediated sustained IL-10 expression also significantly ameliorated hypertensive organ damage to improve survival rate of Dahl salt-sensitive rats.[19] Furthermore, this protein supplementation therapy by rAAV1-mediated muscle transduction was quite effective to prevent vascular remodeling and end-organ damage in the stroke-prone spontaneously hypertensive rat.[20] Interestingly, alpha-sarcoglycan expression with single intramuscular injection of rAAV8 was widely distributed in the hind limb muscle as well as cardiac muscle, and persisted for 7 months with a reversal of the muscle pathology and improvement in the contractile force in the alpha-sarcoglycan-deficient mice.[21] Intravenous administration of rAAV8 into the hind limb in dogs resulted in improved transgene expression in the skeletal muscles lasting over a period of 8 weeks.[22] Moreover, rAAV9 would be administered systemically with excellent cardiac tropism.[23] Further strategies have been attempted to discover novel AAV capsid sequences from primate tissue, which can be used to develop newer-generation rAAVs with a greater diversity of tissue tropism for clinical gene therapy.

1.4. scAAV

Clinical gene therapy often requires rapid transduction with reasonable efficiency. In the case of AAV, second strand synthesis of the vector genome in the nucleus is the rate-limiting step for efficient transduction. Therefore, self-complementary AAV (scAAV) vector would be quite promising to promote efficient transduction regardless of DNA synthesis or annealing. [24] The scAAV vectors can bypass the inter-molecular annealing or second-strand synthesis by using intra-molecular annealing to immediately form transcriptionally active double-stranded DNA (Figure 2). Although immediate and efficient transduction could be observed with scAAV, the maximal insert size of the transgene cassette is reduced to 3.3 kb.[25]

2. Effective production strategies of rAAV

2.1. Principle of production

To gain acceptance as a medical treatment with a dose of over 1×10^{13} genome copies (g.c.)/kg body weight, therapeutic strategies with AAV vectors require a scalable and provident production method. However, the production and purification of recombinant virus stocks with conventional techniques entails cumbersome procedures not suited to the clinical setting. Therefore, development of effective large-scale culture and purification steps are required to meet end-product specifications.

A production protocol of AAV vectors in the absence of a helper virus[13] is widely employed for triple plasmid transduction of human embryonic kidney 293 cells.[1] The adenovirus regions that mediate AAV vector replication (namely, the VA, E2A and E4 regions) were assembled into a helper plasmid. When this helper plasmid is co-transfected into 293 cells along with plasmids encoding the AAV vector genome and *rep-cap* genes, the AAV vector is produced as efficiently as when using adenovirus infection. Importantly, contamination of most adenovirus proteins can be avoided in AAV vector stock made by this helper virus-free method.

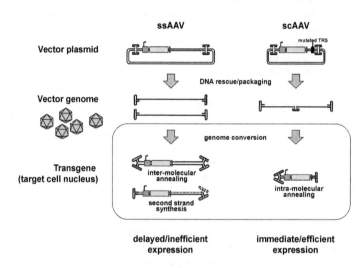

Figure 2. DNA rescue and transduction of a conventional single-stranded AAV (ssAAV) and a self-complementary AAV (scAAV) vector. Full-length ssAAV vector genome of both polarities are rescued from the vector plasmid and individually packaged into the AAV capsids. As a genome conversion in the transduced cell nucleus, the single-to-double stranded conversion of the DNA goes through the inter-molecular annealing or second strand synthesis. In contrast, a scAAV vector with half the size of the ssAAV genome has a mutation in the terminal resolution site (TRS) to form a vector genome with wild-type ITRs at the both ends and mutated ITR at the center of symmetry. After uncoating in the target cell nucleus, this DNA structure can readily fold into transcriptionally active double-stranded form through intra-molecular annealing.

Although various subtypes of the 293 cells harbor the E1 region of the adenovirus type 5 genome, to utilize a 293 cell stably expressing Bcl-xL (293B) has great advantage to support E1B19K function and protect cells from apoptosis.[26] Despite improvements in vector production, including the development of packaging cell lines expressing Rep/Cap or methods to regulate Rep/Cap,[27] maintaining such cell lines remains difficult, as the early expression of Rep proteins is toxic to cells.

We developed a large-scale transfection method of producing AAV vectors with an active gassing system that uses large culture vessels to process labor-effective transfection in a closed system.[28] This vector production system achieved reasonable production efficiency by improving gas exchange to prevent pH drop in the culture medium. Also, vector purification with the dual ion-exchange membrane adsorbers was effective and allowed higher levels of gene transfer *in vivo*.[29] Furthermore, the membrane adsorbers enabled the effective recovery of the AAV vector in the supernatant exosomes of the transduced cells culture.

This rapid and scalable viral purification protocol is particularly promising for considerable *in vivo* experimentation and clinical investigations (Figure 3).

Recent developments also suggest that AAV vector production in insect cells would be compatible with current good manufacturing practice production on an industrial scale.[30]

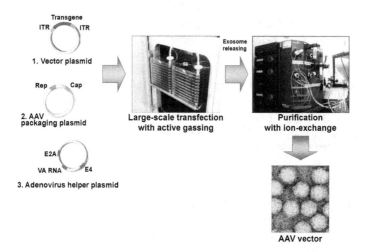

AAV vector

Figure 3. A scalable triple plasmid transfection using active gassing. When (1) a vector plasmid encoding the transgene cassette flanked by ITRs is co-transfected into human embryonic kidney 293 cells with (2) an AAV packaging plasmid harboring *rep-cap* genes and (3) an adenovirus helper plasmid, the AAV vector is produced as efficiently as when using adenovirus infection. A large-scale transduction method to produce AAV vectors with an active gassing system makes use of large culture vessels for labor- and cost-effective vector production in a closed system. Samples containing vector particles are further purified with a quick two-tier CsCl gradient centrifugation and an ion-exchange chromatography to obtain highly purified vector stocks.

2.2. Large-scale production with active gassing

Our protocol utilizes the transfection of 293B cells in one 10-Tray flask (CF10; Nalge Nunc International, Rochester, NY) with a surface area of 6320 cm^2 by using an active gassing at 500 ml/min. Typical transduction procedure is conducted with one or two CF10 to meet downstream purification protocol. Although previous protocols for recombinant virus production in a large culture vessel had the problem of insufficient transduction efficiency because of inadequate gas exchange, this method to use active gassing significantly improves productivity of the vectors and is linearly scalable from the small 225-cm^2 flask.[3]

The 293B cells are cultured in Dulbecco's modified Eagle's medium and Nutrient Mixture F-12 (D-MEM/F-12, Invitrogen, Grand Island, NY) with 10% fetal bovine serum (SIGMA-ALDRICH, St Louis, MO), 100 units/ml penicillin, and 100 µg/ml streptomycin at 37 °C in a 5% CO_2 incubator. Cells are initially plated at 8 x 10^7 cells per CF10 to achieve a monolayer of 20 to 40% confluency when cells attached to surface of the flask. The volume of medium utilized per flask is 1120 ml. Subsequently, cells are grown for 48-72 h until reaching 70-90% confluence and are consequently transfected with appropriate triple plasmids. An aquarium pump (Nisso, Tokyo, Japan) should be used to circulate the gas through the CF10 with 5% CO_2 and humidity in an incubator.

Half of the medium in the CF10 tissue culture flask are exchanged with fresh D-MEM/F-12 containing 10% FBS, 1 h before transfection of the 293 cells. Subsequently, the cells are co-transfected with 650 μg of each plasmid: a proviral vector plasmid, an AAV helper plasmid, as well as an adenoviral helper plasmid, using calcium phosphate co-precipitation. Each plasmid was added to 112 ml of 300 mM $CaCl_2$. This solution was gently added to the same volume of 2 x HBS (290 mM NaCl, 50 mM HEPES buffer, 1.5 mM Na_2HPO_4, pH 7.0) and gently inverted 3 times to form a uniform solution. This solution was immediately mixed with fresh D-MEM/F-12 containing 10% FBS to produce a homogeneous plasmid solution mixture. Subsequently, the medium in the culture flask was replaced with this plasmid solution mixture. At the end of a 6-12 h incubation, the plasmid solution mixture in the culture flask was replaced with pre-warmed fresh D-MEM/F-12 containing 2% FBS.

2.3. Purification phase

The culture supernatant sample for the ion-exchange procedure is processed by centrifugation and filtration. The culture supernatant fluid 72-96 h after the transduction is sampled and then clarified with an appropriate amount of the activated charcoal (Wako Pure Chemical Industries, Osaka, Japan). Insoluble debris is removed by a centrifugation at 3,000 g for 15 min and filtration. The elucidated culture supernatant is enriched with a hollow fiber cross flow membrane (100,000 NMWC, GE Healthcare, Pittsburgh, PA). For the material obtained from a CF10, 5 mM $MgCl_2$ (final concentration) with 2,500-5,000 units of Benzonase nuclease is added to incubate for 30 min at 37 °C. Sequentially, 5 mM EDTA (final concentration) is added to terminate the reaction. Place 38 ml of the sample solution in a semi-sterile ultracentrifuge tube (Ultrabottle #3430-3870; Nalge Nunc, Rochester, NY) and remove the cell debris by centrifugation at 10,000g for 15 minutes at 4 °C to achieve cleared lysates. The sample is quickly concentrated by the brief two-tier CsCl (1.25 and 1.60 g/cm³) step gradient centrifugation for 3 h and then the vector fraction is dialyzed in the MHA buffer (3.3 mM MES 3.3 mM HEPES [pH 8.0], 3.3 mM NaOAc).

Chromatography can be performed using an appropriate FPLC system, such as AKTA explorer 10S (Amersham Biosciences, Piscataway, NJ, USA) equipped with a 50 ml Superloop. The sample which passed through the Mustang™ S membrane (optional treatment, PALL corporation, NY) is dialyzed against MHA buffer and further loaded onto an anion-exchange membrane (acrodisc unit with Mustang™ Q membrane, PALL corporation, equilibrated with MHA buffer) at a rate of 3 ml/min. The membrane is then washed with 10 column volumes of MHA buffer. Bound virus on the Mustang™ Q membrane is eluted over a 50 column volume span with a 0-2 M linear NaCl gradient in MHA buffer and 0.5-1 ml fractions are collected. Recombinant rAAV particle number is determined by quantitative PCR of DNase I-treated stocks with plasmid standards. The final titer of the purified vectors from a CF10 usually ranges around 5 x 10^{13} genome copies (g.c.), although it depends on the vector constructs and transgene.

3. AAV-mediated therapeutic approach to neuromuscular disease

3.1. DMD gene replacement therapy

Duchenne muscular dystrophy (DMD) is the most common form of childhood muscular dystrophy and is an X-linked recessive disorder with an incidence of one in 3500 live male births.[31] DMD causes progressive degeneration and regeneration of skeletal and cardiac muscles due to mutations in the *dystrophin* gene, which encodes a 427-kDa subsarcolemmal cytoskeletal protein.[32] DMD is associated with severe, progressive muscle weakness and typically leads to death between the ages of 20 and 35 years. Due to recent advances in respiratory care, much attention is now focused on treating the cardiac conditions suffered by DMD patients. The approximately 2.5-megabase *dystrophin* gene is the largest gene identified to date, and because of its size, it is susceptible to a high sporadic mutation rate. Absence of dystrophin and the dystrophin-glycoprotein complex (DGC) from the sarcolemma leads to severe muscle wasting. Whereas DMD is characterized by the absence of functional protein, Becker muscular dystrophy, which is commonly caused by in-frame deletions of the *dystrophin* gene, results in the synthesis of an incompletely functional protein.

Successful therapy for DMD requires the restoration of dystrophin protein in skeletal and cardiac muscles. While various viral vectors have been considered for the delivery of genes to muscle fibers, the AAV-based vector is emerging as an appropriate gene transfer vehicle with the most potential for use in DMD gene therapies. As for another candidate vehicle, the gutted adenovirus vector can package 14-kb of full-length *dystrophin* cDNA due to the large deletion in virus genome. Multiple proximal muscles of seven-day-old utrophin/dystrophin double knockout mice (*dko* mice), which typically show symptoms similar to human DMD, were effectively transduced with the gutted adenovirus bearing full-length murine *dystrophin* cDNA.[33] However, further improvements are needed to regulate the virus-associated host immune response before clinical trials can be performed.

A series of truncated *dystrophin* cDNAs containing rod repeats with hinge 1, 2, and 4 were constructed (Figure 4A).[4] Although AAV vectors are too small to package the full-length *dystrophin* cDNA, AAV vector-mediated gene therapy using a rod-truncated *dystrophin* gene provides a promising approoch.[34] The structure and, particularly, the length of the rod are crucial for the function of micro-dystrophin.[35] An AAV type 2 vector expressing micro-dystrophin (DeltaCS1) under the control of a muscle-specific MCK promoter was injected into the tibialis anterior (TA) muscles of dystrophin-deficient *mdx* mice,[36] and resulted in extensive and long-term expression of micro-dystrophin that exhibited improved force generation. Likewise, AAV6 vector-mediated systemic *micro-dystrophin* gene transfer was effective in treating *dko* mice.[37] The potential for ameliorating the pathology of advanced-stage muscular dystrophy by systemic administration of AAV6 vectors encoding a micro-dystrophin expression construct was also demonstrated.[38] Furthermore, AAV9 vector-mediated *micro-dystrophin* transduction of *mdx* mice accomplished prevention of cardiac fibrosis as well as heart failure.[23] The transduction efficiency achieved with rAAV9 was nearly complete, with persistent expression for 74 weeks after transduction (Figure 4BC). Both the strong affinity of the rAAV9 for cardiac tissue and the therapeutic effect of the expressed micro-dystrophin might be involved in the prevention of the degeneration of the cardiomyocytes and cardiac fibrosis.

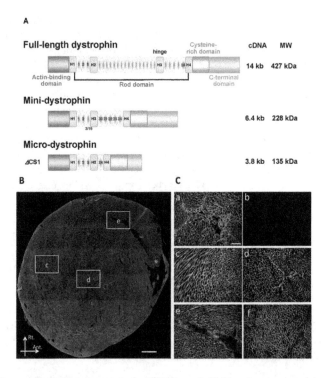

Figure 4. AAV9 vector-mediated *cardiac* transduction. (A) Structures of full-length and truncated dystrophin. Helper-dependent adenovirus vector can package 14-kb of full-length dystrophin cDNA because of the large-sized deletion in its genome. A mini-dystrophin is cloned from a patient with Becker muscular dystrophy, which is caused by in-frame deletions resulting in the synthesis of partially functional protein. A truncated micro-dystrophin cDNAs harboring only four rod repeats with hinge 1, 2, and 4 and a deleted C-terminal domain (delta CS1) is constructed to be packaged in the AAV vector. (B) Transverse section of *mdx* mouse heart at mid-ventricular level 24 weeks after transduction of *micro-dystrophin*, stained with anti-dystrophin antibody NCL-DysB. Scale bar, 500 μm. (C) Expression of dystrophin in C57BL10 hearts at the sarcolemma (a), while it is absent in *mdx* hearts (b). Magnified views of sections from the center of the left ventricle at 28 weeks (c-e) show micro-dystrophin expression in the areas indicated in B (scale bar, 100 μm). At 74 weeks after transduction, *mdx* mice still retain extensive expression of micro-dystrophin (f).

The impact of codon usage optimization on micro-dystrophin expression and function in the *mdx* mouse was demonstrated to compare the function of two different configurations of codon-optimized *micro-dystrophin* genes under the control of a muscle-restrictive promoter

(Spc5-12).[39] Codon optimization of micro-dystrophin significantly increased micro-dystrophin mRNA and protein levels after intramuscular and systemic administration of plasmid DNA or rAAV8. By randomly assembling myogenic regulatory elements into synthetic promoter recombinant libraries, several artificial promoters were isolated whose transcriptional potencies greatly exceed those of natural myogenic and viral gene promoters.[40]

3.2. Intravascular vector administration by limb perfusion

Although recent studies suggest that vectors based on AAV are capable of body-wide transduction in rodents,[21] translating the characteristics into large animals with advanced immune system remains a lot of challenges. Intravascular delivery can be performed as a form of limb perfusion, which might bypass the immune activation of DCs in the injected muscle. [41] We performed limb perfusion-assisted intravenous administration of rAAV8-lacZ into the hind limb of Beagle dogs (Figure 5A).[42] Administration of rAAV8 by limb perfusion demonstrated extensive transgene expression in the distal limb muscles of canine X-linked muscular dystrophy in Japan (CXMD$_J$) dogs without obvious immune responses for the duration of the experiment over four weeks after injection.

3.3. Systemic transduction and immunological issues

In comparison with fully dystrophin-deficient animals, targeted transgenic repair of skeletal muscle, but not cardiac muscle, paradoxically elicits a five-fold increase in cardiac injury and dilated cardiomyopathy.[43] Because the dystrophin-deficient heart is highly sensitive to increased stress, increased activity by the repaired skeletal muscle provides the stimulus for heightened cardiac injury and heart remodeling. In contrast, a single intravenous injection of AAV9 vector expressing micro-dystrophin efficiently transduces the entire heart in neonatal *mdx* mice, thereby ameliorating cardiomyopathy.[44]

Since a number of muscular dystrophy patients can be identified through newborn screening in future, neonatal transduction may lead to an effective early intervention in DMD patients. After a single intravenous injection, robust skeletal muscle transduction with AAV9 vector throughout the body was observed in neonatal dogs.[45] Systemic transduction was achieved in the absence of pharmacological intervention or immune suppression and lasted for at least six months, whereas rAAV9 was barely transduced into the cardiac muscle of dogs. Likewise, *in utero* gene delivery of full-length murine *dystrophin* to *mdx* mice using a high-capacity adenoviral vector resulted in effective protection from cycles of degeneration and regeneration.[46]

Neo-antigens introduced by AAV vectors evoke significant immune reactions in DMD muscle, since increased permeability of the DMD muscle allows leakage of the transgene products from the dystrophin-deficient sarcolemma of muscle fibers.[47] rAAV2 transfer into skeletal muscles of normal dogs resulted in low levels of transient expression, together with intense cellular infiltration, and the marked activation of cellular and humoral immune responses.[48] Furthermore, an *in vitro* interferon-gamma release assay showed that canine splenocytes respond to immunogens or mitogens more strongly than do murine splenocytes. Therefore, co-administration of immunosuppressants, cyclosporine (CSP) and mycophenolate mofetil (MMF) was attempted to improve rAAV2-mediated transduction. The AAV2 capsids can induce a cellular immune response via MHC class I antigen presentation with a cross-presentation pathway,[49] and rAAV2 could also stimulate human dendritic cells (DCs).[50] Whereas the non-immunogenic nature of AAV6 in murine studies, rAAV6 also elicited robust cellular immune responses in dogs.[51] In contrast, other serotypes, such as rAAV8, induce T-cell activation to a lesser degree.[42] The rAAV8-injected muscles showed lowed rates of infiltration of $CD4^+$ and $CD8^+$ T lymphocytes in the endomysium than the rAAV2-injected muscles.[42]

Resident antigen-presenting cells, such as DCs, myoblasts, myotubes and regenerating immature myofibers, should play a substantial role in the immune response against rAAV. Our study also showed that MyD88 and co-stimulating factors, such as CD80, CD86 and type I interferon, are up-regulated in both rAAV2- and rAAV8-transduced dog DCs (Figure 5B).[42]

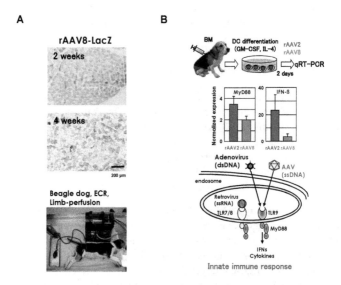

Figure 5. rAAV-mediated transduction of dog. (A) Intravascular vector administration by limb perfusion. A blood pressure cuff is applied just above the knee of an anesthetized CXMD$_j$ dog. A 24-gauge intravenous catheter is inserted into the lateral saphenous vein, connected to a three-way stopcock, and flushed with saline. With a blood pressure cuff inflated to over 300 mmHg, saline (2.6 ml/kg) containing papaverine (0.44 mg/kg, Sigma-Aldrich, St. Louis, MO) and heparin (16 U/kg) is injected by hand over a 10 second period. The three-way stopcock is connected to a syringe containing rAAV8 (1 x 10^{14} vg/kg, 3.8 ml/kg). The syringe is placed in a PHD 2000 syringe pump (Harvard Apparatus, Edenbridge, UK). Five minutes after the papaverine/heparin injection, rAAV8-LacZ is injected at a rate of 0.6 ml/sec. Two minutes after the rAAV injection, the blood pressure cuff is released and the catheter is removed. Four weeks after the transduction, the expression slightly fell off. (B) AAV-mediated stimulation of innate immune response via TLR9/MyD88 pathway. Bone marrow (BM)-derived dendritic cells (DCs) were obtained from humerus bones and cultured in RPMI (10% FCS, p/s) for 7 days with canine GM-CSF and IL-4. DCs were transduced with rAAV2- or rAAV8-*lacZ* (1x10^6 vg/cell for 4 hours, and mRNA levels of MyD88 and IFN-β were analyzed. Untransduced cells were used as a normalization standard to demonstrate relative value of expression. Results are representative of two independent experiments. Error bars represent s.e.m., n = 3.

4. Safety and potential impact of clinical trials

4.1. Clinical trials for muscle transduction

While low immunogenicity was considered a major strength supporting the use of rAAV in clinical trials, a number of observations have recently provided a more balanced view of this procedure.[52] An obvious barrier to AAV transduction is the presence of circulating neutralizing antibodies that prevent the virion from binding to its cellular receptor.[53] This potential threat can be reduced by prescreening patients for AAV serotype-specific neutralizing antibodies or by performing therapeutic procedures such as plasmapheresis before gene transfer. Another challenge recently revealed is the development of a cell-mediated cytotoxic T-cell (CTL) response to AAV capsid peptides. In the human factor IX gene therapy trial in which rAAV was delivered to the liver, only short-term transgene expression was achieved and levels of therapeutic protein declined to baseline levels 10 weeks after vector infusion.[52] This was accompanied by elevation of serum transaminase levels and a CTL response toward specific AAV capsid peptides. To overcome this response, transient immunosuppression may be required until AAV capsids are completely cleared. Additional findings suggest that T-cell activation requires AAV2 capsid binding to the heparan sulfate proteoglycan (HSPG) receptor, which would permit virion shuttling into a DC pathway, as cross-presentation.[54] Exposure to vectors from other AAV clades, such as AAV8, did not activate capsid-specific T-cells.

The initial clinical studies lay the foundation for future studies, providing important information about vector dose, viral serotype selection, and immunogenicity in humans. The first virus-mediated gene transfer for muscle disease was carried out for limb-girdle muscular dystrophy type 2D using rAAV1. The study, consisting of intramuscular injection of virus into a single muscle, was limited in scope and the main conclusion was to establish the safety of this procedure in phase I clinical trials. The first clinical gene therapy trial for DMD began in March 2006.[55] This was a Phase I/IIa study in which an AAV vector was used to deliver micro-dystrophin to the biceps of boys with DMD. The study was conducted on six boys with DMD, each of whom received an injection of mini-dystrophin-expressing rAAV2.5 in a muscle of one arm and a placebo in the other arm. Dystrophin-specific T cells were detected after treatment, providing evidence of transgene expression even when the functional protein was not visualized in skeletal muscle.[56] The potential for T-cell immunity to self and non-self dystrophin epitopes should be considered in designing and monitoring experimental therapies for this disease. Basically, this issue is in common with the treatment of genetic diseases. Although concerns regarding risk of an immune response to the transgene product limited the ability to achieve therapeutic efficacy, rAAV2-mediated gene transfer to human skeletal muscle can persist for up to a decade.[57]

4.2. Gene therapy medicine

After more than two decades of expectations, the field of gene therapy appears close to reaching a regulatory approval by proposing rAAV-mediated muscle transduction. European medicine agency eventually recommends first gene therapy medicine for approval.

(http://www.ema.europa.eu/ema) The European Medicines Agency's Committee for Medicinal Products for Human Use has recommended the authorization of Glybera (rAAV1-expressing LPL S447X variant) for marketing in the European Union. It is intended to treat lipoprotein lipase deficiency in patients with severe or multiple pancreatitis attacks, despite dietary fat restrictions.

5. Challenges and future perspectives

5.1. Immunomodulation to augment clinical benefits

To regulate host immune response against vectors and transgene products, treatments involving immunosuppressants and other strategies have been attempted in the animal models. A brief course of immunosuppression with a combination of anti-thymocyte globulin (ATG), CSP and MMF was effective in permitting AAV6-mediated, long-term and robust expression of a canine micro-dystrophin in the skeletal muscle of a dog DMD model.[58] To establish the feasibility of multiple AAV1 injections for extending the treatment to whole body muscles, the dystrophic *mdx* mouse was repeatedly transduced with AAV1 vector, and the immune response was characterized.[59] By blocking the T-B crosstalk with anti-CD40 Abs and CTLA4/Fc fusion protein, a five-day-long immunomodulation treatment was found to be sufficient for totally abrogating the formation of anti-AAV1 antibodies.

There have been numerous reports to develop the therapeutic potential of mesenchymal stem cells (or mesenchymal multipotent stromal cells MSCs).[60] Because of their immunomodulatory properties, increasing experimental and early clinical observations indicate that allogeneic, and even xenogeneic, MSCs may be useful for tissue transplantation.[61] In fact, the immune tolerance with MSCs is well investigated in various animal studies. Infusion of syngeneic MSCs into a sensitized mouse model of kidney transplantation resulted in the expansion of donor-specific T- regulatory cells into lymphoid organs, prolonged allograft survival and promoted the development of tolerance.[62]

5.2. Pharmacological intervention

The use of a histone deacetylase (HDAC) inhibitor depsipeptide effectively enhances the utility of rAAV-mediated gene therapy.[63] In contrast to adenovirus-mediated transduction, the improved transduction with rAAV induced by the depsipeptide is due to enhanced transgene expression rather than to increased viral entry. The enhanced transduction is related to the histone-associated chromatin form of the rAAV concatemer in the transduced cells. Since various HDAC inhibitors are approved in clinical usage for many diseases to achieve therapeutic benefits, the application of such inhibitors to the rAAV-mediated gene therapy is theoretically and practically reasonable.

5.3. In situ gene therapy

Transplantation of genetically modified vector-producing cells is a possible future treatment for genetic diseases as an *in situ* gene therapy. MSCs are known to accumulate at the site of inflammation or tumors, and therefore can be utilized as a platform for the targeted delivery of therapeutic agents.[64] The MSCs-based targeted gene therapy should enhance the therapeutic efficacy, since MSCs would deliver therapeutic molecules in a concentrated fashion. This targeted therapy can also reduce systemic adverse side effects, because the reagents act locally without elevating their systemic concentrations. We developed the genetically-modified MSCs that produce viral vectors to augment therapeutic efficacy of systemic gene therapy.[65] MSCs isolated from the SD rats bone marrow were transfected with retroviral vector components by nucleofection. As a result, the injection of luciferase-expressing vector-producing MSCs caused significantly stronger signal of bioluminescence at the site of subcutaneous tumors in mice compared with luciferease-expressing non-vector-producing MSCs. [66] Furthermore, tumor-bearing nude mice were treated with the vector-producing MSCs combined with HSV-*tk*/GCV system to demonstrate improved anti-tumor effects. This study suggests the effectiveness of vector-producing MSCs in systemic gene therapy. The therapeutic benefit of this strategy should be further examined by using rAAV-producing MSCs in the various animal models of inflammatory diseases including neuromuscular disorders.

5.4. Capsid modification

A DNA shuffling-based approach for developing cell type-specific vectors is an intriguing possibility to achieve altered tropism. Capsid genomes of AAV serotypes 1-9 were randomly reassembled using PCR to generate a chimeric capsid library.[67] A single infectious clone (chimeric-1829) containing genome fragments from AAV1, 2, 8, and 9 was isolated from an integrin minus hamster melanoma cell line previously shown to have low permissiveness to AAV. Molecular modeling studies suggest that AAV2 contributes to surface loops at the icosahedral threefold axis of symmetry, while AAV1 and 9 contribute to two-fold and five-fold symmetry interactions, respectively.

A versatile rAAV targeting system to redirect rAAV-mediated transduction to specific cell surface receptors would be useful. Insertion of an IgG binding domain of protein A into the AAV2 capsid at amino acid position 587 could permit antibody-mediated vector retargeting, although producing mosaic particles is required to avoid low particle yields.[68] Alternatively, a targeting system using the genetic fusion of short biotin acceptor peptide along with the metabolic biotinylation via a biotin ligase was developed for the purification and targeting of multiple AAV serotypes.[69]

6. Conclusions and outlook

Although an increasing number of scalable methods for purification of rAAV have been described, in order to generate sufficient clinical-grade vector to support clinical trials we need to further improve a large-scale GMP-compatible system for production and purification. To translate gene transduction technologies into clinical practice, development of an effective delivery system with improved vector constructs as well as efficient immunological modulation must be established. A novel protocol that considers all of these issues would help improve the therapeutic benefits of clinical gene therapy.

Acknowledgments

This work was supported by the Grant for Research on Nervous and Mental Disorders, Health Science Research Grants for Research on the Human Genome and Gene Therapy; and the Grant for Research on Brain Science from the Ministry of Health, Labor and Welfare of Japan. This work was also supported by Grants-in-Aid for Scientific Research from the Ministry of Education, Culture, Sports, Science and Technology (MEXT). We would like to thank Dr. James M. Wilson for providing p5E18-VD2/8 and pAAV2/9.

Author details

Takashi Okada

Address all correspondence to: t-okada@ncnp.go.jp

Department of Molecular Therapy, National Institute of Neuroscience, National Center of Neurology and Psychiatry, Ogawa-Higashi, Kodaira, Tokyo, Japan

References

[1] Okada, T., K. Shimazaki, T. Nomoto, T. Matsushita, H. Mizukami, M. Urabe, et al. (2002). "Adeno-associated viral vector-mediated gene therapy of ischemia-induced neuronal death." Methods Enzymol 346: 378-393.

[2] Inagaki, K., S. Fuess, T. A. Storm, G. A. Gibson, C. F. McTiernan, M. A. Kay, et al. (2006). "Robust systemic transduction with AAV9 vectors in mice: efficient global cardiac gene transfer superior to that of AAV8." Mol Ther 14: 45-53.

[3] Ito, T., T. Okada, H. Miyashita, T. Nomoto, M. Nonaka-Sarukawa, R. Uchibori, et al. (2007). "Interleukin-10 expression mediated by an adeno-associated virus vector prevents monocrotaline-induced pulmonary arterial hypertension in rats." Circ Res 101: 734-741.

[4] Yuasa, K., Y. Miyagoe, K. Yamamoto, Y. Nabeshima, G. Dickson and S. Takeda (1998). "Effective restoration of dystrophin-associated proteins in vivo by adenovirus-mediated transfer of truncated dystrophin cDNAs." FEBS Lett 425: 329-336.

[5] Okada, T., J. Ramsey, J. Munir, O. Wildner and M. Blaese (1998). "Efficient directional cloning of recombinant adenovirus vectors using DNA-protein complex." Nucleic Acids Res. 26: 1947-1950.

[6] Okada, T., N. J. Caplen, W. J. Ramsey, M. Onodera, K. Shimazaki, T. Nomoto, et al. (2004). "In situ generation of pseudotyped retroviral progeny by adenovirus-mediated transduction of tumor cells enhances the killing effect of HSV-tk suicide gene therapy in vitro and in vivo." J Gene Med 6: 288-299.

[7] Hammerschmidt, D. E. (1999). "Development of a gutless vector." J Lab Clin Med 134: C3.

[8] Hoshiya, H., Y. Kazuki, S. Abe, M. Takiguchi, N. Kajitani, Y. Watanabe, et al. (2008). "A highly Stable and Nonintegrated Human Artificial Chromosome (HAC) Containing the 2.4 Mb Entire Human Dystrophin Gene." Mol Ther.

[9] Hacein-Bey-Abina, S., A. Garrigue, G. P. Wang, J. Soulier, A. Lim, E. Morillon, et al. (2008). "Insertional oncogenesis in 4 patients after retrovirus-mediated gene therapy of SCID-X1." J Clin Invest 118: 3132-3142.

[10] Kotin, R. M., R. M. Linden and K. I. Berns (1992). "Characterization of a preferred site on human chromosome 19q for integration of adeno-associated virus DNA by non-homologous recombination." Embo J 11: 5071-5078.

[11] Goncalves, M. A., G. P. van Nierop, M. R. Tijssen, P. Lefesvre, S. Knaan-Shanzer, I. van der Velde, et al. (2005). "Transfer of the full-length dystrophin-coding sequence into muscle cells by a dual high-capacity hybrid viral vector with site-specific integration ability." J Virol 79: 3146-3162.

[12] Srivastava, A., E. W. Lusby and K. I. Berns (1983). "Nucleotide sequence and organization of the adeno-associated virus 2 genome." J Virol 45: 555-564.

[13] Matsushita, T., S. Elliger, C. Elliger, G. Podsakoff, L. Villarreal, G. J. Kurtzman, et al. (1998). "Adeno-associated virus vectors can be efficiently produced without helper virus." Gene Ther 5: 938-945.

[14] Graham, F. L., J. Smiley, W. C. Russell and R. Nairn (1977). "Characteristics of a human cell line transformed by DNA from human adenovirus type 5." J Gen Virol 36: 59-74.

[15] Chiorini, J. A., F. Kim, L. Yang and R. M. Kotin (1999). "Cloning and characterization of adeno-associated virus type 5." J Virol 73: 1309-1319.

[16] Nomoto, T., T. Okada, K. Shimazaki, H. Mizukami, T. Matsushita, Y. Hanazono, et al. (2003). "Distinct patterns of gene transfer to gerbil hippocampus with recombinant adeno-associated virus type 2 and 5." Neuroscience Letters 340: 153-157.

[17] Liu, M., Y. Yue, S. Q. Harper, R. W. Grange, J. S. Chamberlain and D. Duan (2005). "Adeno-associated virus-mediated microdystrophin expression protects young mdx muscle from contraction-induced injury." Mol Ther 11: 245-256.

[18] Yoshioka, T., T. Okada, Y. Maeda, U. Ikeda, M. Shimpo, T. Nomoto, et al. (2004). "Adeno-associated virus vector-mediated interleukin-10 gene transfer inhibits atherosclerosis in apolipoprotein E-deficient mice." Gene Ther 11: 1772-1779.

[19] Nonaka-Sarukawa, M., T. Okada, T. Ito, K. Yamamoto, T. Yoshioka, T. Nomoto, et al. (2008). "Adeno-associated virus vector-mediated systemic interleukin-10 expression ameliorates hypertensive organ damage in Dahl salt-sensitive rats." J Gene Med 10: 368-374.

[20] Nomoto, T., T. Okada, K. Shimazaki, T. Yoshioka, M. Nonaka-Sarukawa, T. Ito, et al. (2009). "Systemic delivery of IL-10 by an AAV vector prevents vascular remodeling and end-organ damage in stroke-prone spontaneously hypertensive rat." Gene Ther 16: 383-391.

[21] Nishiyama, A., B. N. Ampong, S. Ohshima, J. H. Shin, H. Nakai, M. Imamura, et al. (2008). "Recombinant adeno-associated virus type 8-mediated extensive therapeutic gene delivery into skeletal muscle of alpha-sarcoglycan-deficient mice." Hum Gene Ther 19: 719-730.

[22] Ohshima, S., J. H. Shin, K. Yuasa, A. Nishiyama, J. Kira, T. Okada, et al. (2009). "Transduction Efficiency and Immune Response Associated With the Administration of AAV8 Vector Into Dog Skeletal Muscle." Mol Ther 17: 73-91.

[23] Shin, J. H., Y. Nitahara-Kasahara, H. Hayashita-Kinoh, S. Ohshima-Hosoyama, K. Kinoshita, T. Chiyo, et al. (2011). "Improvement of cardiac fibrosis in dystrophic mice by rAAV9-mediated microdystrophin transduction" Gene Ther. 18: 910-919.

[24] McCarty, D. M., P. E. Monahan and R. J. Samulski (2001). "Self-complementary recombinant adeno-associated virus (scAAV) vectors promote efficient transduction independently of DNA synthesis." Gene Ther 8: 1248-1254.

[25] Wu, J., W. Zhao, L. Zhong, Z. Han, B. Li, W. Ma, et al. (2007). "Self-complementary recombinant adeno-associated viral vectors: packaging capacity and the role of rep proteins in vector purity." Hum Gene Ther 18: 171-182.

[26] Yamaguchi, T., T. Okada, K. Takeuchi, T. Tonda, M. Ohtaki, S. Shinoda, et al. (2003). "Enhancement of thymidine kinase-mediated killing of malignant glioma by BimS, a BH3-only cell death activator." Gene Ther 10: 375-385.

[27] Okada, T., H. Mizukami, M. Urabe, T. Nomoto, T. Matsushita, Y. Hanazono, et al. (2001). "Development and characterization of an antisense-mediated prepackaging cell line for adeno-associated virus vector production." Biochem Biophys Res Commun 288: 62-68.

[28] Okada, T., T. Nomoto, T. Yoshioka, M. Nonaka-Sarukawa, T. Ito, T. Ogura, et al. (2005). "Large-scale production of recombinant viruses by use of a large culture vessel with active gassing." Hum Gene Ther 16: 1212-1218.

[29] Okada, T., M. Nonaka-Sarukawa, R. Uchibori, K. Kinoshita, H. Hayashita-Kinoh, Y. Nitahara-Kasahara, et al. (2009). "Scalable purification of adeno-associated virus sero-

type 1 (AAV1) and AAV8 vectors, using dual ion-exchange adsorptive membranes." Hum Gene Ther 20: 1013-1021.

[30] Cecchini, S., A. Negrete and R. M. Kotin (2008). "Toward exascale production of recombinant adeno-associated virus for gene transfer applications." Gene Ther 15: 823-830.

[31] Emery, A. E. (1991). "Population frequencies of inherited neuromuscular diseases--a world survey." Neuromuscul Disord 1: 19-29.

[32] Hoffman, E. P., R. H. Brown, Jr. and L. M. Kunkel (1987). "Dystrophin: the protein product of the Duchenne muscular dystrophy locus." Cell 51: 919-928.

[33] Kawano, R., M. Ishizaki, Y. Maeda, Y. Uchida, E. Kimura and M. Uchino (2008). "Transduction of full-length dystrophin to multiple skeletal muscles improves motor performance and life span in utrophin/dystrophin double knockout mice." Mol Ther 16: 825-831.

[34] Wang, B., J. Li and X. Xiao (2000). "Adeno-associated virus vector carrying human minidystrophin genes effectively ameliorates muscular dystrophy in mdx mouse model." Proc Natl Acad Sci U S A 97: 13714-13719.

[35] Sakamoto, M., K. Yuasa, M. Yoshimura, T. Yokota, T. Ikemoto, M. Suzuki, et al. (2002). "Micro-dystrophin cDNA ameliorates dystrophic phenotypes when introduced into mdx mice as a transgene." Biochem Biophys Res Commun 293: 1265-1272.

[36] Yoshimura, M., M. Sakamoto, M. Ikemoto, Y. Mochizuki, K. Yuasa, Y. Miyagoe-Suzuki, et al. (2004). "AAV vector-mediated microdystrophin expression in a relatively small percentage of mdx myofibers improved the mdx phenotype." Mol Ther 10: 821-828.

[37] Gregorevic, P., J. M. Allen, E. Minami, M. J. Blankinship, M. Haraguchi, L. Meuse, et al. (2006). "rAAV6-microdystrophin preserves muscle function and extends lifespan in severely dystrophic mice." Nat Med 12: 787-789.

[38] Gregorevic, P., M. J. Blankinship, J. M. Allen and J. S. Chamberlain (2008). "Systemic microdystrophin gene delivery improves skeletal muscle structure and function in old dystrophic mdx mice." Mol Ther 16: 657-664.

[39] Foster, H., P. S. Sharp, T. Athanasopoulos, C. Trollet, I. R. Graham, K. Foster, et al. (2008). "Codon and mRNA sequence optimization of microdystrophin transgenes improves expression and physiological outcome in dystrophic mdx mice following AAV2/8 gene transfer." Mol Ther 16: 1825-1832.

[40] Li, X., E. M. Eastman, R. J. Schwartz and R. Draghia-Akli (1999). "Synthetic muscle promoters: activities exceeding naturally occurring regulatory sequences." Nat Biotechnol 17: 241-245.

[41] Hagstrom, J. E., J. Hegge, G. Zhang, M. Noble, V. Budker, D. L. Lewis, et al. (2004). "A facile nonviral method for delivering genes and siRNAs to skeletal muscle of mammalian limbs." Mol Ther 10: 386-398.

[42] Ohshima, S., J. H. Shin, K. Yuasa, A. Nishiyama, J. Kira, T. Okada, et al. (2008). "Transduction Efficiency and Immune Response Associated With the Administration of AAV8 Vector Into Dog Skeletal Muscle." Mol Ther.

[43] Townsend, D., S. Yasuda, S. Li, J. S. Chamberlain and J. M. Metzger (2008). "Emergent dilated cardiomyopathy caused by targeted repair of dystrophic skeletal muscle." Mol Ther 16: 832-835.

[44] Bostick, B., Y. Yue, Y. Lai, C. Long, D. Li and D. Duan (2008). "Adeno-associated virus serotype-9 microdystrophin gene therapy ameliorates electrocardiographic abnormalities in mdx mice." Hum Gene Ther 19: 851-856.

[45] Yue, Y., A. Ghosh, C. Long, B. Bostick, B. F. Smith, J. N. Kornegay, et al. (2008). "A single intravenous injection of adeno-associated virus serotype-9 leads to whole body skeletal muscle transduction in dogs." Mol Ther 16: 1944-1952.

[46] Reay, D. P., R. Bilbao, B. M. Koppanati, L. Cai, T. L. O'Day, Z. Jiang, et al. (2008). "Full-length dystrophin gene transfer to the mdx mouse in utero." Gene Ther 15: 531-536.

[47] Yuasa, K., M. Sakamoto, Y. Miyagoe-Suzuki, A. Tanouchi, H. Yamamoto, J. Li, et al. (2002). "Adeno-associated virus vector-mediated gene transfer into dystrophin-deficient skeletal muscles evokes enhanced immune response against the transgene product." Gene Ther 9: 1576-1588.

[48] Yuasa, K., M. Yoshimura, N. Urasawa, S. Ohshima, J. M. Howell, A. Nakamura, et al. (2007). "Injection of a recombinant AAV serotype 2 into canine skeletal muscles evokes strong immune responses against transgene products." Gene Ther.

[49] Li, C., M. Hirsch, A. Asokan, B. Zeithaml, H. Ma, T. Kafri, et al. (2007). "Adeno-associated virus type 2 (AAV2) capsid-specific cytotoxic T lymphocytes eliminate only vector-transduced cells coexpressing the AAV2 capsid in vivo." J Virol 81: 7540-7547.

[50] Zhang, Y., N. Chirmule, G. Gao and J. Wilson (2000). "CD40 ligand-dependent activation of cytotoxic T lymphocytes by adeno-associated virus vectors in vivo: role of immature dendritic cells." J Virol 74: 8003-8010.

[51] Wang, Z., J. M. Allen, S. R. Riddell, P. Gregorevic, R. Storb, S. J. Tapscott, et al. (2007). "Immunity to adeno-associated virus-mediated gene transfer in a random-bred canine model of Duchenne muscular dystrophy." Hum Gene Ther 18: 18-26.

[52] Manno, C. S., G. F. Pierce, V. R. Arruda, B. Glader, M. Ragni, J. J. Rasko, et al. (2006). "Successful transduction of liver in hemophilia by AAV-Factor IX and limitations imposed by the host immune response." Nat Med 12: 342-347.

[53] Scallan, C. D., H. Jiang, T. Liu, S. Patarroyo-White, J. M. Sommer, S. Zhou, et al. (2006). "Human immunoglobulin inhibits liver transduction by AAV vectors at low AAV2 neutralizing titers in SCID mice." Blood 107: 1810-1817.

[54] Vandenberghe, L. H., L. Wang, S. Somanathan, Y. Zhi, J. Figueredo, R. Calcedo, et al. (2006). "Heparin binding directs activation of T cells against adeno-associated virus serotype 2 capsid." Nat Med 12: 967-971.

[55] Rodino-Klapac, L. R., L. G. Chicoine, B. K. Kaspar and J. R. Mendell (2007). "Gene therapy for duchenne muscular dystrophy: expectations and challenges." Arch Neurol 64: 1236-1241.

[56] Mendell, J. R., K. Campbell, L. Rodino-Klapac, Z. Sahenk, C. Shilling, S. Lewis, et al. (2010). "Dystrophin immunity in Duchenne's muscular dystrophy." N Engl J Med 363: 1429-1437.

[57] Buchlis, G., G. M. Podsakoff, A. Radu, S. M. Hawk, A. W. Flake, F. Mingozzi, et al. (2012). "Factor IX expression in skeletal muscle of a severe hemophilia B patient 10 years after AAV-mediated gene transfer." Blood 119: 3038-3041.

[58] Wang, Z., C. S. Kuhr, J. M. Allen, M. Blankinship, P. Gregorevic, J. S. Chamberlain, et al. (2007). "Sustained AAV-mediated Dystrophin Expression in a Canine Model of Duchenne Muscular Dystrophy with a Brief Course of Immunosuppression." Mol Ther 15: 1160-1166.

[59] Lorain, S., D. A. Gross, A. Goyenvalle, O. Danos, J. Davoust and L. Garcia (2008). "Transient immunomodulation allows repeated injections of AAV1 and correction of muscular dystrophy in multiple muscles." Mol Ther 16: 541-547.

[60] Nitahara-Kasahara, Y., H. Hayashita-Kinoh, S. Ohshima-Hosoyama, H. Okada, M. Wada-Maeda, A. Nakamura, et al. (2012). "Long-term engraftment of multipotent mesenchymal stromal cells that differentiate to form myogenic cells in dogs with Duchenne muscular dystrophy." Mol Ther 20: 168-177.

[61] Chiu, R. C. (2008). "MSC immune tolerance in cellular cardiomyoplasty." Semin Thorac Cardiovasc Surg 20: 115-118.

[62] Casiraghi, F., N. Azzollini, M. Todeschini, R. A. Cavinato, P. Cassis, S. Solini, et al. (2012). "Localization of Mesenchymal Stromal Cells Dictates Their Immune or Proinflammatory Effects in Kidney Transplantation." Am J Transplant. (in press)

[63] Okada, T., R. Uchibori, M. Iwata-Okada, M. Takahashi, T. Nomoto, M. Nonaka-Sarukawa, et al. (2006). "A histone deacetylase inhibitor enhances recombinant adeno-associated virus-mediated gene expression in tumor cells." Mol Ther 13: 738-746.

[64] Studeny, M., F. C. Marini, J. L. Dembinski, C. Zompetta, M. Cabreira-Hansen, B. N. Bekele, et al. (2004). "Mesenchymal stem cells: potential precursors for tumor stroma and targeted-delivery vehicles for anticancer agents." J Natl Cancer Inst 96: 1593-1603.

[65] Okada, T. and K. Ozawa (2008). "Vector-producing tumor-tracking multipotent mesenchymal stromal cells for suicide cancer gene therapy." Front Biosci 13: 1887-1891.

[66] Uchibori, R., T. Okada, T. Ito, M. Urabe, H. Mizukami, A. Kume, et al. (2009). "Retroviral vector-producing mesenchymal stem cells for targeted suicide cancer gene therapy." J Gene Med 11: 373-381.

[67] Li, W., A. Asokan, Z. Wu, T. Van Dyke, N. DiPrimio, J. S. Johnson, et al. (2008). "Engineering and selection of shuffled AAV genomes: a new strategy for producing targeted biological nanoparticles." Mol Ther 16: 1252-1260.

[68] Muzyczka, N. and K. H. Warrington, Jr. (2005). "Custom adeno-associated virus capsids: the next generation of recombinant vectors with novel tropism." Hum Gene Ther 16: 408-416.

[69] Arnold, G. S., A. K. Sasser, M. D. Stachler and J. S. Bartlett (2006). "Metabolic biotinylation provides a unique platform for the purification and targeting of multiple AAV vector serotypes." Mol Ther 14: 97-106.

Chapter 10

Retroviral Genotoxicity

Dustin T. Rae and Grant D. Trobridge

Additional information is available at the end of the chapter

1. Introduction

Gene therapies have enormous potential to cure human disease. In recent years, hematopoietic stem cell (HSC) gene therapy has advanced tremendously, due in part to years of intense research to develop effective vectors and efficient ex vivo transduction protocols. In early clinical trials, inefficient gene transfer resulted in either a lack of therapeutic benefit or short-lived therapeutic benefit [1-3]. Advances in preclinical animal models, led to improved gene transfer in human clinical trials, where long-term efficacy has now been achieved. HSC gene therapy has been used to correct several monoallelic genetic diseases [4], such as X-linked severe combined immune-deficiency (SCID X-1) [5], chronic granulomatous disease (CGD) [6-8], adenine deaminase deficiency (ADA-SCID) [9-12], Wiskott-Aldrich syndrome [13-14], and X-linked adrenoleukodysrophy [15,16]. Recently HSC gene therapy has also been used to treat glioblastoma [17], X-linked hyper-immunoglobulin M syndrome (HIGM), and familial haemophagocyticlymphohistiocytosis syndrome (HLH) [18]. These successes are in large part due to advances in ex vivo transduction protocols and improvements with recombinant vector technologies. The French SCID-X1 HSC gene therapy trial marked a major turning point in the field when nine of the ten patients treated exhibited therapeutic benefit. However, following this exciting achievement the field was dealt a major setback when it was initially reported, that two patients from the study had developed vector-mediated leukemia resulting from the treatment [19]. This was the first vector-mediated malignancy reported in a HSC gene therapy clinical trial. Four boys ultimately developed leukemia as a side effect of the gene therapy procedure [5]. Three of the four boys were successfully treated with chemotherapy, but one patient died due to vector-mediated T cell leukemia. In these patients, vector-mediated dysregulation of host genes led to leukemia, and this unwanted adverse side effect is currently a major challenge for HSC gene therapy. The effect of the integrated viral vector on host gene expression resulting in an altered phenotype is known as genotoxicity.

Genotoxicity is a result of retroviral mediated delivery of the integrated form of the retroviral vector genome known as the vector provirus into the host genome. Integration of the vector provirus into a host chromosome, by definition, alters the host DNA. In cases where a retrovirus or retroviral vector provirus has dysregulated host gene expression, insertional mutagenesis is said to have occurred. However, it is important to remember that provirus integration always results in mutation of the host genome, regardless of whether the vector provirus exerts an effect on host gene expression. The oncogenic properties of replication-competent retroviruses were well known prior to the development of retroviral vectors for gene therapy. However, vectors that are used in gene therapy have been engineered so that they do not have the ability to replicate, only to insert their genome into a target cell. These vectors are thus referred to as replication-incompetent. In numerous preclinical and clinical studies conducted prior to the SCID-X1 trial, malignancies were not observed when using replication-incompetent vector systems [20]. It was therefore assumed that the potential for malignant transformation from a replication-incompetent vector was very low. Unfortunately, it has now been clearly shown in the French SCID-X1 trial and in subsequent HSC gene therapy trials, that genotoxicity is indeed a problem for replication-incompetent vectors. Here we review the mechanisms of vector-mediated genotoxicity in HSC gene therapy and describe efforts in the field to reduce genotoxicity which is currently a major challenge in the field [21, 22].

2. Why integrating vectors are used for HSC gene therapy

Why use integrating vectors for HSC gene therapy if we know that retroviral vectors mutagenize the genome and therefore carry a risk to induce genotoxicity? The answer is that provirus integration to HSCs is currently the only way to efficiently and stably deliver transgenes to the billions of mature blood cells produced every day in the body. Our mature blood cells are generated from a relatively small pool of self-renewing long term-repopulating HSCs in the bone marrow through a process known as hematopoiesis (Figure 1). During hematopoiesis, long-term repopulating stem cells provide lifelong supplies of the mature cells of each blood cell lineage via massive expansion of transit-amplifying cells that include multi-potent and lineage restricted progenitors. By permanently modifying a long term re-populating HSC via proviral integration into the HSC genome we can ensure that all progeny produced from these gene-modified cells will inherit the transgene during mitosis. Thus, the mature blood cells that arise during hematopoiesis from gene-modified HSCs and their daughter transit amplifying cells all inherit the transgene. Using retroviral vectors to efficiently deliver a therapeutic transgene via integration of the vector provirus into a HSC is currently the only effective approach for HSC gene therapy. While there have been reports of some success with adenovirus and other non-integrating approaches in small animal models, to date only integrating vectors have been used successfully for HSC gene therapy in large animal models and in clinical trials.

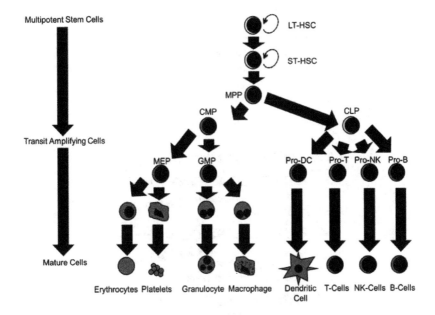

Figure 1. Human Hematopoiesis. Long-term-hematopoietic stem cells (LT-HSCs) are a self-renewing population of stem cells that reconstitute the blood system throughout the entirety of our life span. Short-term-HSCs, reconstitute our blood system for only limited periods. The short-term-HSCs differentiate into multipotent progenitors (MPPs), which have the ability to differentiate into several transit amplifying cell lineages. Common lymphoid progenitors (CLPs) differentiate into (Pro- Dendritic Cell, Pro-T, Pro-NK, and Pro-B) lymphoid progenitor cells. Finally, these progenitors give rise to the mature lymphoid class cells of the blood system (T- lymphocytes, B-lymphocytes, and natural killer (NK) cells). Common myeloid progenitors (CMPs), give rise to granulocyte-macrophage progenitors (GMPs) and mega-karyocyte-erythroid progenitors (MEPs) that differentiate into :(macrophages, granulocytes, megakaryocytes, and er-ythroid) myeloid class progenitors. Finally, these progenitors give rise to the mature myeloid class cells of the blood system.

3. Retroviruses as insertional mutagens

We now know that the use of retroviral vectors for HSC gene therapy, though highly effi-cient, can dysregulate host genes near the vector provirus and ultimately lead to malignant transformation. The ability of replicating retroviruses to cause tumorigenesis is well estab-lished. In 1911, Peyton Rous showed that a sarcoma growing on a domestic chicken could be transferred to another chicken by exposing the healthy bird to a cell-free filtrate [23]. This filterable agent is now known to be the Rous sarcoma retrovirus. Since this report, many ret-roviruses have been discovered that cause diverse malignancies. There are several mecha-nisms whereby retroviruses can cause malignancy. Varmus et al. showed that acutely transforming onco-retroviruses capture and deliver cellular oncogenes, which allow these viruses to efficiently, convert target cells into a malignant phenotype [24]. It is important to note that oncogene capture does not occur at a detectable frequency with current replica-tion-incompetent vectors used in gene therapy. Yet several mechanisms remain for cellular transformation from replication-incompetent retroviral vector proviruses (Figure 2). Despite the risks associated with malignant transformation from retroviral vectors via insertional mutagenesis, for several severe hematopoietic diseases the therapeutic benefit of HSC gene therapy outweighs the risks. Currently, major efforts are underway to further our under-standing of genotoxic events and to improve vector safety by reducing their genotoxic po-tential [18, 25, 26].

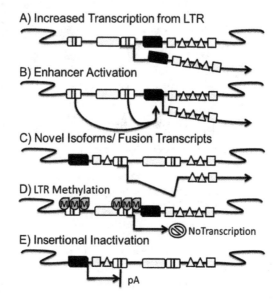

Figure 2. Mechanisms of Retroviral Mutagenesis. The black boxes represent promoters, and grey squares represent exons. A) The proviral 3' LTR can drive transcription of nearby cellular gene at an increased rate. B) Proviral LTR en-hancers can activate a nearby promoter, increasing transcription of cellular genes. C) Transcription from 5' LTR in con-junction with proviral cryptic splice sights creates novel isoforms and fusion transcripts of both cellular and viral genes. D) Proviral LTR methylation, induces epigenetic changes, silencing proviral genes and nearby cellular genes. E) Proviral integration can disrupt cellular gene expression by causing premature polyadenylation (pA) signaling.

4. Overview of ex vivo HSC gene therapy

It is important when studying genotoxicity to consider how the target cells are manipulated during the gene transfer process. HSC gene therapy is conceptually straightforward but re-quires culture of stem cells under the appropriate ex vivo conditions. A patient's cells are collected and enriched for repopulating stem cells using the CD34 marker. The CD34 pro-tein is a member of the sialomucin family, and is expressed in early HSCs [27]. The CD34 marker allows for rapid enrichment of HSCs, typically via column enrichment using CD34 antibody-conjugated magnetic beads. CD34-enriched cells that include repopulating HSCs are then exposed to the vector containing the therapeutic gene in an ex vivo transduction process. Following ex vivo transduction, gene modified cells must be infused into the patient. Correction of the disease phenotype will occur if enough gene-modified repopulating cells engraft. Engraftment requires that gene modified cells survive, home to the bone marrow, and proliferate sufficiently to repopulate the blood system.

Early preclinical HSC gene therapy studies in mice demonstrated high gene transfer rates. However, early clinical trials using similar approaches and culture conditions had inefficient gene transfer [28, 29]. Large animal models such as the dog and non-human primates more accurately model human HSC gene therapy and have since been used to establish the conditions for efficient ex vivo transduction [30]. More effective ex vivo gene protocols were developed, that resulted in higher gene transfer efficiencies while maintaining efficient engraftment. These improvements included defining cytokine support and the extracellular matrix CH-296 fibronectin fragment [5, 31, 32]. Together these advances contributed to the success of HSC gene therapy clinical trials such as the French SCID-X1 trial, and now efficient transduction of human CD34+ cells can be routinely achieved using retroviral vectors. These improved gene transfer efficiencies also factored into the observed genotoxicity. For example, two patients in the French SCID-X1 trials were estimated to have a total of 4.3×10^6 and 11.3×10^6 CD34+γC + cells/kg body weight gene modified cells respectively [5]. Thus in each of these patients many proviral integrants exist with the potential to dysregulate many nearby genes, including proto-oncogenes.

5. The SCID-X1 trials as an example of genotoxicity in HSC gene therapy

SCID-X1 is a fatal X-linked inherited mutation of the IL2RG locus harboring the gamma c (γC) cytokine receptor common subunit [5]. Inactivating mutations in this gene prevent proper cellular communication and maturation of lymphoid progenitor cells. The loss of cellular signaling in lymphoid progenitors prevents the development of mature T, NK, and B cells. Many SCID-X1 patients fail to thrive or suffer morbidity and mortality in early life because of impaired immune function, which leaves them susceptible to life-threatening infection. Allogeneic HSC transplantation has been used to treat SCID-X1, but many patients do not have suitable donors. In addition, graft versus host disease is a major source of mortality for patients treated by this approach. Graft versus host disease occurs when transplanted (allogeneic) immune cells from a donor recognize the host recipient tissue as foreign and attack these cells. SCID-X1 HSC gene therapy using the γC transgene has a lower mortality rate and a higher treatment efficacy compared to conventional allogeneic bone marrow transplants [25], and is currently the only therapeutic choice for patients without a suitable donor. Prior to the French study, preclinical studies conducted in both murine and canine models corrected SCID-X1 deficiency was with no reported adverse events [20, 31, 33, and 34].

In the French SCID-X1 trial, four of the ten patients developed T-cell leukemia from insertional mutagenesis from the murine moloney leukemia virus (MLV)-based vector [5, 25]. Careful molecular analysis of leukemic cells showed that the MLV provirus integrated near the proto-oncogene, LMO2, and suggested that viral enhancer elements in the provirus contributed to leukemia (Figure 2B) [25]. The SCID-X1 trials were the first HSC gene therapy clinical trial where vector-mediated insertional mutagenesis led to cancer. In this trial, MLV vector LTR enhancers activated LMO2 expression, resulting in T-cell LMO2 dependent proliferation (Figure 2B). LMO2 is normally silenced in mature T-cells, and when viral enhancers turn on expression, LMO2 drives T-cell proliferation by dysregulating transcription networks that affect the cell cycle. This promotes cell cycle escape and can result in higher proliferation rates compared to normal cells [35]. Leukemic transformation was a result of provirus integration near LMO2 with additional proviral integrants near other proto-oncogenes that resulted in expansion of cells with these mutations [5, 19].

6. Clonal expansion in the SCID-X1 trials

As evidenced in the French SCID-X1 trial, retroviral vector integration can dysregulate nearby host genes, thus affecting cell growth and survival. Once integrated, elements in the provirus, particularly enhancers in the LTR, can dysregulate nearby gene expression through several mechanisms (Figure 2). Aberrant gene expression can dysregulate host cell genes and regulatory networks involved with cell growth, including proto-oncogenes. A survival advantage can occur through the activation of proto-oncogenes giving cells a proliferative advantage or "go signal". Alternatively, tumor suppressors can be inactivated, causing a proliferative advantage with uncontrolled cellular division from the lack of a "stop signal". To date the genotoxicity described in HSC gene therapy trials has been through activation of growth promoting genes and proto-oncogenes, rather than inactivation of tumor suppressors. This is because activation requires a single integration into only one allele whereas inactivation of a tumor suppressor requires a second event, either a second integration or a loss of heterozygosity at that allele, to inactivate tumor suppressor activity. Tumor suppressors have however been identified in preclinical mouse studies [36-37]. These vector mediated mutations along with additional accumulating mutagenic events in expanding gene-modified repopulating cells can ultimately result in tumorigenesis. The proviral promoter and enhancer elements have been shown to act up to a distance of 500 Kb upstream and downstream of the site of proviral integration [38]. In the SCID-X1 trials where patients developed T-cell leukemia, the integration sites of dominant repopulating clones near the genes LMO2, BMI1, HMGA2, SEPT9, RUNX2, and RUNX3 gave rise to cells with a proliferative advantage or survival advantage over competitor repopulating cells. These advantages eventually led to an over-representation of these clones (Figure 3) [5].

We now know how vector-mediated dysregulation of these different genes may have contributed to clonal expansion and frank leukemia. LMO2 or Lim only 2 is a proto-oncogene that regulates early progenitor expansion during hematopoiesis [39]. LMO2 oncogenic properties were first observed in mature gene-modified T-cells, where it is not normally expressed [39]. However, after proviral integration events, resulting in activation of LMO2, these gene-modified T-cells begin to expand from dysregulation of transcriptional regulatory pathways. In 2010, Oram et al. demonstrated that LMO2 expression in T cells activates FLI1 and ERG enhancers, known to be involved in blood stem/progenitor cells. These gene products of FLI1 and ERG in turn activate the enhancer of the HHEX/PRH gene locus, which has been shown to act in early progenitor cell expansion and formation of T-lineage acute lymphoblastic leukemia (T-ALL) [35]. LMO2 overexpression has also been demonstrated to reduce or eliminate cell cyclin dependent kinase (CDK) inhibitors promoting escape of the G1 cell cycle checkpoints during cellular division [40]. Once aberrantly expressed within a cell, LMO2 promotes cell cycle progression via multiple mechanisms, giving the cell a proliferative advantage.

Additional proto-oncogenes were activated in the French SCID-X1 patients. The BMI1 proto-oncogene normally functions in self-renewal and maintenance of hematopoietic primitive stem cells [40, 41]. Like LMO2, dysregulation of BMI-1 via enhancer activation results in clonal expansion. Additional mechanisms mediate clonal expansion, such as the high mobility group AT-hook2 (HMGA2) which can provide a proliferative advantage when the endogenous gene is truncated via insertional mutagenesis. Truncation results in the loss of regulatory target sequences within the protein mRNA preventing degradation by the endogenous miRNA let7. These miRNA elements normally function to regulate HMGA2 via RNA interference using the RNA induced silencing complex (RISC) machinery [42]. Truncated HMGA2 mRNA is not degraded thus continuing activation of gene networks involved with cell proliferation, and cell-cycle progression [42]. Another mechanism that can contribute to clonal expansion is the aberrant expression of septin proteins. SEPT9 functions as a microtubule regulator and plays an important function in cytokinesis and chromosome segregation, thus affecting genomic stability [43, 44]. When aberrantly expressed, SEPT9 causes dysregulated cytokinesis or cell division resulting in missegregation of chromosomes [43, 44]. Genomic instability then results from SEPT9 dysregulation, leading to the accumulation of chromosomal deletions or amplifications from missegregation of chromosomes. These events in conjunction with additional mutations can enhance cell proliferation and survival.

Two additional genes identified near vector proviruses in the SCID-X1 trial were RUNX family members RUNX2 and RUNX3. RUNX proteins (RUNX 1, 2, 3) are a family of RUNT homology domain containing α-subunits that form heterodimeric transcription factors that mediate hematopoietic differentiation and expansion in conjunction with β subunit core binding factor (CBF). Aberrant expression of the RUNX proteins in mouse models hinders myeloid class progenitor differentiation capacity and represses expression of several target genes including Csf1R, Mpo, Cebpd, and the cell cycle inhibitor Cdkn1a [45]. Repression of these genes blocks hematopoietic stem cell differentiation leading to an accumulation of undifferentiated cells. These cells cannot pass the differentiation block to repopulate the depleted blood cell niche. The lack of differentiated mature cells continues to generate proliferative signaling pathways that further stimulate mutant HSC expansion. The expanded undifferentiated blast cells accumulate in the bone marrow, disrupting normal blood cell production, and can eventually give rise to various cytopenias and leukemic blast crisis.

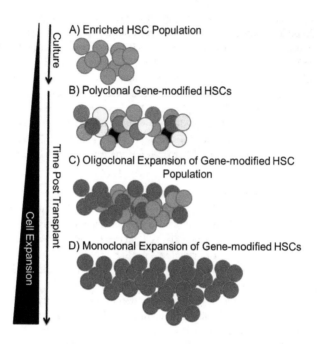

Figure 3. Clonal Expansion. A) Patient derivedCD34⁻ enriched hematopoietic stem cells (HSC) population prior to ex vivo vector exposure. Untransduced cells are blue. B) Polyclonal proviral integration distribution in vector treated HSCs. This is an ideal proviral distribution, which HSC gene therapy would ideally maintain after infusion into patients. However, due to genotoxicity and selection pressures in vivo C) Oligoclonal expansion can be observed, where some clones expand. In some cases, D) individual clones may harbor a proviral integration near genes promoting a proliferative or survival advantage, which may eventually contribute to malignancy.

In summary, our current understanding of genotoxicity is that vector proviruses dysregulate the expression of key regulators of cell cycle, cell survival, genomic stability, proliferative gene networking and cellular differentiation. This leads to an over-representation of gene-modified clones with these mutations in the peripheral blood (PB) and bone marrow (BM) which is referred to as clonal expansion (Figure 3). Clonal expansion can lead to additional mutations that can eventually cause frank leukemia. The leukemias observed in the French SCID-X1 trial refocused the gene therapy field to better understand the mechanisms of vector dysregulation of host genes, with the ultimate goal of reducing the risk of genotoxicity.

7. Risk factors for clonal expansion

It is important to remember that the SCID-X1 trials are one example of clonal expansion in a specific disease setting using a specific vector type with a specific transgene. Several factors can influence clonal expansion including the type of vector, vector design, the therapeutic transgene and the disease setting. For example the transgene in and of itself may provide a selective advantage to cells through its expression. This was true in the SCID-X1 trials, where expression of the corrective γC transgene gave cells a proliferative advantage allowing reconstitution of the lymphoid cell population from a modest number of gene modified HSCs [5]. To determine the mechanisms behind these expansion events investigators must first characterize the integration sites of the vectors being used to deliver the therapeutic transgene. This allows identification of nearby genes that may have been dysregulated leading to clonal expansion.

8. Vector integration sites in expanded repopulating clones allow clonal tracking

To understand the risk of genotoxicity we need to identify where different vectors tend to integrate. Conveniently, integrated vector proviruses serve as molecular tags to identify integration sites and to track specific clones in order to study clonal expansion. Sequencing the unique vector-chromosome junctions can identify where in the genome the virus has integrated. Analysis of vector insertion sites has allowed researchers to compile comprehensive integration profiles for specific virus types and assess the safety of viral vectors based on the regions of preferred or recurrent integration.

Long term tracking of gene-modified cells is necessary to monitor potential adverse events that may occur over time resulting in clonal expansion. By identifying the spectrum of vector integration sites in repopulating cells, the clonality of repopulating cells can be estimated and the expansion of specific clones can be monitored. Long-term tracking may also provide insight into specific mechanism of clonal expansion, such as emergent LMO2 expansion in SCID-X1 trials, and will direct novel approaches to reduce genotoxic effects [46]. It has become an important area of study to understand where retroviruses integrate in the human genome, thus affecting their safety for use in HSC gene therapy approaches.

9. The integration profile of retroviruses and its relation to genotoxicity

Identifying the integration profiles of different vector types has provided important data on the relative genotoxic risk associated with different vectors. Following the leukemias observed in the SCID-X1 trial, integration site distributions were described for different retroviral vectors being developed for gene therapy. Viral integration sites for HIV-1, MLV and foamy virus (FV) vectors were reported and each exhibits a specific and unique integration profile. HIV-1 based vectors showed preferences for integration within actively transcribed genes [47] whereas MLV vectors tends to integrate within transcription start sites near CpG islands [48-50]. FV vectors also preferentially integrate near transcription start sites and CpG islands but less frequently than MLV vectors and integrate less frequently in genes than HIV vectors. The propensity of MLV-based vectors to integrate preferentially very close to promoter regions was of significant concern since this may increase the risk of dysregulating proto-oncogenes. The integration profiles were found to be largely independent of the route of entry [47, 51, 52] and target cell type [49, 53, 54] although characteristics such as cell cycle of the target cell can play a minor role in the profile [49,54].

The factors that contribute to the integration profile of viruses and viral vectors are greatly influenced by a compliment of host proteins that interact with a poorly defined retroviral pre-integration complex (PIC). The PIC is a complex of proteins associated with the viral genome, and during infection, the PIC must migrate to the nucleus to mediate integration of the reverse-transcribed viral DNA to generate the vector provirus. This process and the associated proteins that affect it have been studied using various methods [55-57]. Viral Gag and integrase proteins have been shown to interact with chromatin, affectively tethering the PIC to specific chromosomal regions, thus directing integration [57, 58]. Studies have compared the contributions of the viral integrase and Gag proteins using MLV-HIV chimeras, and shown that both play important roles in integration site specificity [57]. The HIV lens-epithelium-derived growth factor (LEDGF) is a host derived tethering protein that has been demonstrated to associate with the PIC and chromatin affecting HIV-1 integration patterns. This host protein has a strong binding affinity for HIV integrase proteins, which are associated with the lentiviral PIC [59]. The tethering of the PIC to LEDGF protects the PIC from host enzymatic defenses [56], promotes chromatin binding [57, 60], and directs integration site distribution [61]. Unique to foamy virus biology, the c-terminal end of the Gag protein contains glycine-arginine motifs known as a GR boxes [62]. These boxes direct viral packaging [63, 64] and nuclear localization [62, 64]. In addition to these features, a 13 amino acid motif called the chromatin-binding site (CBS) has been characterized [58]. This CBS contains a functional binding domain for core histones H2A/H2B that is thought to tether the PIC to the chromatin after translocation into the nucleus [58]. Host chromatin tethering proteins often associate with the PIC complex and affect integration site distributions. Better characterization of cell-virus interaction should enhance our understanding of viral integration patterns. This has potentially led to novel approaches to direct vector integrations to "safe harbor" chromosomal regions, that do not have genes that can lead to clonal expansion when dysregulated.

10. Methods for integration site analysis

Many methods exist for generating retroviral insertion site data. PCR based techniques include ligation mediated PCR (LM-PCR Figure 4A), Linear amplification-mediated PCR (LAM-PCR Figure 4B), and non-restrictive LAM-PCR (nrLAM-PCR Figure 4C). LM-PCR relies on frequently cutting restriction enzymes to generate fragments that contain the provirus: chromosome junction. These fragments are then ligated to linkers, and after several rounds of PCR, the resulting products are sequenced. LAM-PCR uses an LTR-specific primer in several rounds of 'linear' amplification where the LTR: chromosome junction is amplified. Nested PCR is then used to produce products that can be directly sequenced or transformed into bacteria and sequenced. nrLAM-PCR is similar to LAM-PCR but uses random shearing rather than digestion of DNA with restriction enzymes prior to linker ligation and sequencing, thus avoiding restriction site bias and is currently the gold standard in the field.

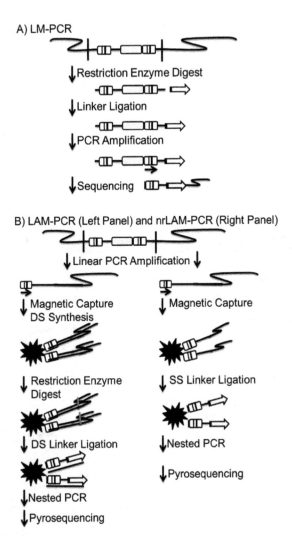

A) LM-PCR

↓ Restriction Enzyme Digest

↓ Linker Ligation

↓ PCR Amplification

↓ Sequencing

B) LAM-PCR (Left Panel) and nrLAM-PCR (Right Panel)

↓ Linear PCR Amplification ↓

↓ Magnetic Capture   ↓ Magnetic Capture
DS Synthesis

↓ Restriction Enzyme   ↓ SS Linker Ligation
Digest

↓ DS Linker Ligation   ↓ Nested PCR

↓ Nested PCR   ↓ Pyrosequencing

↓ Pyrosequencing

Figure 4. PCR Based LTR: Chromosome Junction Sequencing. A) Demonstration of ligation-mediated PCR, where genomic DNA is cut by restriction enzyme digestion, ligated to a linker, and amplified before sequencing of oligos with an LTR specific primer. B) Left Panel: Linear-amplification-mediated PCR (LAM-PCR) amplifies regions of genomic DNA containing integrated vector proviruses using an LTR specific primer. The resulting oligos are captured on magnetic beads and double strand synthesis is performed, followed by restriction enzyme digestion and ligation of a double stranded linker. Nested PCR is then used and the resulting products sequenced. Right Panel: Non-restrictive linear-amplification-mediated PCR (nrLAM-PCR) amplifies genomic DNA with integrated vector proviruses with an LTR specific primer. The resulting products are enriched on magnetic beads, followed by single strand linker ligation. Nested PCR is then employed and the products are sequenced.

One limitation of the above methods is that PCR bias can affect the frequency of detected integration sites [65, 66]. Another method that has been used is shuttle vector rescue technology, which eliminates PCR-based bias [67, 68, and 54]. In shuttle vector rescue, vector plasmids encode a bacterial origin of replication and selection gene. DNA fragments that contain the shuttle vector LTR: chromosome junction are ligated and then transformed into bacteria. These bacteria can then be grown as colonies to amplify plasmid clones of each potential insertion site in the absence of PCR based skewing (Figure 5). Plasmid DNA is then extracted from bacterial colonies and sequenced with an LTR specific primer. In all of the above methods, aligning the genomic sequence immediately next to the proviral LTR to a published genome databases allows for identification of the proviral integration site. It will be interesting to compare the shuttle vector approach to nrLAM-PCR in animal models to provide information on any potential bias from either technique.

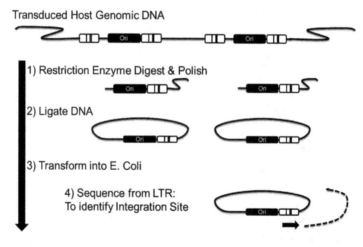

Figure 5. Plasmid Shuttle Vector Rescue. Genomic DNA is presented with vector integrations showing the proviral 5′ LTR, the genetic element encoding a bacterial origin of replications (Ori), and the vector provirus 3′LTR. Vector exposed cells are lysed and genomic DNA harboring integrated vector proviruses collected. The genomic DNA harboring proviral integrants is fragmented by restriction enzyme digest, and then self-ligated to form plasmids which may contain portions of the provirus encoding a bacterial origin of replication and an antibiotic selection gene. These plasmids are then transformed into E. coli. E. coli transformed with plasmids containing the bacterial origin and antibiotic resistance gene will form colonies. Sequencing the colony plasmids identifies proviral LTR: chromosome junctions.

11. Animal models to study genotoxicity: Tumor prone mouse models

Animal models allow the in vivo study of the genotoxicity of HSC gene therapy approaches, within specific disease contexts. These studies are critical because while in vitro genotoxicity assays can provide important information on the relative genotoxicity of different vectors [50], only animal models can assess genotoxic effects on in vivo hematopoiesis. Tumor prone mouse models have provided important data on the relative genotoxicity of different vectors systems and have identified genes and gene networks involved in vector-mediated malignant transformation [69]. The advantage of tumor prone mice is that the frequency of clonal expansion and tumorigenesis resulting from vector-mediated genotoxic events is increased, thereby allowing readout of vector-mediated malignancy within the life span of a mouse.

Several studies have focused on gammaretroviral and lentiviral vectors; testing vectors with hybrid LTRs from both viral systems to identify the elements responsible for different genotoxicities. These studies, in conjunction with tumor-prone mouse models, have informed vector design modifications. Enhancer deletion, use of internal housekeeping promoters, and deletions of vector cryptic splice sites can be used to reduce genotoxic events and improve safety [69]. The tumor prone cdkn2a-/- mouse model has been used to compare retroviral insertional oncogenic potential using MLV and HIV-based vectors in in vivo genotoxicity assays [70]. These assays demonstrated HIV- based lentiviral vectors exhibited an improved safety profile compared to MLV based vectors. The Cdkn2a locus controls cell senescence and has been shown to prevent cell transformation. Inactivation of this gene promotes malignancy and has been implicated in almost all types of human cancer [71, 72]. These studies have compared the genotoxic contribution of vector components such as strong LTR promoters. They have also shown the ability of self-inactivating LTR designs to reduce genotoxicity.

Although these studies primarily identify activated proto-oncogenes, it is also possible to identify dysregulated tumor suppressors using retroviral mutagenesis screens [73-75]. Proviruses can downregulate nearby host gene transcription via host cell methylation of the proviral LTR that also leads to methylation of the nearby host genes. Identification of the vector provirus location and nearby host genes can be used to identify haplo-insufficiencies related to malignancy. Recent observations of viral LTR methylation causing proviral transgene silencing can now be used to identify down regulation of host genes near the methylated proviral integration sites [75]. The vector LTR methylation events and subsequent silencing of host genes can identify potential tumor suppressors related to vector-mediated genotoxicity. A recent study used methylation specific PCR and methylated DNA immunoprecipitation assays to analyze methylated proviral integrations in mutagenized mouse tumors [75]. In this study the identification of the methylated and downregulated gene PTP4A3 in MLV vector-mutagenized murine leukemia samples, suggests that haplo-insufficiency may be involved in retroviral genotoxicity [75]. This study also suggests that future studies may identify vector-mediated haploinsufficiency genes that contribute to genotoxicity.

12. Large animal models of genotoxicity

Large animal models allow long term monitoring of HSC genotoxicity due to the longer life span of large animals such as dogs and nonhuman primates relative to mice. These models are important to assess the long-term risks associated with malignant transformation following insertional mutagenesis from clonal expansion and long-term selection pressures. In two non-human primate studies, the distribution of MLV-based gammaretroviral and SIV and HIV-1 based lentiviral integration sites were evaluated over long periods [76, 77]. Clonal expansion or malignant transformation was not observed. However, integrants were observed at higher than expected frequencies near growth promoting genes and proto-oncogenes. This suggests that repopulating cells with integrations near these genes can influence survival of those clones. These studies can shed light on potential mechanisms of clonal expansion and can allow comparison of different vector types. However, these studies in normal animals using vectors with a reporter gene that is not expected to provide a selective growth advantage did not predict the clonal expansion observed in the SCID-X1 trial. This suggests that large animal models of specific disease settings such as the SCID-X1 dog model [34] will be important to test improved vectors designed to reduce genotoxicity in a specific disease setting.

Another important contribution of large animal models has been to improve our understanding of the effects of ex vivo culture on clonal expansion. It has been shown in a nonhuman primate model that genotoxicity can be significantly influenced by the culturing conditions of gene-modified cells ex vivo. In this study, only six days of culture increased the incidence of specific clones with gamma retroviral vector integrations near MDS/ EVI1 locus associated with a leukemic phenotype [78]. To monitor the potential effects of ex vivo culturing condition and in vivo selection on gene-modified repopulating cells, clonal tracking methods must be employed.

13. Tracking of genetically modified clones

The above studies have identified mechanisms of genotoxicity and clonal expansion. During clinical trials, it is important to monitor potential clonal expansion in order to understand genotoxicity and to anticipate potential adverse events [79]. As an example, dysregulation of HMGA2 in a clinical trial for β-thalassemia resulted in clonal expansion of gene-modified cells that has provided a therapeutic benefit without malignancy to date [80]. β-thalassemia is a genetic deficiency that hinders β-globin production and patients with this mutation are reliant upon continued blood transfusions to restore normal blood globin levels. Before HSC gene therapy the only therapeutic available was allogeneic transplant, however the procedure is high risk and patient limited due to a lack of matched donors. Thus, patients risk transplant rejection or development of graft versus host disease. To achieve therapeutic benefit using HSC gene therapy, lineage specific transgene expression in erythrocytes is required, promoting appropriate β-globin expression. Therapeutic benefit was achieved in two gene therapy patients resulting from a partially dominant clone harboring proviral insertions near HMGA2 [80]. The authors of this study conclude the clone with HMGA2 may remain homeostatic or eventually progress through multistep leukemogenesis, indicating a strong need for continued gene-marking studies and clonal tracking of these gene-modified cells in vivo [80].

14. MDS1/EVI1, PRDM16, SETBP1 in trial for CGD

Chronic Granulomatous disease (CGD) is an x-linked inherited immunodeficiency resulting from a mutation in one of the NADPH oxidase genes [87]. The gp91phox protein accounts for 70% of cases [81]. The gp91phox transgene has been used in corrective HSC gene therapy clinical trials [81]. Unlike SCID-X1 gene-modified cells, CGD gene-modified cells do not exhibit a proliferative advantage from transgene expression. The lack of conditioning or selection of gene-modified cells contributed to a loss of therapeutic benefit and detection of gene-modified cells. Patients in the initial trials had low marking with gene expression of the corrected transgene for short periods of therapeutic benefit. Adverse genotoxic events developed 2 ½ years after the initial therapy, with clonal expansion and leukemic transformation [7, 82]. Clonal analysis found activation of MDS1/EVI1, PRDM16, and SETBP1 proto-oncogenes [81]. One of the patients died in treatment from complications arising from the leukemia, the other patient survived after receiving an additional allogeneic transplant. In this study there was inefficient engraftment and short-term transgene expression, with vector silencing via vector LTR methylation (Figure 2D) [83]. Further improvements to enhance engraftment and selection of gene-modified cells after infusion are needed for HSC gene therapy to treat CGD.

15. CCND2 and MDS1/EVI1 trial for Wiskott-Aldrich

HSC gene therapy has also been used in the treatment of Wiskott-Aldrich syndrome (WAS), an X-linked recessive immune disorder. In this study, patients underwent conditioning with busulfan to enhance the engraftment of gene-modified cells [84] Patients exhibited therapeutic benefit, with resolution of disease symptoms, although clonal skewing was detected for clones that harbored vector integration sites near CCND2 and MDS1/EVI1 [84]. Despite the high success of WAS HSC gene therapy in nine of the ten patients treated, patient 2 was reported to have experienced vector-derived genotoxic events after more than 3 years of therapeutic benefit [84], ultimately resulting in T-cell leukemia. The leukemia was a result of proviral integration near the gene LMO2, and this patient has since been treated with chemotherapy resulting in remission [85-87].

Clonal tracking in vivo has recently been employed in a study where patients with glioblastoma were given gene-modified hematopoietic repopulating repopulating stem cells carrying a methylguanine methyltransferase mutant (MGMT-P140K) [17]. In this approach gene-modified hematopoietic repopulating cells expressing this mutant enzyme are resistant to O6-benzylguanine (O6BG). This allows treatment of the glioblastoma solid tumor with O6BG and an alkylating agent. By protecting the hematopoietic system from chemotherapy-mediated hematopoietic toxicity, higher doses of chemotherapy can be used to treat the glioblastoma. In patients undergoing chemotherapy, gene-modified cells were monitored to track potential clonal expansion and to assess patient safety. Repopulating cells were tracked and their retroviral integration sites monitored at several different time points, pre- and post-chemotherapeutic treatment. Throughout the course of chemotherapy treatment, over 12,000 unique retroviral insertion sites (RISs) were present in the three treated patients. The heterogeneity of RISs suggests a highly polyclonal engraftment of gene-modified repopulating cells. During tracking two patients exhibited clonal expansion, with prominent clones appearing with vector proviruses in PRDM16 (PR domain-containing 16), Set binding protein 1(SETBP1), and high-mobility group A2 (HMGA2) genes.

In summary, it is clear that HSC gene therapy is an efficacious therapeutic approach, able to treat debilitating and often fatal genetic deficiencies. However, the observed clonal expansion in these early clinical trials presents a major concern in the field. There is a need for vectors with an improved safety profile that are less likely to dysregulate genes and lead to clonal expansion.

16. Next-generation vectors: Reducing genotoxicity

Extensive efforts are underway to develop vector systems with safer integration profiles and reduced genotoxic effect. One approach is to retarget vector integration using tethering proteins that redirect the PIC. Other efforts focus on reducing genotoxicity by producing vectors less likely to dysregulate nearby genes. Such vectors include self-inactivating LTRs, which have deleted enhancer elements or U3 regions, preventing enhancer mediated expression of nearby genes. Newer vectors are also able to regulate context dependent transgene expression using insulators and repressor elements to prevent viral promoters from activating genes near the site of insertion [88]. Recently investigators have also identified insertional effects mediating alternative splicing, producing aberrant splice variants and protein fusion products causing oncogenesis [89, 90]. Modifying the vector-borne cryptic splice sites in vector backbones can create safer vectors reducing aberrant splice variant, reducing post-translational dysregulation of gene expression (Figure 2 C), [89, 91-93]. In addition, vector and host miRNAs have recently been explored. An example of miRNA control was demonstrated using miRNA let7 control elements, regulating expression of transgenes in stem cells versus somatic cells. Silencing of the transgenes occurs in somatic mature cells by miRNA cleavage sites. When let7 target sequence is matured and expressed, cleavage of the transgene containing the target sequence occurs [94]. In pluripotent cells, let7 is not expressed, thus the target sequences are not cleaved and full-length transgene is expressed [94]. This technology could potentially direct HSC gene therapy over a major hurdle, by reducing vector-born genotoxicity through transgene expression in a highly controlled, cell specific context. These miRNA technologies have the ability to restrict transgene expression to a specific cell type and are even able to restrict transgene expression within a specific differentiation stage of that cell type, allowing a more specific control of transgene delivery, dosage, and expression [95]. Incorporation of miRNA technologies can improve vector efficacy and safety, ultimately reducing or limiting vector-born genotoxic events.

17. Chromatin insulators

Chromatin insulators are being developed to reduce the propensity of integrated vector proviruses to dysregulate host gene expression. Insulators are DNA elements that repress the activity of enhancers on promoters. The chicken hypersensitive site-4 (cHS4) insulator contains five DNA binding elements within a 250 bp fragment known as the dominant DNase hypersensitive site [96, 97]. A 650 bp cHS4 element has been characterized in conjunction with a 400 bp element from cHS4 that can sufficiently block enhancer activation [98]. Additional insulators have been described for sea urchin sns5 insulator and an adeno-associated (AAVS1) viral insulator DHS-S1 [99, 100].

The cHS4 insulator has been used in several retroviral vector systems [80,99, 101-106]. Initial studies with cHS4 lentiviral vectors were shown to be effective in reducing genotoxicity [107]. Their use in erythrocytes gave encouraging results, albeit with low titers. In addition, this study also demonstrated the effects of insulator failure after a reduction of cHS4 element repeats, which was reported to have contributed to insertional mutagenesis and expansion of clones harboring HMGA2 mutations [80]. Sea urchin sns5 is a 462 bp insulator region that was demonstrated to function in gamma retroviral vectors by maintaining chromatin position affects [100]. This element also contains a previously identified insulator region of 265 bp found to block enhancer-activated directional transcription in human cells [108, 109]. The DHS-S1 viral insulator has been demonstrated to increase transgene expression 1000-fold from an elongation factor 1-alpha (EF1α) promoter in muscle cells, but was not studied for its ability to block transactivation of host genes [99]. Insulators can potentially serve several major functions, by protecting against vector silencing, moderating vector variegation or uniformity of expression, and protecting nearby host genes from enhancer activation. Additional studies should help better characterize the efficacy of insulated vectors

18. Incorporation of cell-type specific control elements

Incorporation of cell-type specific control elements such as erythrocyte specific enhancer-promoter has been used to control transgene expression [110]. The use of a lineage specific promoter ensures that transgene expression only occurs within the lineage from which the promoter is active. Moreover, avoiding expression of the transgene in other cell types with which the promoter is not active. The premise of lineage-restricted promoters for HSC gene therapy is that they may eliminate or reduce genotoxicity resulting from dysregulation of genes in stem/progenitor cells. This is accomplished by activating transgene expression only in a cell lineage with which transgene expression is required for therapeutic benefit. This approach might protect primitive cells from dysregulation, as the promoter is not expressed until differentiation into the target cell type. This is an attractive area of research for diseases that characteristically are exhibited in one lineage of the blood system such as hemaglobino-pathies. This approach was used in a thalassemia trial, where a β-locus-control-region-derived promoter was used [80]. The transgene is delivered to long term repopulating HSCs, but the promoter is not active. Only after erythroid differentiation would the enhancer become active, resulting in transgene expression in erythrocytes. This may reduce the occurrence of proto-oncogene activation in stem/progenitor cells. Other lineage specific promoters are being studied, including B cell lineage specific promoters [111]. When a lineage specific promoter is not a viable option, vectors may need to be targeted to specific regions of the chromatin, where vector insertion is at a much lower risk of causing malignancy.

19. Re-targeting of retroviral vectors

Efforts have been made to target retroviral proviruses to specific chromosomal locations. LEDGF, a host cell protein that interacts with HIV Gag has been used to effect tethering and targeting of viral integration Gijsbers et al [112]. In this study, cells were modified to express LEDGF protein containing a chromatin-interacting domain of chromobox homolog 1 (CBX1), which binds di- and tri- methylated regions of histone 3 (H3) in heterochromatic regions of the genome [112]. H3s are located pericentric to regions of heterochromatin, which is safer in terms of insertional mutagenesis as genes in these regions are normally silent. However, the reporting of significant retargeting of integration sites to heterochromatin is encouraging.

In addition, authors reported that transgene expression was not affected by targeting to these transcriptionally unfavorable heterochromatic sites [112]. These exciting experiments have demonstrated that vectors containing Gag and Pol C termini with adapted or unique binding domains could direct insertional distribution [113]. However, LEDGF cannot be modified in HSC gene therapy and alternative tethering approaches must be devised.

Additional tethering proteins have been studied and need to be fully characterized to expand targeted integration locations in in vivo approaches [113]. In future studies use of appropriate tethers for modified integration site preference may reduce genotoxicity and may provide a better understanding of virus and host interactions affecting viral integration. In addition, even with vector systems that have incorporated these safety mechanisms, genotoxic events may arise and methods to ablate the gene-modified cells will be useful to avoid malignancy.

20. Approaches to ablate expanded cell clones

Several approaches exist to ablate or control expanded clones after insertionally activated oncogenesis has occurred. Conditional selection systems have been employed to control the longevity and survival of HSC gene-modified clones after infusion. Several conditional promoter systems such as TET on/off and pro-drug inducible expression cassettes have been used to target cancer cells harboring dangerous integrations through vector silencing and suicide gene activation [114].

The tetracycline (Tet) on/off gene expression system utilizes a pro-drug to regulate transgene expression by modifying a Tet repressor protein (TetR). TetR is constitutively expressed and depending on its conformation will either be bound to the tetracycline operator (TetO), or unbound. In a Tet on system, TetR does not bind TetO until administration of the pro-drug, typically doxycycline. Once the pro-drug is administered, TetR actively binds TetO and silences transcription of nearby transgenes. In the absence of the pro-drug TetR cannot bind TetO, and this region of the genome is no longer blocked from transcription, and gene expression resumes. Alternatively, modifications have been made to TetR, allowing it to bind to repressor sequences until it is deactivated by a pro-drug; this system is called Tet off. The Tet on/off system may be used in conjunction with suicide genes to ablate undesired clones.

In gene suicide approaches, HSC gene therapy delivers an active transgene in conjunction with a pro-drug induced suicide gene such as Thymidine Kinase [115]. In the event that transformations result from insertional mutagenesis and clonal expansion, clones harboring integrations can be eliminated or reduced by activating expression of the suicide gene, inducing apoptosis and eliminating clones harboring proviral integrations [26]. Recent clinical trials using an inducible caspase 9 (iCasp9), which remains in an inactivated state until dimerization following treatment with AP1903 small molecule, was reported in four patients with graft versus host disease after gene-modified hematopoietic transfusion [116]. In four patients, a single infusion of AP1903 was reported to have eliminated 90% of gene modified T cells within 30 minutes of administration of the inducing drug AP1903. GVHD and other associated illnesses typically observed after allogeneic bone marrow transplants were not detected up to a year after AP1903 treatment [116]. Thymidine kinase and iCasp9 present effective safety switches to control an array of genotoxic effects arising from HSC gene therapy [26, 117]. Utilizing these safety mechanisms in new vector designs will aid in furthering safety and reducing genotoxic events, and allow for selective ablation of expanded gene-modified clones in vivo.

21. Concluding summary

The use of HSC gene therapy in clinical trials is expanding, and the therapeutic potential is enormous. Following the initial successes with ADA SCID and SCID-X1 additional efficacious therapies were reported for WAS, β-thalassemia, and CGD. Seymour et al. reported that the majority of over 90 patients receiving HSC gene therapy exhibit prolonged clinical benefit, with greater than 90% survival rate despite the occurrence of genotoxic events [46]. Current studies that are underway aim to characterize and reduce genotoxicity. Several approaches have reduced genotoxic events in preclinical studies. With ongoing technological refinement, newer and safer HSC gene therapy vectors are entering, or will soon enter, the clinical arena. These advances are crucial for HSC gene therapy to enter mainstream medicine as an effective and safe therapeutic approach.

Acknowledgements

G.D.T. was supported in part from the National Institutes of Health (AI097100), by funds provided for medical and biological research by the State of Washington Initiative Measure No. 171, and by the Department of Defense Peer Reviewed Cancer Research Program under award number W81XWH-11-1-0576. Views and opinions of, and endorsements by the author(s) do not reflect those of the US Army or the Department of Defense.

Author details

Dustin T. Rae[1] and Grant D. Trobridge[1,2]

*Address all correspondence to: grant.trobridge@wsu.edu

1 Department of Pharmaceutical Sciences, Washington State University, Pullman, Washington, USA

2 School of Molecular Biosciences, Washington State University, Pullman, Washington, USA

References

[1] Malech H, Maples P, Whiting-Theobald N, Linton G, Sekhsaria S, Vowells S, et al. Prolonged production of NADPH oxidase-corrected granulocytes after gene therapy of chronic granulomatous disease. Proc. Natl. Acad. Sci. 1997; 94(22): p. 12133-12138.

[2] Malech H, Horwitz M, Linton G. Extended production of oxidase normal neutrophils in X-linked chronic granulomatous disease (CGD) following gene therapy with gp91phos transduced CD34+ cells. Blood. 1998; 92((suppl 10)): p. 690a.

[3] Barese CN, Goebel WS, Dinauer MC. Gene therapy for chronic granulomatous disease. Expert Opinion on Biological Therapy. 2004; 4(9): p. 1423-1434.

[4] Bleijs DA. Gene Therapy Net. [Online].; 2012 [cited 2012 June 18. Available from: http://www.genetherapynet.com/.

[5] Hacein-Bey-Abina S, Garrigue A, Wang G, Soulier J, Lim A, Morillon E, et al. Insertional oncogenesis in 4 patients after retrovirus-mediated gene therapy of SCID-X1. J. Clin. Invest. 118:3132–3142 (2008). doi:10.1172/JCI35700. 2008; 118(9): p. 3132-3142.

[6] Segal BH, Veys P, Malech H, Cowan MJ. Chronic Granulomatous Disease: Lessons from a Rare Disorder. Biol Blood Marrow Transplant. 2011; 17(1): p. s123-s131.

[7] Stein S, Ott M, Schultze-Strasser S, Jauch A, Burwinkel B, Kinner A, et al. Genomic instability and myelodysplasia with monosomy 7 consequent to EVI1 activation after gene therapy for chronic granulomatous disease. Nat Med. 2010; 16(2): p. 198-204.

[8] Kang EM, Malech HL. Gene Therapy for Chronic Granulomatous Disease. In Friedmann T, editor. Methods in Enzymology. San Diego, CA: Academic Press; ELSEVIER; 2012. p. 125-154.

[9] Aiuti A, Cattaneo F, Galimberti S, Benninghoff U, Cassani B, Callegaro L, et al. Gene therapy for severe combined immunodeficiency due to adenosine deaminase deficiency. N. Engl.J. med. 2009; 360(5): p. 447-458.

[10] Aiuti A, Slavin S, Aker M, Ficara F, Deola S, Mortellaro A, et al. Correction of ADA-SCID by stem cell gene therapy combined with nonmyeloablative conditioning. Science. 2002; 296(5577): p. 2410-2413.

[11] Aiuti A, Cassani B, Andolfi G, Mirolo M, Biasco L, Recchia A, et al. Multilineage hematopoietic reconstituion without clonal selection in ADA-SCID patients treated with stem cell gene therapy. J Clin Invest. 2007; 117(8): p. 2233-2240.

[12] Blaese RM, Culver KW, Miller AD, Carter CS, Fleisher T, Clerici M, et al. T lymphocyte-directed gene therapy for ADA- SCID: initial trial results after 4 years. Science. 1995; 270(5235): p. 475–480.

[13] Charrier S, Dupré L, Scaramuzza S, Jeanson-Leh L, Blundell M, Danos O, et al. Lentiviral vectors targeting WASp expression to hematopoietic cells, efficiently transduce and correct cells from WAS patients. Nature: Gene Therapy. 2007; 14(5): p. 415-428.

[14] Zanta-Boussif M, Charrier S, Brice-Ouzet A, Martin S, Opolon P, Thrasher A, et al. Validation of a mutated PRE sequence allowing high and sustained transgene expression while abrogating WHV-X protein synthesis: application to the gene therapy of WAS. Nature; Gene Therapy. 2009; 16(5): p. 605-619.

[15] Cartier N, Hacein-Bey-Abina S, Bartholomae C, Veres G, Schmidt M, Kutschera I, et al. Hematopoietic stem cell gene therapy with a lentiviral vector in X-linked adrenoleukodystrophy. Science. 2009; 326(5954): p. 818-823.

[16] Biffi A, De Palma M, Quattrini A, Del Carro U, Amadio S, Visigalli I, et al. Correction of metachromatic leukodystrophy in the mouse model by transplantation of genetically modified hematopoietic stem cells. J. Clin. Invest. 2004; 113(8): p. 1118-1129.

[17] Adair JE, Beard BC, Trobridge Gd, Neff T, Rockhill JK, Daniel L. Silbergeld MMM, et al. Extended Survival of Glioblastom Patients After Chemoprotective HSC Gene Therapy. Sci. Transl. Med. 2012; 4(133): p. 133ra57.

[18] Booth C, Gaspar BH, Thrasher AJ. Gene therapy for primary immunodeficiency. Curr. Opin. Pediatr. 2011; 23(6): p. 659-666.

[19] Hacein-Bey-Abina S, Von KC, Schmidt M, McCormack M, Wulffraat N, Leboulch P, et al. LMO2-associated clonal T cell proliferation in two patients after gene therapy for SCID-X1. Science. 2003; 302(5644): p. 415-419.

[20] Scobie L, Hector R, Grant L, Bell M, Nielsen A, Meikle S, et al. A novel model of SCID-X1 reconstitution reveals predisposition to retrovirus-induced lymphoma but no evidence of gamma C gene oncogenicity. Mol Ther. 2009; 17(8): p. 1483.

[21] Nienhuis AW. Development of gene therapy for blood disorders. American Society of Hematology; BLOOD. 2008; 111(9): p. 4431-4444.

[22] Olga K, Martijn B, Baum C. The Genomic risk of somatic gene therapy. Seminars in Cancer Biology. 2010; 20(4): p. 269-278.

[23] Rous R. Transmission of a malignant new growth by means of a cell-free filtrate. JAMA. 1983; 250(11): p. 1445-1449.

[24] Varmus H, Weiss R, Friis R, Levinson W, Bishop J. Detection of avian tumor virus-specific nucleotide sequences in avian cell DNAs (reassociation kinetics-RNA tumor viruses-gas antigen-Rous sarcoma virus, chick cells). Proc. Natl. Acad. Sci. USA. 1972; 69(1): p. 20-24.

[25] Sheridan C. Gene therapy finds its niche. Nature biotechnology. 2011; 29(2): p. 121-128.

[26] Rivie're I, Dunbar CE, Sadelain M. Hematopoietic stem cell engineering at a crossroads. BLOOD. 2012; 119(520): p. 1107-1116.

[27] Nielsen J, McNagny K. Novel functions of the CD34 family. J of Cell Science. 2008; 121(Pt 22): p. 3682-3692.

[28] Brenner M, Rill D, Holladay M, Heslop H, Moen R, Buschle M, et al. Gene marking to determine whether autologus marrow infusion restores long-term haemopoiesis in cancer patients. Lancet. 1993; 342(8880): p. 1134-1137.

[29] Brenner M, Rill D, Moen R, Krance R, Mirro JJ, Anderson W, et al. Gene-marking to trace origin of relapse after autologous bone-marrow transplant. Lancet. 1993; 341(8837): p. 85-86.

[30] Horn PA, Morris JC, Neff T, Hiem HP. Stem Cell Gene Transfer- Efficacy and Safety in Large Animal Studies. Mol Ther. 2004; 10(3): p. 417-431.

[31] Di Santo JP, Kuhn R, Muller W. Common Cytokine Receptor Y chain (Yc)- Dependent Cytokines: Understanding in vivo Functions by Gene Targetting. immunological Reviews. 1995; 148.

[32] Kiem H, Andrews R, Morris J, Peterson L, Heyward S, Allen J, et al. Improved gene transfer in baboon marrow repopulating cells using recombinant human fibronectin fragment in combination with interleukin-6, stem cell factor, FLT-3 ligand, and megakaryocyte growth and evelopment factor. Blood. 1998; 92(6): p. 1878-1886.

[33] Ting-De Ravin S, Kennedy D, Naumann N, Kennedy J, Choi U, Hartnett B, et al. Correction of canine X-linked severe combined immunodeficiency by in vivo retroviral gene therapy. Blood. 2006; 107(8): p. 3091-3097.

[34] Kennedy D, Hartnett B, Kennedy J, Vernau W, Moore P, O'Malley T, et al. Ex vivo γ-retroviral gene therapy of dogs with X-linked severe combined immunodeficiency and the development of a thymic T cell lymphoma. Veterinary Immunology and Immunopathology. 2011; 142(1-2): p. 36-48.

[35] Oram S, Thoms J, Pridans C, Janes M, Kinston S, Anand S, et al. A previously unrecognised promoter of LMO2 forms part of a transcriptional regulatory circuit mediating LMO2 expression in a subset of T-acute lymphoblastic leukemia patients. Oncogene. 2010; 29(43): p. 5796-5808.

[36] Kool J, Berns A. High-throughput insertional mutagenesis screens in mice to identify oncogenic networks. Nat. Rev. Cancer. 2009; 9(6): p. 389-399.

[37] Suzuki T, Minehata K, Akagi K, Jenkins N, Copeland N. Tumor supresor gene identification using retroviral insertional mutagenesis in Blm-deficient mice. Embo. J. 2006; 25(14): p. 3422-3431.

[38] Kustikova O, Fehse B, Modlich U, Yang M, Düllmann J, Kamino K, et al. Clonal Dominance of Hematopoietic Stem Cells Triggered by Retroviral Gene Marking. Science. 2005; 308(5725): p. 1171.

[39] Warren A, Colledge W, Carlton M, Evans M, Smith A, Rabbitts T. The oncogenic cysteine-rich LIM domain protein rbtn2 is essential for erythroid development. Cell. 1994; 78(1): p. 45-57.

[40] Lessard J, Sauvageau G. Bmi-1 determines the proliferative capacity of normal and leukemic stem cells. Nature. 2003; 423(6937): p. 255-260.

[41] Park I, Qian D, Kiel M, Becker M, Pihalja M, Weissman I, et al. Bmi-1 is required for maintenance of adult self-renewing hematopoietic stem cells. Nature. 2003; 423(6937): p. 302-305.

[42] Kazuhiko I, Philip J, Bessler M, Bessler M. 3¢UTR-truncated Hmga2 cDNA causes MPN-like hematopoiesis by conferring a clonal growth advantage at the level of HSC in mice. Blood. 2011; 117(22): p. 5860-5869.

[43] Peterson EA, Stanbery L, Li C, Kocak H, Makarova O, Petty EM. SEPT9_i1 and Genomic Instability: Mechanistic Insights and Relevance to Tumorigenesis. GENES, CHROMOSOMES & CANCER. 2011; 50(11): p. 940–949.

[44] Cerveira N, Santos J, Teixeira M. Structural and Expression Changes of Septins in Myeloid Neoplasia. Critical Re3views in Oncogenesis. 2009; 15(1-2): p. 91-115.

[45] Kuo YH,. Zaidi SK, Gornostaeva S, Komori T, Stein GS, and Lucio H. Runx2 induces acute myeloid leukemia in cooperation with Cbfb -SMMHC in mice. Blood. 2009; 113(14): p. 3323-3332.

[46] Seymour LW, Thrasher AJ. Gene therapy matures in the clinic. Nature Biotechnolo-
      gy. 2012; 30(7): p. 588-593.

[47] Schröder A, Shinn P, Chen H, Berry C, Ecker J, Bushman F. HIV-1 integration in the
      human genome favors active genes and local hotspots. Cell. 2002; 110(4): p. 521-529.

[48] Tsukahara T, Agawa H, Matsumoto S, Matsuda M, Ueno S, Yamashita Y, et al. Mur-
      ine leukemia virus vector integration favors promoter regions and regional hot spots
      in human T-cell line. Biochemical and Biophysical Research Communications. 2006;
      345(3): p. 1099-1107.

[49] Mitchell R, Beitzel B, Schroder A, Shinn P, Chen H, Berry C, et al. Retroviral DNA
      integration: ASLV, HIV, and MLV show distinct target site preferences. PLoS Biol.
      2004; 2(8): p. E234.

[50] Wu X, Li Y, Crise B, Burgess S. Trasncription start regions in the human genome are
      favored targets for MLV integration. Science. 2003; 300(5626): p. 1749-1751.

[51] Barr S, Ciuffi A, Leipzig J, Shinn P, Ecker J, Bushman F. HIV integration site selec-
      tion: targeting in macrophages and the effects of different routes of viral entry. Mol
      Ther. 2006; 14(2): p. 218-225.

[52] Aiken C. Pseudotyping human immunodeficiency virus type 1 (HIV-1) by the glyco-
      protein of vestcular stomattits virus targets HIV-1 entry to an endocytic pathway and
      suppresses both the requirment for Nef and the sensitivity to cyclosporin. A. J Virol.
      1997; 71(8): p. 5871-5877.

[53] Narezkina A, Taganov K, Litwin S, Stoyanova R, Hayashi J, Seeger C, et al. Genome-
      wide analyses of avian sarcoma virus integration sites. J Virol. 2004; 78(21): p.
      11656-11663.

[54] Trobridge G, Miller D, Jacobs M, Allen J, Kiem H, Kaul R, et al. Foamy virus vector
      integration sites in normal human cells. Proc Natl Acad SCI USA. 2006; 103(5): p.
      1498-1503.

[55] Brass A, Dykxhoorn D, Benita Y, Yan N, Engelman A, Xavier R, et al. Identification of
      host proteins required for HIV infection through a functional genomic screen. Sci-
      ence. 2008; 319(5865): p. 921-926.

[56] Llano M, Delgado S, Vanegas M, Poeschla E. Lens epithelium-derived growth
      factor/P75 prevents proteasomal degredation of HIV-1 integrase. J Biol Chem. 2004;
      279(53): p. 55570-55577.

[57] Lewinski M, Yamashita M, Emerman M, Ciuffi A, Marshall H, Crawford G, et al. Ret-
      roviral DNA integration: viral and cellular determinants of target-site selection. PLoS
      pathog. 2006; 2(6): p. e60.

[58] Tobaly-Tapiero J, Bittoun P, Lehmann-Che J, Delelis O, Giron M, de Thé H, et al.
      Chromatin Tethering of Incoming Foamy Virus by the Structural Gag Protein. Traffic
      2008. 2008; 9(10): p. 1717-1727.

[59] Cherepanov P, Maertens G, Proost P, Devreese B, Van Beeumen J, Engelborghs Y, et al. HIV-1 integrase forms stable tetramers and associates with LEDGF/p75 protein in human cells. J Biol Chem. 2003; 278(1): p. 373-381.

[60] Emiliani S, Mousnier A, Busschots K, Maroun M, Van Maele B, Tempé D, et al. Integrase mutants defective for interaction with LEGF/p75 are impaired in chromosome tethering and HIV-1 replication. J Biol Chem. 2005; 280(27): p. 25517-25523.

[61] Ciuffi A, Llano M, Poeschla E, Hoffmann C, Leipzig J, Shinn P, et al. A role of LEGF/p75 in targetting HIV DNA integration. Nat Med. 2005; 11(12): p. 1287-1289.

[62] Schliephake A, Rethwilm A. Nuclear localization of foamy virus Gag precursor protein. J Virol. 1994; 68(8): p. 4946–4954.

[63] Stenbak C, Linial M. Role of the C terminus of foamy virus Gag in RNA packaging and Pol expression. J Virol. 2004; 78(17): p. 9423–9430.

[64] Yu S, Edelmann K, Strong R, Moebes A, Rethwilm A, Linial M. The carboxyl terminus of the human foamy virus Gag protein contains separable nucleic acid binding and nuclear transport domains. J Virol. 1996; 70(12): p. 8255–8262.

[65] Gabriel R, Eckenberg R, Paruzynski A, Bartholomae C, Nowrouzi A, Arens A, et al. Comprehensive genomic access to vector integration in clinical gene therapy. Nat Med. 2009; 15(12): p. 1431-1436.

[66] Biasco L, Baricordi C, Aiuti A. Retroviral Integrations in Gene Therapy Trials. Molecular Therapy. 2012; 20(4): p. 709-716.

[67] Berger SA, Bernstein A. Characterization of a Retrovirus Shuttle Vector Capable of Either Proviral Integration or Extrachromosomal Replication in Mouse Cells. MOLECULAR AND CELLULAR BIOLOGY. 1975; 5(2): p. 305-312.

[68] Cepko CL, Roberts BE, Mulligan RC. Construction and Applications of a Highly Transmissible Murine Retrovirus Shuttle Vector. Cell. 1984; 37(3): p. 1053-1062.

[69] Montini E, Cesana D, Schmidt M, Sanvito F, Bartholomae C, Ranzani M, et al. The genotoxic potential of retroviral vectors is strongly modulated by vector design and integration site selection in a mouse model of HSC gene therapy. J. Clin. Invest. 2009; 119(4): p. 964-975.

[70] Montini E, Cesana D, Schmidt M, Sanvito F, Ponzoni M, Bartholomae C, et al. Hematopoietic stem cell gene transfer in a tumor-prone mouse model uncovers low genotoxicity of lentiviral vector integration. Nat. Biotechnol. 2006; 24(6): p. 687-696.

[71] Sherr CJ. Principles of tumour supression. Cell. 2004; 116(2): p. 235-246.

[72] Sherr CJ. The INK4a/ARF network in tumour supression. Nat. Rev. Mol. Cell Biol. 2001; 2(10): p. 731-737.

[73] Greenman CD. Haploinsufficient Gene Selection in Cancer. Science. 2012; 337(6090): p. 47-48.

[74] Solimini N, Xu Q, Mermel C, Liang A, Schlabach M, Luo J, et al. Recurrent Hemizygous Deletions in Cancers May Optimize Proliferative Potential. Science. 2012; 337(6090): p. 104-108.

[75] Beekman R, Valkhof M, Erkeland S, Taskesen E, Rockova V, Peeters J, et al. Retroviral Integration Mutagenesis in Mice and Comparative analysis in Human AML Identify Reduced PTP4A3 Expression as a Prognostic Indicator. PLoS one. 2011; 6(10): p. e26537-e26537.

[76] Beard B, Dickerson D, Beebe K, Gooch C, Fletcher J, Okbinoglu T, et al. Comparison of HIV-derived lentiviral and MLV-based gammaretroviral vector integration sites in primate repopulating cells. J mole Ther. 2007; 15(7): p. 1356-1365.

[77] Hematti P, Hong B, Ferguson C, Adler R, Hanawa H, Sellers S, et al. Distinct genomic integration of MLV and SIV vectors in primate hematopoietic stem and progenitor cells. PLoS Biol. 2004; 2(12): p. e423.

[78] Sellers S, Gomes T, Larochelle A, Lopez R, Adler R, Krouse A, et al. Ex vivo expansion of retrovirally transcuded primate CD34+ cells results in over representation of clones with MDS1/EVI1 insertion sties in the myeloid lineage after tranplantation. Mol Ther. 2010; 18(9): p. 1633-1639.

[79] Tey SK, Brenner Mk. The Continuing Contribution of Gene Marking to Cell and Gene Therapy. Molecular Therapy. 2007; 15(4): p. 666-677.

[80] Cavazzana-Calvo M, Payen E, Negre O, Wang G, Hehir K, Fusil F, et al. Transfusion independence and HMGA2 activation after gene therapy of human beta-thalassaemia. Nature. 2010; 467(7313): p. 318-322.

[81] Kang H, Bartholomae C, Paruzynski A, Arens A, Kim S, Yu S, et al. Retroviral gene therapy for X-linked Chronic Granulomatus Disease: Results from Phase I/II Trial. Mol.Ther. 2011; 19(11): p. 2092-2101.

[82] Ott M, Schmidt M, Schwarzwaelder K, Stein S, Siler U, Koehl U, et al. Correction of X-linked chronic granulomatous disease by gene therapy, augmented by insertional activation of MDS1-EVI1, PRDM16 or SETBP1. Nat Med. 2006; 12(4): p. 401-409.

[83] Segal BH, Veys P, Malech H, Cowan aMJ. Chronic Granulomatous Disease: Lessons from a Rare Disorder. Biol Blood Marrow Transplant. 2011; 17(1 suppl): p. S123-S131.

[84] Boztug K, Schmidt M, Schwarzer A, P B, Avedillo Díez I, Dewey RA, et al. Stem-cell gene therapy for the Wiskott-Aldrich syndrome. N Engl J Med. 2010; 363: p. 1918-1927.

[85] Braun CJ, Boztug K, Schmidt M, Albert MH, Schwarzer A, Paruzynski A, et al. 165 Efficacy of Gene Therapy for Wiskott-Aldrich-Syndrome. In 53 rd ASH Anual Meeting and Exposition; 2011; Elizabeth Ballroom DE (Manchester Grand Hyatt San Diego).

[86] Galya A, Thrasher AJ. Gene therapy for the Wiskott–Aldrich syndrome. Current Opinion in Allergy and Clinical Immunology. 2011; 11(6): p. 545-50.

[87] Stefan Zorn. Effective Gene Therapy for Children with Wiskott-Aldrich-Syndrome, a Severe Inborn Immunodeficiency Disease. 2010..

[88] Bushey A, Dorman E, Corces V. Chromatin insulators; regulatory mechanisms and epigentic inheritance. MOl Cell. 2008; 32(1): p. 1-9.

[89] Moiani A, Paleari Y, Sartori D, Mezzadra R, Miccio A, Cattoglio C, et al. Lentiviral vector integration in the human genome induces alternative splicing and generates aberrant transcripts. J. Clin. Invest. 2012; 122(5): p. 1653-1666.

[90] Nilsen T, Maroney P, Goodwin R, Rottman F, Crittenden L, Raines M, et al. c-ervB activation in ALV-induced erythroblastosis: novel RNA processing and promoter insertion result in expression of aminotruncated EGF receptor. Cell. 1985; 41(3): p. 719-726.

[91] Cattoglio C, Pellin D, Rizzi E, Maruggi G, Corti G, Miselli F, et al. High-definition mapping of retroviral integration sites identifies avtice regulatory elements in human multipotent hematopoietic progenitors. Blood. 2010; 116(25): p. 5507-5517.

[92] Maruggi G, Porcellini S, Facchini G, Perna S, Cattoglio C, Sartori D, et al. Transcriptional enhancers induce insertional gene deregulation independantly from the vector type and design. Mol. Ther. 2009; 17(5): p. 851-856.

[93] Almarza D, Bussadori G, Navarro M, Mavilio F, Larcher F, Murillas R. Risk assessment in skin gene therapy: viral-celluar fusion transcripts generated by proviral transcriptional read-through in Keratinocytes transduced with self-inactivating lentiviral vectors. Gene Ther. 2011; 18(7): p. 674-681.

[94] Di Stefano B, Maffioletti S, Gentner B, Ungaro F, Schira G, Naldini L, et al. A miRNA-based System for Selecting and Maintaining the Pluripotent State in Human Induced Pluripotent Stem Cells. Stem Cells. 2011; 29(11): p. 1-18.

[95] Brown B, Naldini L. Exploiting and antagonizing microRNA regulation for therapeutic and experimental applications. Nat. Rev. Genet. 2009; 10(8): p. 578-585.

[96] Wallace J, Felsenfeld G. We gather together: insulators and genome organization. Current opinion in genetics & development. 2007; 17(5): p. 400-407.

[97] Gaszner M, Felsenfeld G. Insulators: exploiting transcriptional and epigenetic mechanisms. Nat Rev Genet. 2006; 7(9): p. 703-713.

[98] Arumugam P, Urbinati F, Velu C, higashimoto T, Grimes H, Malik P. The 3' region of the chicken hypersensitive site-4 insulator has properties similar to its core and is required for fill insulator activity. PloS one. 2009; 4(9): p. e6995.

[99] Ogata T, Kozuka T, Kanda T. Identification of an insulator in AAVS1, a preferred region for integration of adeno-associated virus DNA.. Journal of virology. 2003; 77(16): p. 9000-9007.

[100] D'Apolito D, Baiamonte E, Bagliesi M, Di Marzo R, Calzolari R, Ferro L, et al. The sea urchin sns5 insulator protects retroviral vectors from chromosomal position effects by maintaining active chromatin structure. Mol Ther. 2009; 17(8): p. 1434-1441.

[101] Li C, Emery D. The cSH4 chromatin insulator reduced gammaretroviral vector silencing by epigenetic modification of integrated provirus. Gene Therapy. 2008; 15(1): p. 49-53.

[102] Evans-Galea M, Wielgosz M, Hanawa H, Srivastava D, Nienhuis A. Supression of clonal dominance in cultured human lymphoid cells by addition of the cHS4 insulator to a lentiviral vector. Mol Ther. 2007; 15(4): p. 801-809.

[103] Li C, Xiong D, Stamatoyannopoulos G, Emery D. Genomic and functional assays demonstrate reduced gammaretroviral vector genotoxicity associated with use of the cHS4 chromatin insulator. Mol Ther. 2009; 17(4): p. 716-724.

[104] Aker M, Tubb J, Groth A, Bukovsky A, Bell A, Felsenfeld G, et al. Extended corse sequences from the cSH4 insulator are necessary for protecting retroviral vectors for silencing position effects. Human Gene Therapy. 2008; 18(4): p. 333-343.

[105] Arumugam P, Scholes J, Perelman N, Xia P, Yee J, Malik P. Improved human betaglobin expression from self-inactivating lentiviral vectors carrying the chicken hypersensitive site-4 (cSH4) insulator element. Mol Ther. 2007; 15(10): p. 1863-1871.

[106] Malik P, Arumugam P, Yee J, Puthenveetil G. Successfull correction of the human Cooley's anemia beta-thalassemia major phenotype using a lentiviral vector flanked by the chicken hypersensitive site 4 chromatin insulator. Ann N Y Acad Sci. 2005; 1054: p. 238-249.

[107] Hanawa H, Yamamoto M, Zhao H, Shimada T, Persons DA. Optimized lentiviral vector improves titers and transgene expression of vectors containing the chicken B-globin locus HS4 insulator element. Mol. Ther. 2009; 17(4): p. 667-674.

[108] Palla F, Melfi R, Anello L, Di Bernardo M, Spinelli G. Enhancer blocking activity located near the 3' end of the sea urchin early H2A histone gene. Proceedings of the National Academy of Sciences of the United States of America. 1997; 94(6): p. 2272-2277.

[109] Melfi R, Palla F, Di Simone P, Alessandro C, Cali L, Anello L, et al. Functional characterization of the enhancer blocking element of the sea urchin early histone gene cluster reveals insulator properties and three essential cis-acting sequence. J Mol Biol. 2000; 304(5): p. 753-763.

[110] Cassani B, Montini E, Maruggi G, Ambrosi A, Mirolo M, Selleri S, et al. Integration of retroviral vectors induces minor changes in the transcriptional activity of T cells from ADA-SCID patients treated with gene therapy. Blood. 2009; 114(17): p. 3546-3456.

[111] Sather B, Ryu B, Stirling B, Garibov M, Kerns H, Humblet-Baron S, et al. Development of B-lineage predominant lentiviral vectors for use in genetic therapies for B cell disorders. Mol Ther. 2011; 19(3).

[112] Gijsbers R, Ronen K, Vets S, Malani N, De Rijck J, McNeely M, et al. LEDGF hybrids efficiently retarget lentiviral integration into heterochromatin. Mol ther. 2010; 18(3): p. 552-560.

[113] Yi Y, Hahm S, Lee K. Retroviral Gene Therapy: Safety Issues and Possible Solutions. Current Gene Therapy. 2005; 5(1): p. 25-35.

[114] Curtin J, Candolfi M, Xiong W, Lowenstein P, Castro M. Turning the gene tap off; implications of regulating gene expression for cancer therapeutics. Mol Cancer Ther. 2008; 7(3): p. 439-449.

[115] Lupo-Stanghellini M, Provasi E, Bondanza A, Ciceri F, Bordignon C, Bonini C. Clinical impact of suicide gene therapy in allogeneic hematopoietic stem cell transplantation. Hum Gene Ther. 2010; 21(3): p. 241-250.

[116] Sadelain M. Eliminating Cells Gone Astray. n engl j med. 2011; 365(18): p. 1735-1736.

[117] Ellis J, Baum C, Benvenisty N, Mostoslavsky G, Okano H, Stanford W, et al. Benefits of utilizing genemodified iPSCs for clinical applications. Cell Stem Cell. 2010; 7(4): p. 429-430.

Permissions

The contributors of this book come from diverse backgrounds, making this book a truly international effort. This book will bring forth new frontiers with its revolutionizing research information and detailed analysis of the nascent developments around the world.

We would like to thank Francisco Martín Molina, for lending his expertise to make the book truly unique. He has played a crucial role in the development of this book. Without his invaluable contribution this book wouldn't have been possible. He has made vital efforts to compile up to date information on the varied aspects of this subject to make this book a valuable addition to the collection of many professionals and students.

This book was conceptualized with the vision of imparting up-to-date information and advanced data in this field. To ensure the same, a matchless editorial board was set up. Every individual on the board went through rigorous rounds of assessment to prove their worth. After which they invested a large part of their time researching and compiling the most relevant data for our readers. Conferences and sessions were held from time to time between the editorial board and the contributing authors to present the data in the most comprehensible form. The editorial team has worked tirelessly to provide valuable and valid information to help people across the globe.

Every chapter published in this book has been scrutinized by our experts. Their significance has been extensively debated. The topics covered herein carry significant findings which will fuel the growth of the discipline. They may even be implemented as practical applications or may be referred to as a beginning point for another development. Chapters in this book were first published by InTech; hereby published with permission under the Creative Commons Attribution License or equivalent.

The editorial board has been involved in producing this book since its inception. They have spent rigorous hours researching and exploring the diverse topics which have resulted in the successful publishing of this book. They have passed on their knowledge of decades through this book. To expedite this challenging task, the publisher supported the team at every step. A small team of assistant editors was also appointed to further simplify the editing procedure and attain best results for the readers.

Our editorial team has been hand-picked from every corner of the world. Their multi-ethnicity adds dynamic inputs to the discussions which result in innovative outcomes. These outcomes are then further discussed with the researchers and contributors who give their valuable feedback and opinion regarding the same. The feedback is then collaborated with the researches and they are edited in a comprehensive manner to aid the understanding of the subject.

Apart from the editorial board, the designing team has also invested a significant amount of their time in understanding the subject and creating the most relevant covers. They scrutinized every image to scout for the most suitable representation of the subject and create an appropriate cover for the book.

The publishing team has been involved in this book since its early stages. They were actively engaged in every process, be it collecting the data, connecting with the contributors or procuring relevant information. The team has been an ardent support to the editorial, designing and production team. Their endless efforts to recruit the best for this project, has resulted in the accomplishment of this book. They are a veteran in the field of academics and their pool of knowledge is as vast as their experience in printing. Their expertise and guidance has proved useful at every step. Their uncompromising quality standards have made this book an exceptional effort. Their encouragement from time to time has been an inspiration for everyone.

The publisher and the editorial board hope that this book will prove to be a valuable piece of knowledge for researchers, students, practitioners and scholars across the globe.

List of Contributors

Cian M. McCrudden and Helen O. McCarthy
School of Pharmacy, Queen's University Belfast, Northern Ireland, UK

Ana C. Calvo, Pilar Zaragoza and Rosario Osta
Laboratory of Genetics and Biochemistry (LAGENBIO-I3A), Aragon's Institute of Health Sciences (IACS), Faculty of Veterinary School, University of Zaragoza, Spain

Christopher D. Porada and Graça Almeida-Porada
Wake Forest Institute for Regenerative Medicine, Winston-Salem, NC, USA

Hélio A. Tomás, Ana F. Rodrigues, Paula M. Alves and Ana S. Coroadinha
Instituto de Tecnologia Química e Biológica, Universidade Nova de Lisboa, Oeiras, Portugal
Instituto de Biologia Experimental Tecnológica, Oeiras, Portugal

Matthew H. Wilson
Michael E. DeBakey VA Medical Center, Baylor College of Medicine, Houston TX, USA
Interdepartmental Program in Translational Biology & Molecular Medicine, Baylor College of Medicine, Houston TX, USA
Department of Medicine-Nephrology Division, Baylor College of Medicine, Houston TX, USA
Center for Cell and Gene Therapy, Baylor College of Medicine, Houston TX, USA

Sunandan Saha
Interdepartmental Program in Translational Biology & Molecular Medicine, Baylor College of Medicine, Houston TX, USA
Department of Medicine-Nephrology Division, Baylor College of Medicine, Houston TX, USA

Ines Dufait and Karine Breckpot
Department of Physiology–Immunology, Medical School, Free University of Brussels, Belgium

Therese Liechtenstein, Alessio Lanna, Roberta Laranga, Antonella Padella and David Escors
Division of Infection and Immunity, Rayne Institute, University College London, United Kingdom

Christopher Bricogne and Frederick Arce
UCL Cancer Institute, University College London, United Kingdom

Grazyna Kochan
Structural Genomics Consortium Oxford, University of Oxford, Old Road Campus Research Building, United Kingdom

Cleo Goyvaerts and Karine Breckpot
Laboratory of Molecular and Cellular Therapy, Department of Immunology-Physiology, Vrije Universiteit Brussel, Jette, Belgium

Therese Liechtenstein, Christopher Bricogne and David Escors
Division of Infection and Immunity, Rayne Institute, University College London, London, UK

Shigeki Kato and Kazuto Kobayashi
Department of Molecular Genetics, Institute of Biomedical Sciences, Fukushima Medical University School of Medicine, Fukushima, Japan

Kenta Kobayashi
Section of Viral Vector Development, National Institute of Physiological Sciences, Okazaki, Japan

Ken-ichi Inoue and Masahiko Takada
Systems Neuroscience Section, Primate Research Institute, Kyoto University, Inuyama, Japan

Takashi Okada
Department of Molecular Therapy, National Institute of Neuroscience, National Center of Neurology and Psychiatry, Ogawa-Higashi, Kodaira, Tokyo, Japan

Grant D. Trobridge
Department of Pharmaceutical Sciences, Washington State University, Pullman, Washington, USA
School of Molecular Biosciences, Washington State University, Pullman, Washington, USA

Dustin T. Rae
Department of Pharmaceutical Sciences, Washington State University, Pullman, Washington, USA

Printed in the USA
CPSIA information can be obtained
at www.ICGtesting.com
JSHW011451221024
72173JS00005B/1035

9 781632 421968